Little, Brown's Paperback Book Series

Basic Medical Sciences

Albers, Agranoff, Katzman, & Siegel	Basic Neurochemistry
Colton	Statistics in Medicine
Hine & Pfeiffer	Behavioral Science
Levine	Pharmacology
Peery & Miller	Pathology
Selkurt	Physiology
Sidman & Sidman	Neuroanatomy
Snell	Clinical Anatomy for Medical Students
Snell	Clinical Embryology for Medical Students
Valtin	Renal Function
Watson	Basic Human Neuroanatomy

Clinical Medical Sciences

Clark & MacMahon	Preventive Medicine
Eckert	Emergency-Room Care
Grabb & Smith	Plastic Surgery
Green	Gynecology
Judge & Zuidema	Methods of Clinical Examination
Keefer & Wilkins	Medicine
MacAusland & Mayo	Orthopedics
Nardi & Zuidema	Surgery
Thompson	Primer of Clinical Radiology
Ziai	Pediatrics

Nursing Sciences

DeAngelis	Basic Pediatrics for the Primary Health Care Provider
Sana & Judge	Physical Appraisal Methods in Nursing Practice
Selkurt	Basic Physiology for the Health Sciences

Manuals and Handbooks

Arndt	Manual of Dermatologic Therapeutics
Children's Hospital Medical Center, Boston	Manual of Pediatric Therapeutics
Condon & Nyhus	Manual of Surgical Therapeutics
Friedman & Papper	Problem-Oriented Medical Diagnosis
Gardner & Provine	Manual of Acute Bacterial Infections
Massachusetts General Hospital	Manual of Nursing Procedures
Neelon & Ellis	A Syllabus of Problem-Oriented Patient Care
Papper	Manual of Medical Care of the Surgical Patient
Shader	Manual of Psychiatric Therapeutics
Spivak & Barnes	Manual of Clinical Problems in Internal Medicine: Annotated with Key References
Wallach	Interpretation of Diagnostic Tests
Washington University Department of Medicine	Manual of Medical Therapeutics
Zimmerman	Techniques of Patient Care

Little, Brown and Company
34 Beacon Street
Boston, Massachusetts 02106

Manual of
Psychiatric
Therapeutics

Manual of Psychiatric Therapeutics

Practical Psychopharmacology and Psychiatry

Edited by
Richard I. Shader, M.D.

Associate Professor and Director, Psychopharmacology Research Laboratory, Harvard Medical School at the Massachusetts Mental Health Center; Director of Training and Education, Massachusetts Mental Health Center, Boston

Little, Brown and Company
Boston

Preface

Advances in clinical psychopharmacology over the past twenty years have brought both changes in the care of the emotionally ill and a reexamination of psychiatric nosology. It is the purpose of this manual to offer clinicians and students an overview of contemporary clinical therapeutics. A manual of this type emphasizes the generalizations that can be made about diagnosis and patient care. It does not, and cannot, go into such detail as to make clinical judgment and experience unnecessary. Direct responsibilities for patient care and a grasp of the pertinent basic, theoretical, and clinical literature are essential for comprehensive and competent clinical work. Special attention should be paid to the application to children of procedures derived from clinical experience with adults.

Standards and guidelines for clinical therapeutics are continually evolving. We include current recommendations from the Food and Drug Administration in various chapters. Many physicians worry about the extensive lists of side effects contained in package inserts and about using drugs only for approved indications. The Commissioner of the Food and Drug Administration states that the package insert contains "conventional knowledge" and emphasizes that the package insert is not law (*Resident and Staff Physician* 20:65–69, 1974). He assumes that "physicians using a drug for a condition or in dose forms other than those described in the insert will do so knowingly and for rational reasons." We would add to this that since the package insert is considered conventional knowledge, the prescribing physician should be aware of its message, including contraindications, warnings, precautions, and the listing of side effects. Only then can a clinician adequately weigh the benefits and risks and in the light of this conventional knowledge proceed to prescribe. He can also give his patient a proper perspective about what to expect, without causing undue alarm.

Good clinical practice should include the use of test doses in the presence of experienced personnel to identify, for example, unwanted hypotensive responses and hidden contraindications (i.e., a patient placed on propanolol who does not acknowledge a past history of asthma) and to make possible treatment of any sudden allergic responses. Clinicians should document in their charts such issues as informed consent (particularly about deviations from conventional practices or when the ratio of risk to benefit is high) and patient and family history of past and present experiences with medications. Charts should be flagged to identify patients with known unwanted responses to drugs. An awareness of potential drug interactions is an important dimension of prescriptive practice. Clinicians also should make every effort to maximize patients' compliance with the medication regimen, for example, by using the smallest possible number of dosage units and by setting dosage schedules of once or twice daily when this is compatible with known pharmacokinetic properties of the drugs prescribed.

I wish to thank many colleagues and friends, whose comments have been useful during the evolution of this manual, in particular Drs. Niroo Gupta, Ralph Jacobsen, Jerome Jaffe, Donald Jasinski, David Lewis, W. Leigh Thompson, and Abraham Wickler, for their help in the preparation of Chapter 13. Special thanks go to Mrs. Margaret Jonah and Miss Eugenia Romanos for their assistance in the preparation of many manuscripts and to Mrs. Linda Shadgett and Mr. Jerold Harmatz for their editorial skills. I also thank the *American Journal of Psychiatry,* the *Journal of Nervous and Mental Disease,* the *Journal of Hospital and Community Psychiatry,* and the J. B. Lippincott Company for permission to reprint certain charts and tables. I thank Dr. Elliot Mishler for the photograph in Chapter 6. Lastly, I thank Lin Richter of Little, Brown and Company.

R.I.S.

Newton Centre, Massachusetts

Contents

Contributing Authors

Eric D. Caine, M.D.

Clinical Fellow in Psychiatry, Harvard Medical School; Resident in Psychiatry, Massachusetts Mental Health Center, Boston

Magda Campbell, M.D.

Associate Professor of Psychiatry and Director, Children's Psychopharmacology Unit, New York University School of Medicine, New York University Medical Center, New York

Samuel Gershon, M.D.

Professor of Psychiatry and Director, Neuropsychopharmacology Research Unit, New York University School of Medicine, New York University Medical Center, New York

Alan I. Green, M.D.

Research Consultant, Special Action Office for Drug Abuse Prevention, Office of the President of the United States, Washington, D.C.; Clinical Fellow in Psychiatry, Harvard Medical School; Resident in Psychiatry, Massachusetts Mental Health Center, Boston

David J. Greenblatt, M.D.

Assistant Professor of Medicine, Harvard Medical School; Assistant in Medicine, Massachusetts General Hospital, Boston

Jerold S. Harmatz, B.A.

Associate in Psychiatry (Psychology) and Research Psychologist, Psychopharmacology Research Laboratory, Harvard Medical School at the Massachusetts Mental Health Center, Boston

Anthony H. Jackson, M.D.

Clinical Fellow in Psychiatry, Harvard Medical School; Resident in Psychiatry, Massachusetts Mental Health Center, Boston

Donald F. Klein, M.D.

Professor of Psychiatry, School of Medicine, Health Sciences Center, State University of New York at Stony Brook; Director of Research, Department of Psychiatry, Long Island Jewish—Hillside Medical Center, Glen Oaks, New York

Roger E. Meyer, M.D.

Associate Professor of Psychiatry, Harvard Medical School; Director, Harvard—Boston University Center for Biobehavioral Studies in the Addictions Boston

Carl Salzman, M.D.

Assistant Professor of Psychiatry and Co-Director, Psychopharmacology Rese Laboratory, Harvard Medical School at the Massachusetts Mental Health Cen Assistant Clinical Director (Day Hospit Massachusetts Mental Health Center, Boston

Joseph J. Schildkraut, M.D.

Professor of Psychiatry, Harvard Medical School; Director, Neuropsychopharmacology Laboratory, Harvard Medical School at the Massachusetts Mental Health Center, Boston

Richard I. Shader, M.D.

Associate Professor of Psychiatry and Director, Psychopharmacology Researc Laboratory, Harvard Medical School at the Massachusetts Mental Health Cen Director of Training and Education, Massachusetts Mental Health Center, Boston

Theodore Shapiro, M.D.

Associate Professor of Psychiatry and Director of Child Psychiatry, Bellevue Hospital, New York University School of Medicine, New York University Medical Center, New York

David Spiegel, M.D.

Clinical Fellow in Psychiatry, Harvard Medical School; Resident in Psychiatry, Massachusetts Mental Health Center, Boston

Joe P. Tupin, M.D.

Professor and Vice Chairman, Department of Psychiatry, and Chief, Consultation Service, University of California, Davis, School of Medicine, Davis, California

Bessel van der Kolk, M.D.

Clinical Fellow in Psychiatry, Harvard Medical School; Resident in Psychiatry, Massachusetts Mental Health Center, Boston

Paul H. Wender, M.D.

Professor in Psychiatry, College of Medicine, The University of Utah, Salt Lake City

Manual of
Psychiatric
Therapeutics

1

Psychotropic Drugs in the General Hospital

David J. Greenblatt
Richard I. Shader

Numerous surveys of drug use in hospitalized medical and surgical patients suggest that psychoactive agents are among the most widely prescribed drugs. It is an irony of medical practice that physicians' attention to the pharmacologic properties and rational administration of psychotropic drugs does not begin to parallel the magnitude of their use. In most teaching hospitals, house officers and staff physicians now administer digitalis glycosides, antiarrhythmics, antihypertensives, analgesics, antibiotics, corticosteroids, and anticoagulants based on consideration of known pharmacokinetic parameters, possible adverse effects, potential drug interactions, and in some cases, blood concentrations of the drug in question. For many commonly used psychotropic agents, such data are available but frequently are not utilized by prescribing physicians. It is no surprise that psychoactive agents are frequently misused and that adverse reactions to these drugs contribute greatly to iatrogenic morbidity in hospitalized patients.

A vast number of sedatives, hypnotics, and tranquilizers confront the house officer. He cannot and need not attempt to understand the pharmacology of each in detail. Within each drug category there are many agents with closely similar or identical properties. In such cases, an understanding of a single drug within the category is sufficient. Enlightened hospital formulary committees recently have been reducing the number of available drugs whose properties do not differ significantly. This measure usually enhances rational drug use by making physician education easier. It is unnecessary for a hospital pharmacy to stock seven penicillinase-resistant semisynthetic penicillin derivatives; it is equally unnecessary to require house officers to choose from among seven piperazine phenothiazines with similar pharmacologic properties. This chapter will consider aspects of psychopharmacology that are relevant to the physician's care of medical and surgical patients.

I. **Practical Pharmacology of Psychotropic Drugs**

    A. **Principles of classification** The meaning of terms such as sedative, hypnotic, and tranquilizer is often unclear or ambiguous. The most important pharmacologic distinctions lie between the

Table 1-1. Sedative-Hypnotics and Tranquilizers: Basic Pharmacologic Differences

Properties	Sedative-Hypnotics	Tranquilizers
Antipsychotic effects	No	Yes
Antianxiety effects	In low to moderate doses	In low doses
Sleep-inducing effects	In high doses	Normal subjects: drowsiness produced by some drugs, not others
		Psychotic patients: all drugs can produce improved sleep
General-anesthesia-like effects	In very high doses	No
Habituation and addiction	Yes	No
Extrapyramidal effects	No	Yes
Antiemetic effects	No	Yes
Alpha-adrenergic blocking effects	No	Yes
Dopaminergic blocking effects	No	Yes
Seizure threshold	Elevated	Lowered

sedative-hypnotics and the tranquilizers. In this chapter **sedative-hypnotics** include sleep-inducing (hypnotic) agents and antianxiety drugs (synonymous with minor tranquilizers, sedatives, or anxiolytics). **Tranquilizers** are antipsychotic drugs (synonymous with major tranquilizers and neuroleptics) and include the phenothiazines, butyrophenones, thioxanthenes, and dihydroindolones. The major differences between these two classes of drugs (summarized in Table 1-1) are as follows:

1. **Sedative-hypnotics** are general CNS depressants. They have antianxiety effects in low doses, produce sleep in high doses, and cause a comatose or general-anesthesia-like state in very high doses. All of these drugs can produce some degree of tolerance, habituation, and addiction, although the addiction potentials of the various drugs are not identical. Sedative-hypnotics have negligible autonomic nervous system effects, and they have no important influence on organ system function other than those effects mediated through the CNS.

2. **Tranquilizers** have a specific capacity to diminish or reverse the disordered thought processes that occur in schizophrenic or psychotic patients. Sedative or sleep-inducing effects of major tranquilizers in nonpsychotic individuals vary with the drugs — some produce dose-related drowsiness and sedation, while others do not. In psychotic patients, however, any of the major tranquilizers can appear to have calming effects and to promote sleep when disordered thought contributes to agitation or insomnia or both. A general-anesthesia-like state does not occur at any

dose. Habituation and addiction do not occur. Major tranquilizers produce a variety of autonomic, extrapyramidal motor, and organ system effects that are of concern to physicians in nonpsychiatric hospitals.

B. **Hypnotic drugs** Hypnotic agents are a subcategory of sedative-hypnotics. Their pharmacologic properties are not strikingly different from those of the sedative or antianxiety agents. The hypnotics are deliberately used in doses large enough to induce sleep. Most of the available hypnotic agents are relatively lipid-soluble drugs. After oral administration, absorption is rapid and complete. The drugs are biotransformed in the liver to inactive metabolites. Elimination half-lives are relatively short, thus minimizing the chances of residual morning drowsiness following sleep-inducing doses.

All nonproprietary hypnotic drugs are equally effective sleep-inducing agents *when given in adequate doses.* A drug may appear to be ineffective when in fact the quantity administered was too small. It is not always possible to predict how much is necessary to produce sleep in a given individual. In general, however, the "usual dose range" is conservative. Doses at the middle or high end of the usual dose range are more consistently effective and pose no hazard to most adults. These doses can be given unless there is a specific reason to use smaller quantities. Hypnotic drugs are also similar with respect to toxicity. "Hangover," or unwanted morning drowsiness, occurs with approximately equal frequency after all sleep-inducing agents. Symptomatic hangover is reported in 5 to 10 percent of hospitalized persons who receive hypnotics. Impaired psychomotor function and electroencephalographic (EEG) abnormalities can be demonstrated in a much larger fraction.

1. **Considerations for choosing among hypnotic drugs** Since available hypnotic drugs do not differ significantly in efficacy or in unwanted effects, hospital physicians must use other guidelines for choosing among drugs:

   a. **The character of the drug-induced sleep state** Normal individuals spend about 25 percent of total sleep time in the dreaming state of sleep. Rapid eye movements (REM) can be detected during dreaming; hence "REM sleep" is used synonymously with "dreaming sleep." All hypnotic drugs probably alter either the character or the duration of REM sleep. This effect appears to be greatest with the barbiturates and glutethimide, which reduce dreaming time from 25 percent to 10 or 15 percent of the total sleep duration. The consequences of partial dream deprivation produced by certain hypnotic drugs are not clear. Most individuals seem to tolerate repeated nightly use of REM-inhibiting drugs without apparent ill effects. Some patient with ischemic heart disease have nocturnal anginal pain or ventricular arrhythmias that correspond to dreaming. In cases like these, REM suppression might be of theoretical benefit. It appears, however, that the brain becomes aware of a "dreaming debt" when REM-suppressing hypnotics are used repeatedly. After REM-inhibiting drugs are discontinued, dreaming time *increases* to supranormal levels ("REM rebound") and remains increased for up to five weeks. Nightmares and insomnia often occur during REM rebound, and can be sufficiently unpleasant as to cause patients to resume using the drug. When hypnotics are given in the hospital, the rebound phenomenon may occur after the patient is discharged. Whenever REM rebound is of clinical concern, physicians would be wise to prescribe hypnotic drugs that cause minimal interference with REM sleep.

b. **The potential for drug interactions** This is of great importance in hospitalized patients. Polypharmacy is common on medical wards — surveys show that an average of eight or more drugs per patient are administered — and the possibilities for drug interactions are almost uncountable.

Physicians can anticipate that hypnotic drugs will produce CNS depression in addition to that caused by other concurrently administered CNS depressants, whether opiates, antianxiety agents, or general anesthetics. Other, more insidious drug interactions also occur. The most important are those caused by *enzyme induction* or by *protein-binding displacement* (see Chapter 16). Barbiturates and glutethimide are potent enzyme-inducers; they stimulate the activity of hepatic microsomal drug-metabolizing enzymes. Other drugs, such as coumarin anticoagulants, may become less effective and require increased dosage when barbiturates or glutethimide are given concurrently. Protein-binding displacement occurs when chloral derivatives are metabolized to trichloroacetic acid (TCA), which is tightly bound to serum albumin. Administration of a chloral derivative can cause acute potentiation of other protein-bound drugs (warfarin, diphenylhydantoin, tolbutamide) because TCA displaces them from their binding sites. Hospital physicians must exercise care when administering hypnotics that can potentiate or antagonize the action of other drugs. Benzodiazepine hypnotics appear not to cause enzyme induction or protein-binding displacement.

c. **The potential for habituation and abuse** The addicting liability and abuse potential of hypnotic drugs vary widely. Barbiturates, glutethimide, and methaqualone are frequently abused, while benzodiazepines (flurazepam, nitrazepam) are only rarely abused. The importance of this consideration can be minimized when the drugs are given to hospitalized patients, since dosage and frequency of administration are controlled by the medical staff. It is important to remember, however, that hospital wards are not immune to illicit drug traffic. Treatment of sedative-hypnotic dependence is discussed in Chapter 12.

2. **Specific hypnotic agents** The following hypnotic drugs are commonly listed in hospital formularies. Pertinent data are summarized in Appendix I.

a. **Barbiturates** Derivatives of barbituric acid are ususally divided into short-, intermediate-, and long acting categories. With respect to onset of action and efficacy, these divisions are of no consequence provided adequate hypnotic doses are given. It appears, however, that long-acting agents can accumulate in the body when used repeatedly.

All barbiturates depress the respiratory drive, and all are strong enzyme-inducing agents. REM sleep likewise is significantly depressed by all derivatives. Because of these disadvantages, there is seldom reason to select barbiturates as hypnotics for hospitalized patients except when economic considerations cannot be put aside.

(1) **Short-acting barbiturates** The recommended starting dose of *secobarbital* or *pentobarbital* is 100 mg. In most patients 200 mg can be safely given. Because it is less protein-bound, pentobarbital has a slightly higher relative potency than secobarbital. Otherwise the two drugs do not differ significantly. Biotransformation of both is virtually complete.

(2) **Intermediate-acting barbiturates** *Butabarbital* and *amobarbital* are best given in initial doses of 100 mg.

(3) **Long-acting barbiturates** Unlike the shorter-acting derivatives, a significant proportion (30 percent) of a dose of *phenobarbital* is excreted unchanged by the kidney. In addition, phenobarbital is less lipid-soluble and less strongly protein-bound than other barbiturates. The recommended hypnotic dose is 100 mg.

b. **Chloral derivatives** All chloral derivatives are rapidly biotransformed to trichloroethanol (TCE), which is the pharmacologically active molecule. TCE is then detoxified to trichloroacetic acid (TCA). This molecule is tightly protein-bound and
can displace other drugs that are bound to serum albumin.
Clinically important potentiation of the anticoagulant warfarin
occurs when chloral derivatives are administered concurrently.
Enzyme induction is not known to occur to a significant degree
in humans.

Most chloral derivatives are gastric irritants and can exacerbate gastritis or peptic ulcer disease. The effects on REM
sleep are not clear. Some studies reveal REM depression at
usual clinical doses, while others do not.

Usually 1 gram of *chloral hydrate* is required for hypnotic
purposes; many individuals need more. The recommended
starting dose of *chloral betaine* is 1.74 gm and of *trichloroethyl
phosphate* (triclofos), 1.5 gm.

c. **Piperidinedione derivatives**

(1) **Glutethimide** is a potent enzyme-inducer, respiratory
depressant, and REM suppressor. Because of high lipid-
solubility, absorption from the gastrointestinal tract and
subsequent tissue distribution is rapid. The hypnotic
dose is 500 mg. There are no known advantages associated
with the use of this drug.

(2) The usual hypnotic dose of **methyprylon** is 300 mg. The
drug is an REM depressant; enzyme-inducing properties
have not been adequately studied in humans.

d. **Ethchlorvynol** Ethchlorvynol is a tertiary alcohol derivative
of acetylene. Doses of 750 mg are approximately equivalent in
hypnotic efficacy to 100 mg of a short-acting barbiturate. Enzyme induction has been suggested in some reports, but it has
not yet been evaluated in well-controlled studies. The effects
on REM sleep are not known. At least one case of fatal thrombocytopenia has been attributed to ethchlorvynol. Prolongation
of sedative effects has been reported in patients with renal
failure.

e. **Methaqualone** Dose-dependent REM depression occurs with
methaqualone. The recommended starting dose is 300 mg.
Enzyme induction occurs in animals, but effects in humans are
not established. Methaqualone abuse recently has become quite
popular. The drug can produce tingling or paresthesias of the
extremities ("buzz"), which some individuals find pleasurable.

f. Benzodiazepines Benzodiazepine derivatives have the significant advantage of producing no important enzyme induction in humans. It also appears that hypnotic doses of benzodiazepines are less likely to depress the respiratory drive than are equivalent doses of barbiturates. Two derivatives are currently in wide use:

(1) **Flurazepam** is available in the United States. Thirty milligrams is the recommended hypnotic dose; 30 mg is more consistently effective than 15 mg and is no more toxic. Most studies show that REM sleep is relatively unimpaired provided doses do not exceed 30 mg.

(2) **Nitrazepam,** although not available for clinical use in the United States at the present time, is used in most other parts of the world. A 5 mg dose is usually sufficient. Unlike flurazepam, nitrazepam depressed dreaming in most studies. Anecdotal reports suggest that some individuals are troubled by nightmares following nitrazepam use; it is not clear whether this association is real or coincidental. Repeated use of nitrazepam can lead to drug accumulation.

g. Antihistamines Certain antihistaminic drugs have nonspecific sedative properties at usual therapeutic doses and as such are not really hypnotics. Using antihistamines for sleep induction exploits a secondary pharmacologic property for therapeutic purposes. Like other hypnotics, these drugs are metabolized in the liver. The myth that antihistamines are milder or safer or less toxic than other hypnotics is totally unfounded. If anything, antihistamines have a *greater* toxic potential because of their anticholinergic properties. Acute toxic delirium resembling "atropine psychosis" can occur in certain individuals — particularly the elderly — after hypnotic doses of these drugs.

Three antihistamine derivatives are commonly used as hypnotics. The usual dose of each is 50 to 100 mg.

(1) **Diphenhydramine,** an ethanolamine derivative related to dimenhydrinate (Dramamine).

(2) **Promethazine,** a phenothiazine antihistamine having no antipsychotic properties.

(3) **Hydroxyzine.**

h. Drug cocktails For unknown reasons, the sale of fixed hypnotic drug combination products continues to flourish. Evidence of their superiority over single hypnotics is lacking. Many such prep arations are available. Two of the most popular are:

(1) **Tuinal,** containing 25 to 100 mg each of secobarbital and amobarbital per capsule.

(2) **Mandrax,** containing 250 mg of methaqualone and 25 mg of diphenhydramine in each capsule. This preparation is not available in the United States.

i. **Proprietary hypnotics** Over-the-counter hypnotics have no role in rational therapeutics, particularly in hospitalized patients. Most proprietary preparations contain a combination of scopolamine and methapyrilene (see Appendix IV), both of which have weak sedative properties and can be sold without prescription. Their hypnotic efficacy is not established.

C. **Sedatives (antianxiety agents, minor tranquilizers, anxiolytics)** The objective of antianxiety drug therapy is to reduce anxiety without inducing drowsiness or sleep. While some drugs are reported to have more selective and specific action on the symptoms of anxiety than other agents, no currently available antianxiety agent is completely symptom-specific in its action. Dose-dependent, nonspecific CNS depression occurs with sedative drugs. It is no surprise that the pharmacologic properties of antianxiety agents resemble or are identical to those of the hypnotics. In some cases hypnotic drugs are given in reduced dosage for daytime sedation.

Nearly all antianxiety agents have an addicting potential. Most have muscle-relaxant and anticonvulsant properties. Some also are enzyme-inducers. Unlike the hypnotic drugs, of which *all* are effective in adequate dosage, differences in efficacy can be demonstrated among antianxiety agents. These differences have been documented largely in drug trials on anxious neurotic outpatients. Unfortunately, few if any studies deal with the pharmacologic treatment of anxiety in hospitalized nonpsychotic patients.

Important pharmacokinetic differences exist among antianxiety agents. Some are rapidly biotransformed to inactive products; with others, metabolic transformation is relatively slow, and the metabolites themselves can have psychopharmacologic activity. When drugs are slowly biotransformed, significant drug accumulation can occur with repeated dosage. The degree of accumulation depends on the dosage, frequency of administration, and the metabolic half-life of the drug. Antianxiety agents usually are given in multiple daily doses, but once- or twice-daily doses may be sufficient when the drug has a long half-life. Effective oral dose ranges vary widely. Adequate sedation occurs in some patients after very small doses; in others, it seems that the drugs "hardly touch them" even after large doses. No single dosage schedule can be recommended. Therapy must be carefully individualized by the prescribing physician.

The following antianxiety agents are available in most hospital formularies. Pertinent data are summarized in Appendix II.

1. **Barbiturates** Intermediate- and long-acting barbiturates frequently are used in reduced dosage as daytime sedatives. Their superiority over placebo is weak, and symptomatic drowsiness or somnolence is a common unwanted effect. Enzyme induction and physical dependence can occur with barbiturates. The possibility of drug accumulation — particularly of phenobarbital — is important.

2. **Propanediols**

   a. **Meprobamate** appeared in 1955 with alleged specific antianxiety effects. Controlled studies, however, subsequently showed that meprobamate is only weakly superior to placebo and no more effective than various barbiturates. Meprobamate has a short to intermediate duration of action, so multiple daily doses should be used. The usual total dosage is 1.6 gm per day. Addiction occurs readily at as little as twice the usual daily dosage. Enzyme induction occurs in animals but probably is not important in humans.

   b. The pharmacokinetics of **tybamate** are not well understood. Usual doses are 750 mg to 2.0 gm per day. Addiction has not been reported to date.

   c. Other propanediol derivatives include **phenaglycodol** and **cthina mate.** The latter drug is used primarily as a hypnotic.

3. **Benzodiazepines** Benzodiazepine derivatives appear to have more specific antianxiety action than barbiturates or meprobamate. Superiority over placebo and most other drugs used to treat anxiety is established with some consistency. Clinically significant enzyme induction does not occur in humans with any of the benzodiazepines tested to date. Very high doses and prolonged exposure are necessary to produce physiologic addiction.

   a. **Chlordiazepoxide** is effective in the dose range of 15 to 100 mg per day. Many individuals require 30 to 60 mg per day. Injectable solutions must be freshly prepared and used immediately, since chlordiazepoxide isomerizes to a relatively inactive product when light-exposed or when dissolved in water.

Chlordiazepoxide is a long-acting drug. Its two major metabolites have significant psychopharmacologic activity. Owing to accumulation of the parent drug and its active products, drowsiness can occur in some patients after several days of continuous therapy.

b. **Diazepam** has higher relative potency than chlordiazepoxide. The dose range of diazepam is 6 to 40 mg per day, with 8 to 20 mg being effective in many individuals. There is no consistent evidence that diazepam has greater efficacy than chlordiazepoxide.

Since diazepam is relatively lipid-soluble and water-insoluble, the parenteral preparation employs a nonaqueous solvent (propylene glycol). The solution can cause pain and phlebitis when injected intravenously. Dilution of the parenteral preparation with water or saline results in precipitation of the drug.

Like chlordiazepoxide, diazepam is slowly metabolized to an active product. The demethylated metabolite is inactivated at an even slower rate. Repeated dosage of diazepam produces significant accumulation of the drug and its demethylated derivative. Because of its lipid solubility, diazepam sometimes appears to "wear off" quickly even after large doses. The effect is due to extensive tissue uptake and distribution and can give a false impression of a short duration of action, leading to repetition of high dosage.

c. The dose range of **oxazepam** is 30 to 120 mg per day. Efficacy is similar to other benzodiazepines. Unlike chlordiazepoxide and diazepam, however, oxazepam has a short to intermediate duration of action and has no active metabolites. Cumulative effects are therefore much less important. A parenteral preparation is not available.

d. **Clorazepate** is a relatively new benzodiazepine, having similar efficacy to other derivatives. Its pharmacokinetics have not been well studied. It appears, however, that clorazepate is rapidly hydrolyzed to the demethylated metabolite of diazepam. Long duration of action and cumulative effects can therefore be anticipated. The usual dose range of clorazepate is 11.25 to 60.0 mg per day. A parenteral preparation is not available.

4. **Antihistamines** Nonspecific sedative effects of certain antihistamines are sometimes exploited for daytime sedation. *Hydroxyzine* is the most commonly used. The choice of hydroxyzine as an antianxiety agent occasionally can be rationalized, particularly

when pruritic dermatoses are present and are thought to be exacerbated by emotional stress.

5. **Beta-adrenergic antagonists** Anxiety can be manifest through excessive beta-adrenergic activity: tachycardia, palpitations, sweating, tremor, agitation, breathlessness, fatigue. Some studies show that beta-adrenergic blocking agents can provide relief of these symptoms in anxious individuals. These drugs do not have sedative-hypnotic pharmacologic properties; rather they antagonize the peripheral manifestations of anxiety.

Propranolol is effective at doses of 30 to 120 mg per day. The drug is contraindicated in patients with asthma or uncompensated congestive heart failure. The treatment of anxiety with propranolol is not approved by the Food and Drug Administration.

6. **Major tranquilizers** The pharmacology of major tranquilizers is discussed in Section I.D. The antianxiety effects of these drugs in nonpsychotic humans remains a mystery. Animal studies uniformly fail to demonstrate fear-attenuating properties.

Major tranquilizers are no more effective than benzodiazepines in anxious nonpsychotic patients. Side effects and hazards of major tranquilizer therapy are much greater. For this reason there is seldom, if ever, justification for using these drugs to treat anxiety in patients who are not under the care of a psychiatrist.

D. **Tranquilizers (major tranquilizers, antipsychotics, neuroleptics)**
Major tranquilizers produce dopamine receptor blockade and are uniquely effective in reversing aspects of the disordered thought process in the psychotic patient. Despite wide differences in relative potency (see Table 4-10), all major tranquilizers are equally effective antipsychotic agents when given in adequate dosage. However, nonpsychiatric physicians seldom treat schizophrenic patients and generally use the drugs in smaller doses for other purposes. Internists and surgeons in general hospitals must be aware of the numerous therapeutic and toxic pharmacologic properties of neuroleptic drugs before they can be used rationally.

Antipsychotic drugs are nonaddicting and do not produce general anesthesia. There are differences among drugs in antiemetic effects, adrenergic and cholinergic blocking properties, propensity to produce involuntary movements, and nonspecific sedative effects in nonpsychotic individuals. Organ system toxicity — involving heart, liver, skin, and eye — is well documented but occurs less frequently. The decision to administer a major tranquilizer to a nonpsychotic hospitalized patient must reflect consideration of the numerous possible hazards.

The five major classes of antipsychotic drugs are *phenothiazines, butyrophenones, thioxanthenes, dihydroindolones, and dibenzoxazepines.* The *rauwolfia* derivatives, although historically the first of the "tranquilizing" drugs, now are seldom used except for antihypertensive therapy. Pertinent data on major tranquilizers are summarized in Appendices III and V.

1. **Phenothiazines** Phenothiazine derivatives have a tricyclic structure. The middle ring is heterocyclic, containing nitrogen and sulfur atoms. An electron-withdrawing substituent must be present in the 2-position on one of the aromatic rings for the compound to have antipsychotic effects. Other pharmacologic properties are determined largely by the substituent on the nitrogen atom in the heterocyclic ring. These are of three major types:

   a. **Dimethylaminopropyl substitutions** Phenothiazines with this aliphatic side chain are strongly sedating when given to non-psychotic individuals in doses of 25 to 100 mg. They also are potent dopaminergic and alpha-adrenergic antagonists and can produce debilitating postural hypotension, which can be made worse by administration of epinephrine. Antiemetic and anticholinergic effects are also significant. Involuntary movements (extrapyramidal symptoms, EPS) occur in a large number of middle-aged and elderly patients who receive the drugs for several weeks or more. The syndrome may be one of agitation and restlessness (akathisia) or may resemble parkinsonism. In a small number of recipients, reversible cholestatic jaundice may occur. Many reports have associated sudden death in otherwise healthy individuals with dimethylaminopropyl phenothiazine therapy. A causal relationship has not been demonstrated but appears likely. Profound hypotension, cardiac arrhythmias, aspiration, and extreme hypothermia or hyperthermia are among possible mechanisms of sudden death.

   The three aliphatic phenothiazines in common use are:

      (1) **Chlorpromazine** Nonpsychotic individuals should receive an initial dose of no more than 100 mg orally or 50 mg intramuscularly. Usually doses of half the indicated size will be adequate for antiemetic purposes. Although sustained-action capsules are available, their value is questionable because chlorpromazine has a long duration of action.

(2) **Triflupromazine** has higher relative potency than chlorpromazine (see Table 4-10) but otherwise is pharmacologically similar.

(3) **Promazine** does not have an electron-withdrawing group on the 2-position; hence it has minimal antipsychotic properties. Sedative and antiemetic effects, however, are significant. Dosage is the same as with chlorpromazine.

b. **Piperidino substitutions** Phenothiazines with this type of substitution have relative potencies similar to those of dimethylaminopropyl derivatives (see Table 4-10). Antiemetic properties, however, are negligible. Sedative and alpha-adrenergic blocking effects are also less profound. Piperidine phenothiazines *infrequently* produce involuntary movements. There is increasing concern regarding possible cardiotoxic effects. Most patients receiving moderate to high doses develop electrocardiographic changes resembling those in hypokalemia; these changes are benign. However, sudden and catastrophic cardiac arrhythmias have been reported a number of times. It is not known how often the piperidine phenothiazines produce these arrhythmias, nor even whether the drugs are causally responsible. Sudden deaths have also been attributed to piperidine phenothiazines.

The three piperidine derivatives currently available are:

(1) **Thioridazine** Only oral preparations are available. The usual initial dose is 50 mg. Pigmentary retinopathy occurs often enough with daily doses of 800 mg or more that this dose ceiling should be heeded.

(2) **Mesoridazine** Oral and parenteral preparations are available. The usual initial dose is 25 to 50 mg.

(3) **Piperacetazine** The initial dose is 20 to 50 mg.

c. **Piperazine substitutions** Phenothiazines with this side chain have the highest relative potency (see Table 4-10) and the strongest antiemetic effects. Sedation and alpha-adrenergic antagonism are minimal. Piperazine derivatives can produce parkinsonian-like symptoms similar to the effects of continuous chlorpromazine therapy. Of greater concern, however, are the acute dystonic reactions that can occur in young patients even after small initial doses. These frightening acute spasms of muscle groups — usually of the eye, tongue, neck, or back — may require emergency parenteral treatment with anticholinergic drugs.

The use of piperazine phenothiazines in nonpsychotic patients is usually for antiemetic purposes. It should be remembered that they are of little value in vomiting due to vestibular disorders, as in motion sickness, Ménière's disease, or labyrinthitis. Commonly used drugs are prochlorperazine, trifluoperazine, perphenazine, fluphenazine, carphenazine, butaperazine, and acetophenazine (see also Appendix III).

2. **Butyrophenones** bear no structural similarity to phenothiazines, but they have pharmacologic properties closely resembling piperazine phenothiazines. Butyrophenone derivatives have high relative potency (see Table 4-10), are strong antiemetics, and cause minimal sedation in nonpsychotic individuals. Anticholinergic and antiadrenergic effects also are minimal, but dopaminergic blocking properties are strong. Acute dystonic reactions are relatively common. The suggested initial dosage of *haloperidol* is 2.5 to 5.0 mg. *Droperidol* is used almost exclusively by anesthesiologists as a premedicant and induction agent.

3. **Thioxanthenes** Antipsychotic drugs of the thioxanthene class closely resemble phenothiazines in structure and function. Claims of reduced toxicity and greater efficacy are not substantiated. The two derivatives available for use are:

   a. **Chlorprothixene,** with a dimethylaminopropyl side chain, has pharmacologic properties similar to chlorpromazine. The usual initial dose is 25 to 50 mg orally or 12.5 to 25 mg parenterally.

   b. **Thiothixene** has a piperazine substitution and resembles the piperazine group of phenothiazines. Initial doses of 2 to 4 mg are recommended.

4. **Dihydroindolones** *Molindone* is a dihydroindolone compound structurally unrelated to the phenothiazines, thioxanthenes, and butyrophenones. However, its pharmacologic profile in humans and animals is similar to that produced by these other classes of drugs. The clinical effects of molindone most closely resemble those produced by piperazine phenothiazines and thioxanthenes and by haloperidol, although clinical trials to date suggest that early acute dystonias may be less common with molindone. Clinical experience with this compound has not been extensive.

5. **Dibenzoxazepines** *Loxapine succinate* is a newly marketed antipsychotic with a tricyclic structure. Other clinical and pharmacologic properties: sedative, anticholinergic, and extrapyramidal effects. Experience with this drug to date is minimal. Initial doses of 10 or 20 mg are recommended.

II. **Use of Psychotropic Drugs in the General Hospital** Many situations arise on medical and surgical wards in which the use of a psychotropic drug may be considered. This section presents a review of these situations and a guide to rational pharmacologic management.

A. **Insomnia** Most hospitalized patients have difficulty falling asleep or staying asleep or both. Possible reasons are numerous. Some are mechanical: for example, noise in the corridors, a suffering patient in the next bed, or medical personnel giving medications, taking vital signs, drawing blood samples, or starting IVs. Emotional factors also can prevent sleep. The novel, frightening hospital environment, separation anxiety (especially for the child), the possibility of serious organic disease, or the prospect of surgery or an uncomfortable diagnostic procedure on the following day all can provoke sufficient emotional discomfort to make sleep difficult. Aspects of the disease process itself can also produce insomnia: somatic pain, pulmonary congestion, respiratory insufficiency, urinary or rectal urgency. Usually a combination of factors is present.

When insomnia is due to such causes as pain or hypoxia, efforts should be directed at treating the underlying cause. Physician reassurance and skillful antianxiety drug therapy (see Section **II.B**) can do much to relieve sleeplessness due to emotional discomfort. Still, many patients are unable to sleep without a hypnotic drug. Flurazepam (Dalmane) usually is a reasonable choice among the drugs listed in Appendix I. Of drugs available at the present time, this agent allows the most nearly physiologic sleep and is the least likely to interact unexpectedly with concurrently administered drugs.

Precautions: Additive CNS depression occurs when hypnotics are coadministered with other depressant drugs. Hypnotics are hazardous when respiratory insufficiency is present. Carbon dioxide narcosis and coma can be precipitated by hypnotics and other CNS depressants when given to patients with chronic obstructive pulmonary disease and carbon dioxide retention. Patients with uremia or hepatic insufficiency also can be extremely sensitive to CNS depressants — occasionally hypnotics precipitate coma in these individuals. Elderly patients sometimes react paradoxically to hypnotics, becoming excited, delirious, and combative rather than drowsy and somnolent. Barbiturates and chloral hydrate are usually implicated, but the reaction probably can occur after any hypnotic drug. Nocturnal confusion in geriatric patients ("sundowning") should *not* be treated with sedative-hypnotics (see Section **II.D**).

B. **Anxiety** can be normal or pathologic, depending on the reality of the perceived threat or danger. The possibility that serious organic disease is present or will be discovered, or the anticipation of a surgical ordeal, is a very real threat. Hence, anxiety in hospitalized patients is usually normal (i.e., appropriate fear in response to a real danger).

Anxiety can adversely influence the disease process because of catecholamine discharge. Sympathetic stimulation of the myocardium increases cardiac work and can precipitate ischemic pain or arrhythmias or both. Enhanced gastric acid secretion can aggravate peptic ulcer disease. Of course, anxiety is also subjectively unpleasant to the patient. The natural course of anxiety in the hospitalized patient and the role of drugs in its treatment are largely unknown. It is likely that symptoms spontaneously become less severe as the duration of hospitalization gets longer through adaptation to the environment and increased knowledge of disease. A high placebo response rate therefore also seems likely. Antianxiety agents, particularly benzodiazepines, are more effective than placebo in anxious neurotic outpatients, but adequately controlled studies of minor tranquilizers in hospitalized patients are lacking. Most general hospital patients seem to respond well to antianxiety drug therapy, although it is not clear if improvement is attributable to active drug, placebo effect, physician reassurance, or spontaneous remission.

Long-acting minor tranquilizers (chlordiazepoxide, diazepam, phenobarbital) need not be given more than two or three times daily. When anxiety also interferes with sleep, one-half to three-quarters of the daily dose can be given at bedtime, obviating the need for an additional hypnotic drug. A reasonable dosage schedule for diazepam, for example, is 5 mg at noon and 10 mg at bedtime. Short- to intermediate-acting drugs (oxazepam, meprobamate) must be given in multiple doses; larger doses can be given at bedtime (e.g., oxazepam, 15 mg tid and 30 mg at bedtime). Benzodiazepines usually are the most reasonable choice of antianxiety agent.

Precautions: The same as in Section **II.A.** Drug accumulation of long-acting antianxiety agents must be anticipated with repeated dosage. For example, if diazepam is given on consecutive days, blood levels of diazepam and its active demethylated metabolite will continuously rise and reach a plateau after five to seven days.

C. **Depression** Chapter 3 discusses in detail the concept and diagnosis of depression. This section deals with the particular issue of depression in general hospital patients.

1. **Categories of depressed patients** The following kinds of depressed patients are commonly seen in general hospital populations:

a. **Previously depressed individuals with coincident medical illness** In many such patients, an improvement in mood occurs when they are hospitalized for medical illness because their attention shifts from interpersonal or vocational troubles to legitimate bodily concerns. People whose strong dependency needs have caused shame or reduced self-esteem can accept the dependent role of the hospitalized patient because it is medically indicated. The lifting of mood often is temporary, particularly if the prognosis for physical health is unfavorable. The suicidal potential of such individuals should be assessed and precautions taken if indicated (e.g., psychiatric consultation, screened windows, removal of sharp objects, special nursing). Of particular concern is the possibility of important drug interactions in patients previously treated with antidepressant drugs (see Chapter 16, Section **V**).

b. **The postsuicidal patient** Medical and surgical care is of first importance for the patient who has attempted suicide. Management of self-poisoning with psychotropic drugs is discussed in Chapter 15.

Most patients who attempt self-harm are depressed. They usually have experienced a recent loss   a loved person, their own bodily integrity, or vocational status — leading to a profound feeling of humiliation, loneliness, or frustration. They may feel rage and anger toward the lost object. Suicide attempts may also occur with no apparent precipitating events in patients with "endogenous" depressions, particularly when they begin to emerge from a depressive episode. Attempts at self-harm can range from "gestures" — manipulative, attention-seeking acts, such as wrist-scratching or ingestion of nonlethal quantities of drugs — to serious, premeditated self-destructive acts.

All postsuicidal patients should have psychiatric consultations once they are medically stable and conscious. The psychiatrist can begin the interview with a statement such as, "You must have been feeling very unhappy to attempt to harm yourself as you did." The events precipitating the suicide attempt are briefly explored, with the physician taking care to convey a sense of serious concern for the patient's survival and for the uniqueness of his problems. In subsequent visits the supportive interaction is established, so that the patient acknowledges the need for further psychiatric intervention when medical recovery is complete.

c. **The previously healthy patient who is depressed about his disease** In such individuals, depression is of the reactive or nonpathologic type. Their loss — bodily health and the self-esteem associated with strength and vigor — is real. The response to somatic treatment (antidepressant drugs, electroconvulsive therapy) in these patients is usually poor. More important is the availability of reassurance and support. Physicians and nurses should answer questions honestly, provide reassurance, and avoid prognostic guesswork. Medical staff, social service, family, and friends should combine to support the patient during his adaptation to illness and the changes in life-style that he faces. Depression usually remits in time as adaptation occurs. In many cases, disability is not nearly so extensive as the patient anticipates at the onset of his illness. Young males with acute myocardial infarction, for example, often became profoundly depressed while in the coronary care unit, as they envision a life as a cardiac cripple; yet many recover fully and return to their former profession and their social and sexual vigor.

d. **Disease-related depression** In contrast to depression in *reaction* to disease, a depressive syndrome can occur as part of the symptom complex inherently associated with the following diseases: thyroid disease (hypothyroidism or hyperthyroidism), Addison's disease, Cushing's syndrome, hyperaldosteronism, systemic lupus erythematosus, uremia, parathyroid disease (hypoparathyroidism or hyperparathyroidism), disseminated carcinomatosis. The possibility that any of these diseases is causing or contributing to depression should be ruled out.

e. **Drug-related depression** The following drugs have the potential to induce a depressive syndrome: reserpine, propranolol; methyldopa, diazepam, clonidine, corticosteroids.

2. **Pharmacotherapy of depression** If depression is prolonged, disablingly severe, or interferes with medical therapy, hospital physicians may wish to administer antidepressant drugs with the guidance of a psychiatric consultant.

The two major groups of **tricyclic antidepressants** are the dibenza zepine derivatives (imipramine, desipramine) and the dibenzocycloheptene derivatives (amitriptyline, nortriptyline, protriptyline). All have similar antidepressant activity. Nonspecific sedative effects of the drugs vary from strong (amitriptyline) to weak (protriptyline). Doxepin, a tricyclic drug with a dibenzoxepin structure, is purported to have antianxiety as well as antidepressant effects. Evidence to support this contention is weak. However, doxepin may be useful for treating depressed hypertensive patients who also are receiving guanethidine-like antihypertensive drugs (see Chapter 16, Section **V. D**), since doxepin appears not to antagonize their antihypertensive effects.

Table 1-2. Pertinent Data on Tricyclic Antidepressants

Generic Name	Trade Name(s)	Preparations Available	Initial Daily Dose (mg)	Usual Maintenance Dose (mg)
Dibenzazepines				
Imipramine	Tofranil Tofranil P-M Imavate SK-Pramine Presamine	Tablets or capsules: 10 mg, 25 mg, 50 mg, 75 mg, 100 mg, 125 mg, 150 mg Injection: 12.5 mg/ml	75	150
Desipramine	Norpramin Pertofrane	Tablets or capsules: 25 mg, 50 mg	75	150 to 200
Dibenzocycloheptenes				
Amitriptyline	Elavil	Tablets: 10 mg, 25 mg, 50 mg Injection: 10 mg/ml	75	150
Nortriptyline	Aventyl	Capsules: 10 mg, 25 mg Liquid: 10 mg/5 ml	40 to 75	100 to 150
Protriptyline	Vivactil	Tablets: 5 mg, 10 mg	15	30
Dibenzoxepins				
Doxepin	Sinequan Adapin	Capsules: 10 mg, 25 mg, 50 mg, 100 mg	75	150

Table 1-2 gives data on currently available tricyclic antidepressant drugs. Another category of antidepressants, the **monoamime oxidase (MAO) inhibitors,** was not included in this table. MAO inhibitors are more toxic than the tricyclics, and their use as a first approach to pharmacotherapy in general hospital patients is seldom justified. The following important considerations should guide antidepressant drug therapy:

a. The drugs must be given in **adequate dosage.** This usually means reaching a daily dose of 150 mg per day or more of imipramine or its equivalent. Lower doses are not consistently effective. It is reasonable to initiate therapy with the equivalent of 75 mg per day of imipramine, but the dosage should be raised to 150 mg per day as soon as it can be tolerated. Occasional patients need up to 300 mg per day.

b. Tricyclic antidepressants are *long-acting* drugs with **cumulative effects.** They are usually given on a three times a day schedule, but once- or twice-daily administration is equally reasonable. The sedative effects of amitriptyline can be exploited in patients with sleep disturbances by giving two-thirds of the daily dose at bedtime.

c. Tricyclic antidepressants exert important clinical effects on mood only after a significant **lag period.** Usually 7 to 14 days elapse from the beginning of therapy before mood elevation begins to occur. Antidepressant effects seen before this time are attributable to other aspects of the therapeutic milieu.

d. In some patients mild psychomotor excitement — such as tremor, insomnia, or agitation — accompanies tricyclic therapy. This can be controlled by addition of a minor tranquilizer such as chlordiazepoxide (15 to 40 mg/day) or diazepam (6 to 20 mg/day) in low doses.

e. All tricyclic antidepressants have significant **anticholinergic effects,** accounting for frequent complaints of dry mouth. The hazards of this cholinergic blocking property in hospitalized patients, such as in those with prostatic hypertrophy, glaucoma, or intestinal obstruction, should be considered before the drug is given. Myxedematous patients may be particularly susceptible to cholinergic blocking agents.

f. Antidepressants have been reported to cause serious **cardiac arrhythmias.** The causal role of the drugs has not been unequivocally proved, but the possibility warrants careful attention

Tricyclic antidepressants should be avoided or administered with great caution in patients with ischemic heart disease, particularly those with a history of arrhythmias. In seriously depressed patients, electro-convulsive therapy preceded by hyperventilation using 100% oxygen may be a reasonable alternative (see Chapter 6).

g. **Drug interactions** with antidepressants can be of clinical importance. These are discussed in Chapter 16.

D. **Delirium and confusion** The meaning of these terms is vague. *Delirium* usually refers to a reversible global impairment of cognition, with the nature and degree of impairment fluctuating from hour to hour. Patients need not be agitated and combative; depression of consciousness and obtundation are equally possible. The meaning of *confusion* is more limited, signifying impaired intellectual function and disorientation, but with a normal state of arousal. Disorientation is usually to time and place. Recognition of others may be impaired, but when a patient does not recognize himself, traumatic amnesia, psychosis, and hysterical states must be considered. Physicians usually do not contemplate psychotropic drug treatment of delirium or confusion unless the patient is a management problem due to hyperactivity and combativeness.

In general hospital patients, delirium almost always has a treatable organic etiology that often is obvious. Psychotropic drugs should not be given until the cause of delirium is found, or unless excitement cannot be managed by any other means.

The list of causes of delirium is long. Hypoxia, inadequate cerebral perfusion, elevated intracranial pressure, hepatic decompensation, and fever are common etiologies. Delirium can accompany almost any neoplastic, degenerative, or infectious brain disease. Numerous metabolic causes are possible: hyponatremia, hypernatremia, hypercalcemia, thyrotoxicosis, and myxedema. Delirium can be drug-induced (anticholinergic agents, digitalis, lidocaine, corticosteroids). Frequently delirium arises in response to the unique environment of the intensive care unit.

If a remediable cause cannot be found, then delirium can be treated when necessary with parenteral antipsychotic drugs in doses suggested in Appendix III. The sundowning geriatric patient often can be helped by 12.5 to 25 mg of chlorpromazine given intramuscularly; sedative-hypnotic drugs can exacerbate delirium in such cases. Delirium due to withdrawal from addicting drugs, however, is best treated with a sedative-hypnotic, since phenothiazines can precipitate seizures (see Chapter 12). Phenothiazines also are known to exacerbate delirium due to anticholinergic agents.

Precautions: Psychotropic drug treatment of delirium risks maskin the cause of delirium. The numerous possible side effects of antipsychotic drugs have been discussed previously.

E. **Intractable seizures** Some sedative-hypnotic drugs have anticonvulsant activity and are given parenterally in the treatment of intractable seizures. It is not easy to decide when the therapeutic benefits of treating seizures outweigh the hazards of giving combinations of sedative-hypnotic drugs parenterally. Many experienced neurologists feel that hospital physicians do harm far more often than good in their emergency treatment of seizures.

Status epilepticus is usually defined as a series of repeated seizures culminating in death unless terminated by treatment. *Neither a single seizure nor even a series of seizures necessarily constitutes status epilepticus.* Most acute seizure activity is self-limited and does not require emergency drug treatment. It is not easy for a hospital physician to watch convulsive activity and "do nothing" other than protect the patient against injury, aspiration, and biting of the tongue. Yet in this situation observation and restraint rather than immediate pharmacologic intervention is usually the wisest course of action.

Seizures often have an obvious etiology and will cease without anticonvulsant medications once the inciting cause is removed. Hypox inadequate cerebral perfusion, elevated intracranial pressure, cerebral arterial emboli, withdrawal from addicting sedative-hypnotics, lidocaine infusion, administration of phenothiazines or large doses of penicillins, and a variety of metabolic disturbances are potentially remediable causes of seizures commonly observed in general hospitals. Convulsive activity often develops in patients with a known seizure disorder who simply fail to take their maintenance anticonvulsant medications. True status epilepticus is unusual, and unfortunately it often reflects advanced or terminal brain damage due to neoplasms, infection, or trauma.

If the physician feels that seizures require emergency parenteral therapy, an infusion of *diphenylhydantoin (DPH)* is prepared and started immediately. It is not clear whether DPH alone can arrest acute repetitive seizures. However, since these patients will eventually require maintenance DPH therapy, adequate anticonvulsant blood levels should be attained as rapidly as possible. This requires a *loading dose.* One gram of DPH is diluted in 250 to 500 ml 5% dextrose in water and given intravenously over 1 to 4 hours. Simultaneously anticonvulsant sedative-hypnotics are cautiously coadministered. *Diazepam* is the safest of the currently available drugs. It is given intravenously (undiluted) at a rate of 5 mg per minute until seizure activity stops or until a total of 20 to 30 mg has been given. Intra-muscular *phenobarbital* (120 mg) can also be administered.

This approach will terminate seizure activity in a majority of cases. Continuation of convulsions despite treatment is prognostically grave. Intravenous *amobarbital* at a rate of 50 to 100 mg/min can be tried next, with a dose maximum of 1.0 gm. Some patients eventually require curarization, intubation, and assisted ventilation.

Precautions: Hazards are those of administering multiple parenteral CNS depressant drugs to seriously ill patients. Injudicious use of barbi-turates can precipitate apnea and coma. In those with true status epilepticus, the underlying disease process can rapidly terminate in death despite drug therapy. On the other hand, failure to recognize and reverse a remediable cause of convulsive activity is a grave error.

F. **Nausea and vomiting** The hospital physician's attitude toward pharmacologic treatment of nausea and vomiting should be the same as that recommended in the approach to therapy of seizures. Antiemetic drugs are not innocuous. Anyone can attest that nausea and vomiting are subjectively unpleasant. It is unusual, however, for vomiting not to cease spontaneously; only rarely does vomiting per se threaten the patient's health. Premature antiemetic therapy is often precipitated by nursing staff who insist that the symptoms be treated. It is usually best to withhold antiemetic drugs until one is certain that more good than harm will be done.

A cause for emesis can usually be identified. A common cause is toxicity due to other drugs: digitalis, quinidine, potassium chloride, Veratrum alkaloids, opiates, general anesthetics, antineoplastic drugs. Nausea and vomiting can be associated with acute myocardial infarc-tion, gastroenteritis, neoplastic disease of the GI tract, other disseminat-ed malignancies, viral hepatitis, labyrinthine disease, intestinal ob-struction, and elevated intracranial pressure. Obviously removal of the inciting cause is preferable to antiemetic drug therapy whenever possible.

When nausea and vomiting are protracted, produce excessive dis-comfort, and the underlying cause cannot be removed, then the physician may wish to give symptomatic treatment. Intramuscular or rectal administration of drugs are the usual alternatives. Commonly used drugs and their adult doses by either route are given in Table 1-3. When nausea and vomiting are due to labyrinthine disease, major tranquilizers are relatively ineffective, and a drug of the anti-cholinergic-antihistamine category should be used. Differences in efficacy among the anticholinergic-antihistaminic agents are not sub-stantial enough that a drug of choice can be recommended. Anticho-linergic side effects and drowsiness are their major side effects. In

Table 1-3. Drugs Used To Treat Nausea and Vomiting

Generic Name	Trade Name	Intramuscular Dose (mg)	Rectal Dose (mg)
Anticholinergic-antihistamines			
Dimenhydrinate	Dramamine	25 to 50	100
Diphenhydramine	Benadryl	25 to 50	–
Hydroxyzine	Vistaril	25 to 50	–
Promethazine	Phenergan	25 to 50	25 to 50
Scopolamine	–	0.2 to 0.6	–
Trimethobenzamide	Tigan	100 to 200	200
Major tranquilizers			
Chlorpromazine	Thorazine	25 to 50	100
Haloperidol	Haldol	2.5 to 5.0	–
Perphenazine	Trilafon	5 to 10	–
Prochlorperazine	Compazine	5 to 10	25
Promazine	Sparine	25 to 50	–
Thiethylperazine	Torecan	5 to 10	10

vomiting due to nonlabyrinthine causes, major tranquilizers are probably more effective. However, possible side effects are more numerous and more serious than with the anticholinergic-antihistaminics. When nonlabyrinthine vomiting must be controlled as rapidly and effectively as possible, major tranquilizers can be the initial antiemetic administered. In less urgent situations, anticholinergic-antihistamines should be given first, with major tranquilizers held in reserve.

Precautions: Side effects of major tranquilizers have been discussed previously (see Section I.D). Acute dystonic reactions can occur when piperazine phenothiazines or haloperidol are used. Dimethylaminopropyl phenothiazines can cause postural hypotension and excessive sedation. Anticholinergic effects of major tranquilizers and of other antiemetics can be dangerous. Vomiting due to gastric outlet obstruction can actually be made worse. Antiemetics should not be used in inflammatory bowel disease or when intestinal obstruction is present or impending.

Nausea and vomiting are symptoms rather than disease. The inherent risk of symptomatic treatment is that it will mask signs of an evolving disease process.

G. **Fever** Elevated body temperature usually is significant as an indicator of infection or neoplasm. Occasionally fever by itself can be life-threatening. Body temperatures can reach dangerously high levels in severe infection, disseminated malignancy, following exposure to high environmental temperatures, or after general anesthesia. In adults, pyrexia greater than 104° F is poorly tolerated and requires symptom therapy.

Salicylates and mechanical body cooling are the basis of therapy. Phenothiazines impair temperature-regulating mechanisms and can thereby facilitate symptomatic treatment of fever. Chlorpromazine in doses of 25 to 50 mg IM should be given in association with other measures.

Precautions: Hazards of major tranquilizers have been discussed. Temperature overshoot is a potential danger when chlorpromazine is give to facilitate body cooling. If body temperature is not monitored carefully, severe hypothermia can develop. After chlorpromazine administration, cooling techniques should be stopped *before* normal body temperatures are reached — usually in the range of 101° F. The patient should then be observed for the development of hypothermia.

H. Hiccups Intractable hiccups usually respond to the standard doses of antiemetic drugs as given in Table 1-3. Anticholinergic-antihistamines should be tried first. If they fail, then major tranquilizers can be used.

Precautions: Hazards of drug therapy have been discussed. Symptomatic treatment does not preclude the necessity for a thorough search for the etiology of hiccups.

I. Premedication for diagnostic or therapeutic procedures Several diagnostic and therapeutic procedures performed on hospital wards are not painful enough to warrant the risk of general anesthesia but are sufficiently uncomfortable or disquieting to require some sort of psychosedative premedication. These are as follows:

1. Cardioversion Elective direct-current cardioversion can be performed on medical wards without an anesthesiologist present. Digitalis should be withheld for 24 hours prior to the procedure and replaced with quinidine sulfate, 200 to 300 mg PO every 6 hours for 4 doses. The patient should receive nothing by mouth starting at midnight on the day before cardioversion. No premedication is given.

A reliable intravenous line is established, preferably using a short plastic catheter (Jelco or Angiocath). *Diazepam* is the psychosedative of choice, being far less hazardous than and equally as effective as short-acting barbiturates. Diazepam is given rapidly — at a rate of 5 mg (1 ml)/min — until dysarthria is evident. Most patients require 10 to 20 mg, although some need much more. Cardioversion is performed with the patient in a state of light sleep. Shock-induced skeletal muscle contraction is not eliminated. However, the majority of patients have partial or total anterograde amnesia starting from the time of the injection. Patients may ambulate when they are able — usually in 30 minutes to 2 hours —

and they should be warned of probable persistent sedative effects from the drug. They should not operate automobiles or machinery for 24 hours.

Precautions: Cardiovascular or pulmonary complications from intravenous diazepam are exceedingly rare. However, the procedure should be performed in a coronary care unit where resuscitation equipment is available. Intravenous diazepam occasionally causes pain or induration, and in some cases phlebitis is a sequel. Large veins should be used if possible. The commercial preparation of injectable diazepam cannot be diluted — mixing with water or saline results in precipitation of the drug.

2. **Esophagogastroscopy** Intramuscular premedication is advisable for this procedure. A reasonable combination of drugs is meperidine (0.5 to 1.0 mg/kg) and diazepam (0.1 to 0.2 mg/kg) given 45 to 60 minutes before the procedure.

   Intravenous diazepam is used (as in cardioversion) just prior to passage of the instrument. In most cases cooperation is good, and the gastroscope passes without difficulty.

   Precautions: Resuscitation equipment need not be present for this procedure. Hazards of intravenous diazepam are theoretically increased due to prior administration of other CNS depressants. In practice, however, adverse reactions still are exceedingly rare.

3. **Sigmoidoscopy** This procedure, although invariably very uncomfortable if not moderately painful, is usually done without psychosedative premedication. A combination of intramuscular meperidine (0.5 mg/kg) and diazepam (0.1 mg/kg) given 45 to 60 minutes prior to sigmoidoscopy will make the procedure considerably more tolerable and will not interfere with its diagnostic value.

Suggested Readings

Appleton, W. S. Psychoactive drugs: A usage guide. *Dis. Nerv. Syst.* 32:607–616, 1971

DiMascio, A., and Shader, R. I. (Eds.) *Clinical Handbook of Psychopharmacology.* New York: Science House, 1970.

Greenblatt, D. J., and Shader, R. I. The clinical choice of sedative-hypnotics. *Ann. Intern. Med.* 77:91–100, 1972.

Greenblatt, D. J., and Shader, R. I. On the psychopharmacology of beta adrenergic blockade. *Curr. Ther. Res.* 14:615–625, 1972.

Greenblatt, D. J., and Shader, R. I. *Benzodiazepines in Clinical Practice.* New York: Raven, 1974.

Hollister, L. E. *Clinical Use of Psychotherapeutic Drugs.* Springfield, Ill.: Thomas, 1973

Lader, M. The nature of anxiety. *Br. J. Psychiatry* 121:481–491, 1972.

Shader, R. I., DiMascio, A., and associates. *Psychotropic Drug Side Effects: Clinical and Theoretical Perspectives.* Baltimore: Williams & Wilkins, 1970.

Shader, R. I. (Ed.) *Psychiatric Complications of Medical Drugs.* New York: Raven, 1972

2

The Psychopharmacologic Treatment of Anxiety States

Richard I. Shader
David J. Greenblatt

Anxiety is ubiquitous. We function every day against a backdrop of anxiety generated by life's upheavals, stages, and phases. Anxiety is a part of the internal signal system that alerts us to changes in our bodies and in the world around us. It can be adaptive or maladaptive; it can generate concern or overconcern. We experience some degree of anxiety not only when things are wrong but also when things are changed, unexpected — or just novel. It is an essential but at times unpleasant sense of tension, apprehension, or uneasiness that we experience subjectively and can observe in predictable, if idiosyncratic, bodily changes. Most familiar is a pattern including clammy palms, butterflies in the stomach, racing pulse, and pounding in the chest that may occur when we sense imminent danger and are alerted to cope with it. Coping with a threat or danger is usually accomplished through some form of fight or flight. The latter can take many forms, including escape, avoidance, and denial.

There is considerable overlap between anxiety and fear when the threat or danger is external and real. In this context, anxiety has come to mean an exaggerated or excessive response to verifiable danger. Anxiety also is the name given the response when the source of danger is largely unrecognized, obscure, or unknown, or when the response is incongruous with or inappropriate to the objective reality. Anxiety can also occur when one's sense of being able to take protective steps or effective action is blocked.

I. **Types of Anxiety States** The subtypes listed below can be observed singly or in combination. Some of the distinctions may seem arbitrary, but they are consistent with and derived from clinical observation and patients' reports. It is hoped that such distinctions will permit greater specificity in treatment planning. It should also be noted that anxiety states rarely occur in isolation — accompanying depression, anger, somatic complaints, obsessive-compulsive symptoms, or depersonalization are common. Table 2-1 lists some of the many descriptors and symptoms that are mentioned by anxious patients and observed by their physicians.

Table 2-1. Common Objective and Subjective Descriptors and Symptoms Associated with Anxiety States

Abdominal cramps	Nausea
Anorexia	Overconcern
Anxious	Pallor
Apprehensive	Palpitations
Breathless	Panic
Butterflies in the stomach	Phobias
Chest pains	Pupils dilated
Choking sensations	Rapid respirations or respiratory
Clutched up	distress (hyperpnea)
Diarrhea	Restless
Dizziness	Scared for no reason
Dread	Shaky
Dry mouth	Sweating
Easily startled	Syncope
Faintness	Tense
Fearful	Terror
Flushing	Threatened
Fright	Tightness in the chest
Giddy	Tremulous
Headache	Troubled
Heart racing (tachycardia)	Uneasiness
Impending doom feelings	Urge to urinate (and frequent urination)
Jittery	Vertigo
Jumpy	Vomiting
Keyed up	Weakness
Muscle tension	Worried
	Wound up

A. **Situational anxiety** describes a group of reactions to a diversity of stressful stimuli including interviews, tests, and surgery. Such anxiety is usually shortlived and ends once the experience is started or completed. Situational anxiety can represent a fear of the unknown but it can also be colored by a patient's low self-esteem. In these instances irrational fears of rejection, failure, criticism, and social or interpersonal catastrophe may be prominent. Clinical and research experiences suggest that preparing and informing the patient will quiet his situational anxiety if sensitive self-esteem issues or a high degree of irrationality are not involved. Examples include preparation for surgery by preoperative discussions with anesthesiologists, role playing or rehearsal in preparation for job interviews, and assertiveness training. For many patients, their own use of denial and minimization is adequate.

B. **Phobic anxiety** is a form of situational anxiety in which the major method of management is avoidance. In some instances the etiology of the phobia is clearly discernible, and treatment is straightforward. For example, if a child is bitten by a dog and thereafter fears being in the presence of dogs, one suitable treatment may be systematic desensitization — planned, progressive exposure to the fear-inducing stimulus or its facsimile. These carefully planned increments of ex-

posure are augmented by teaching the patient to relax and sometimes by coadministration of antianxiety agents. In cases where
patients fear open spaces, heights, or elevators, the etiology and treatment may be more complex; a phobia of this type can be understood,
at least in part, as the fear of being restricted from access to important persons in one's life (persons upon whom one can depend)
and thus appears to be a form of separation anxiety. Even more
complex are those phobias in which the feared object has a private,
symbolic, or unconscious meaning. These phobias are most likely
to develop in the context of interpersonal conflict, and often they
involve mental mechanisms such as projection, displacement, and
regression. Although desensitization can be symptomatically helpful, as can pharmacotherapy (see Section IV.B), clinical experience
suggests that it is important to supplement these approaches with
other psychotherapeutic techniques designed to help the patient
understand the evolution of his phobic anxiety in terms of his particular life experience.

C. **Anticipatory anxiety** is frequently associated with phobic anxiety
and situational anxiety. It is an arbitrary distinction at times, but
some patients describe fears preceding actual contact with dreaded
objects or situations. These anticipatory feelings may differ in
quantity and quality from phobic or situational fears, and often
they represent fears of the anxiety and panic states aroused by the
dreaded objects rather than fears of the objects per se. The intensity
of anticipatory anxiety is highly variable, ranging from a mild sense
of anticipation to states of extreme vigilance.

D. **Free-floating anxiety** is anxiety that bears no close temporal relationship to precipitating events or fear-inducing stimuli, and desensitization is rarely an effective treatment technique. Careful inquiry sometimes reveals the precipitants of the anxiety (e.g., something triggered
the emergence of forbidden feelings or painful memories; they are
quickly suppressed, but the anxiety remains). It usually varies in
duration from minutes to hours, although some patients describe
it as chronic and persisting over days. Often it can be linked to
irrational fears of illness or injury. We classify cancer phobias under
free-floating anxiety because there is no actual object or situation
that can be avoided, and a reassuring physical examination rarely
brings relief. Cancer and other illness phobias have a large obsessional component, and they usually occur along with other evidence
of obsessional thinking and depression. Such illness phobias do seem
distinct, however, from the somatic delusions that may be apparent
in psychotic depressions. These illness phobias sometimes occur
in individuals who have heard of the illness in someone else.

E. **Traumatic anxiety** is a distinctive type of anxiety that occurs in survivors of tragic and usually unanticipated experiences, such as natural disasters (sudden floods, tornadoes, fires), bombing raids, shipwrecks. It is usually associated with sleep disturbances and nightmares involving the tragic event and with a daytime syndrome (anxiety, restlessness, irritability, headache, overactive startle reflex, feelings of isolation and distrust, sense of inadequacy, and restriction of social contacts and activities) that may include reliving parts of the experience. This type of anxiety is less common in survivors who were able to participate in a helpful or effective manner after the event. Group discussion and grief work can also be valuable (*Social Work* 11:99—104, 1966). Early pharmacologic treatment should be avoided until careful physical examination can be carried out to identify postconcussion syndromes and occult intracranial and extracranial bleeding. If such complications can be ruled out, relief from the stressor and rest (usually assisted by the judicious use of antianxiety agents) are the cornerstones of treatment.

F. **Psychotic terror** can be quite dramatic in the acutely disorganized, frightened, easily startled patient. Paranoia and hallucinations may be prominent. Visual hallucinations in such patients may indicate a toxic psychosis (e.g., amphetamines, anticholinergic substances). Many schizophrenic patients also describe an earlier stage in their decompensations when they feel anxious and fear they are "going crazy." Treatment with antipsychotic drugs is usually indicated, except in some toxic psychoses. Working with patients in states of psychotic terror should include taking care not to be overstimulating. Efforts should be made to provide calm, familiar persons to stay with the patient (see Chapters 4 and 11).

G. **Anxious depression** is a form of anxiety that encompasses a mixed group of patients in whom anxiety, tension, and agitation are accompanied by overt depressive affect. (We prefer not to use this term to refer to patients for whom it is postulated that the overt anxiety results from depression that is not being openly experienced or expressed.) Many of these patients are chronically depressed, with intermittent exacerbations of anxiety symptoms, and they frequently complain of difficulty in falling asleep. Psychotherapy aimed at uncovering and articulating underlying issues of loss, disappointment, or defeat can be quite beneficial; getting patients in touch with their anger and resentment is helpful, since anxiety-bound hostility and guilt may be prominent features. Benzodiazepines are helpful to some, particularly when the sedating properties of these drugs assist patients in achieving adequate sleep. Some respond to tricyclic antidepressants, such as doxepin or amitriptyline. It is possible that some negative results with this latter group of drugs reflect inadequate dosing and blood levels. For example, dosages up to 150 mg/day of amitriptyline may be employed in outpatients, since many patients will show minimal response with dosages in the 50 to 100 mg/day range (*Br. Med. J.* 1:133—138, 1971). Caution in treating elderly patients with anxious depression is urged. Excessive sedation and resulting motor incoordination can have unwanted consequences, as can the anticholinergic, hypotensive, and arrhythmia-inducing properties of the tricyclic antidepressants. Combinations of antipsychotic agents (neuroleptics) and tricyclic antidepressants are also used (e.g., perphenazine and amitriptyline), but there seem to be few advantages unless there are psychotic elements in the presenting clinical picture.

H. **Anxiety in medical conditions** must be included in the clinician's differential diagnostic considerations. Table 2-2 lists medical conditions that may present with overt anxiety symptoms. Treatment should always be directed at the underlying medical condition. The anxiety associated with angina, for example, is best treated with nitroglycerin. Symptomatic treatment may be helpful in some conditions. Neuroleptics such as acetophenazine, fluphenazine, haloperidol, and thioridazine may be beneficial in some patients showing anxiety and agitation associated with cerebral arteriosclerosis and senile dementia (see Chapter 10). Hypoxic states are best treated by increasing oxygenation rather than by employing sedative-hypnotics, anxiolytics, and neuroleptics, which can produce a further degree of respiratory depression. Stress also may be a factor in medical conditions not listed in Table 2-2. For example, some patients with chronic dermatologic conditions, hypertension, and peptic ulcers may

Table 2-2.   Some Conditions that May Present with Prominent Anxiety Symptoms

Angina pectoris
Aspirin intolerance
Bad trips and drug intoxications
Behavioral toxicity from drugs
Caffeinism
Cerebral arteriosclerosis
Epilepsy (particularly psychomotor or temporal lobe epilepsy)
Hyperdynamic beta-adrenergic circulatory state (hyperventilation)
Hypoglycemia; hyperinsulinism
Hypoxic states (obstructive pulmonary disease; asthma)
Pain
Paroxysmal tachyarrhythmias
Pheochromocytoma
Premenstrual tension
Pulmonary embolism
Thyrotoxicosis; hyperthyroidism
Withdrawal from CNS depressant drugs

benefit from antianxiety agents even in the absence of overt anxiety (see D. J. Greenblatt and R. I. Shader, *Benzodiazepines in Clinical Practice,* New York: Raven, 1974; see also Chapter 1).

II. **General Treatment Considerations**   Based on behavioral studies with animals it may be hypothesized that drug treatments for anxiety work by lessening learned (acquired) avoidance responses or by diminishing anticipatory responses to external or imagined danger (or unpleasant) situations.   A decrement in anticipatory anxiety may be accompanied by a reduction in impulsive escape behaviors.   Although avoidance, escape, and denial can be adaptive at times, in most stressful circumstances a reduction of anxiety would permit the patient to make better use of information, insight, and relationships in preparation for coping with future anxiety.   Once the patient is less anxious, he can be helped to develop some perspective about the causes, manifestations (symptoms), and consequences (including unwanted effects on object relationships).   The patient can also learn whether there has been any secondary gain from the anxiety (e.g., does it get others to act in a more caring or giving manner?).

Although a discussion of various theoretical positions about anxiety is beyond the scope of this chapter, a viewpoint suggested by psychoanalytic psychology may assist the physician to build a relationship with the anxious patient: It is important for the physician to be able to listen to the patient's story without becoming anxious himself.   The history-taking should permit the clinician to listen for material suggesting that the patient becomes anxious about impulses that are forbidden or unacceptable or about painful memories or feelings that are threatening to emerge.   Often such sharing of memories, feelings, or impulses with a nonanxious, noncritical clinician will suffice to reduce anxiety.   When the clinician does choose to prescribe medication for the treatment of anxiety, it should not be done as a substitute for human, empathic involvement.

III. **Specific Pharmacologic Approaches**   In this section specific agents are reviewed.   These treatments are most useful for anticipatory, situational, and free-floating anxiety.   Although anxiety states can be acute, they typically are chronic, intermittent, and characterized by multiple exacerbations and remissions.   Drug treatments may be most effective when time-limited.   For example, a regimen may be continued for one to eight weeks and then interrupted until the patient begins to show symptoms again.

A. **Barbiturates** such as amobarbital, butabarbital, and phenobarbital are widely used.   Short-acting barbiturates are not helpful.   Phenobarbital and butabarbital are available in generic forms and are the least expensive antianxiety agents (see Appendix II). Since barbiturates produce generalized CNS depression and in many patients an unacceptable amount of sedation, their specific value in anxiety states is limited. In addition, barbiturates induce hepatic microsomal enzymes that can modify the metabolism of certain drugs taken concurrently (see Chapter 16). Physiological addiction and tolerance can occur. Intentional overdosage is frequently lethal. Barbiturates are seldom indicated for use as oral antianxiety agents.

B. Propanediols Meprobamate was popular for the treatment of anxiety in the late 1950s and early '60s. However, controlled studies do not consistently support the value of meprobamate, and we do not recommend its use (*Am. J. Psychiatry* 127:1297–1303, 1971). Meprobamate has significant addiction potential, and fatal suicides have occurred with some frequency (see Chapter 15). Drowsiness and ataxia are common unwanted effects. Tybamate has not received wide use or study. Early work suggested that withdrawal reactions from tybamate may be less common and less severe, but subsequent study has not yielded consistent results. As with barbiturates, propanediols are seldom indicated for the treatment of anxiety states. (See Appendix II for dosage information.)

C. Antipsychotic agents (neuroleptics) are occasionally prescribed for the treatment of anxiety states in nonpsychotic patients. As suggested in Section I.F, their major use is in psychotic terror, but they may be helpful in certain anxious and agitated elderly patients showing signs of senile dementia, particularly when irascibility and assaultiveness are part of the clinical picture. In addition, there are a few situations in which neuroleptics are indicated in the treatment of nonpsychotic anxious patients (although it is preferable to try benzodiazepines first):

1. Patients in whom anxiety is associated with a high degree of distractibility.
2. Anxious patients with racing thoughts or periods of thought blocking or both.
3. Anxious obsessional patients with strong imagination, considerable magical thinking, and occasionally poor reality testing.
4. Patients for whom other antianxiety regimens have not proved successful.

Although some of these patients may seem prepsychotic, many show no further evidence of disorganization or decompensation. When neuroleptics (see Appendix III) are selected for nonpsychotic patients, their dosages should be kept as low as possible (e.g., oral chlorpromazine or thioridazine: 10 to 25 mg tid as an initial regimen for one week followed by 25 to 75 mg in a single bedtime dose). Unwanted effects even at low dosages, however, may make the use of neuroleptics undesirable; drowsiness, ataxia, dry mouth, blurred vision, weakness, and feelings of unreality are commonly reported by anxious nonpsychotic patients. Although extrapyramidal side effects and hypotension are less common at low dosages, they may still occur. We do not recommend prohylactic use of antiparkinsonian drugs.

D. **Antidepressants** may be helpful in some patients with anxious depressions (see Section I.G). Amitriptyline and doxepin have been used most often because of their sedative properties. Regimens of 25 to 50 mg tid are common, but, as suggested in Section I.G, adequate dosages should be employed to insure that any lack of response is not attributable to underdosing. Anticholinergic and hypotensive side effects can undermine the successful use of antidepressants. Antidepressants have a special use in the treatment of phobic anxiety and spontaneous panic attacks (see Section IV; see also Chapters 1 and 3).

E. **Antihistamines** are still prescribed by some physicians. Their specific value in anxiety states has not been adequately tested. Comparative studies against benzodiazepines are few in number, but they generally support the greater, more consistent efficacy of the benzodiazepines. The antihistamines have weak, nonspecific CNS effects, and they are anticholinergic. Hydroxyzine is the most commonly used drug within this group. It may have a special usefulness in patients with anxiety-related pruritic dermatoses. Marketed as Vistaril and Atarax, hydroxyzine is usually prescribed at oral dosage levels between 30 and 200 mg daily and is available in 10, 25, 50, and 100 mg strengths. (See Appendix II.)

F. **Beta-adrenergic blocking agents** are effective against many of the peripheral somatic manifestations of anxiety — tachycardia, palpitations, tremor, and hyperventilation are particularly susceptible. Anxiety symptoms associated with hyperdynamic beta-adrenergic circulatory state (*Arch. Intern. Med.* 123:1–7, 1969), thyrotoxicosis, and paroxysmal tachyarrhythmias may be benefited by the use of beta-adrenergic blockers in some patients.

   The use of beta-adrenergic blockers in anxiety states for noninvestigational purposes is *not* currently approved in the United States by the Food and Drug Administration. The most commonly studied drug of this group is DL-propranolol (Inderal). Its use is contraindicated in patients whose cardiac compensation depends on sympathetic stimulation. It is also contraindicated in patients with obstructive lung diseases and asthma, and it should be used with caution in patients with diabetes mellitus. Oral dosages of 30 to 120 mg per day in 3 to 4 divided doses are typically employed. (See Appendix II.) Physicians prescribing beta-adrenergic blocking agents should be alert to their potential to cause or exacerbate symptoms of depression (*Curr. Ther. Res.* 14:615–625, 1972).

G. **Benzodiazepines** are among the most widely prescribed drugs in the United States. In comparison to the barbiturates and propanediols, benzodiazepines have shown greater, more consistent efficacy and a wider range of usefulness and cause less unwanted drowsiness (Greenblatt and Shader, *Benzodiazepines in Clinical Practice*). Although they are not the ultimate in antianxiety agents, benzodiazepines are the most effective of currently marketed antianxiety agents. They are not associated with clinically important enzyme induction, they have a very low addiction risk at therapeutic dosages, and they rarely cause serious outcomes in deliberate or accidental overdosages. Typically encountered side effects for these drugs are drowsiness and ataxia. All drugs of this group are likely to act synergistically with other CNS depressants. Occasional patients experience paradoxical rages, perhaps from the release of anxiety-bound hostility when interpersonal frustration is encountered (see Greenblatt and Shader, *Benzodiazepines in Clinical Practice*).

1 **Chlordiazepoxide** is well absorbed from the gastrointestinal tract. Peak blood levels are achieved within 2 to 4 hours after a single dose. Intramuscular absorption can be slow and incomplete, and we suggest oral administration unless the patient's panic or uncooperativeness is sufficiently extreme to preclude oral use. Intravenous administration is rapid but should be undertaken with caution in uncooperative patients. Care should be taken to employ the proper diluent and to insure that the needle is secure in the core of the vein. Small veins should not be used.

In most normal subjects the half-life of chlordiazepoxide is between 6 and 30 hours. Elderly patients and patients with active hepatic dysfunction metabolize the drug more slowly. Active metabolites are produced during biotransformation. Therefore, repeated, frequent dosing can produce cumulative clinical effects. Initial dosage schedules may necessitate three or four daily administrations, but many patients will do adequately on once- or twice- daily dosages initially or after several days of more frequent dosing. Since the drug may accumulate, particularly in the elderly, alternating dosage schedules may be helpful (e.g., 10 mg

PO hs and 5 mg PO hs on alternating days). See Appendix II for dosage forms and ranges.

2. **Diazepam** is also well absorbed from the gastrointestinal tract. In contrast to chlordiazepoxide, it is relatively lipid-soluble and not water-soluble. Intramuscular and intravenous use carry the same concerns as described for chlordiazepoxide. Diazepam has about two to five times the relative potency of chlordiazepoxide, and its half-life is longer (20 to 50 hours). It also has active metabolites; therefore, similar cautions about accumulation are in order. (See Appendix II.)

3. **Oxazepam** is a metabolite of diazepam. However, it has no known active metabolite in humans. It has the shortest half-life of this group of drugs (3 to 21 hours), and in most patients accumulation is not observed. Because of this short half-life, dosing should be more frequent — typical schedules involve doses given 3 or 4 times daily. Oxazepam has the lowest relative potency of this group. (See Appendix II.) No parenteral forms are available.

4. **Clorazepate** is metabolized to an analogue of diazepam and probably accumulates in a manner similar to that for chlordiazepoxide and diazepam. No parenteral forms are available. It is intermediate in relative potency between diazepam and chlordiazepoxide. Once- or twice-daily dosing is successful for many patients. (See Appendix II.) The published literature on this drug is scanty.

IV. **Phobic Anxiety and Spontaneous Panic Attacks**

A. **Description**   These anxiety states are discussed separately because of their characteristic response to psychopharmacologic intervention. Patients who fall in this subgroup are noted for their specific situational and phobic fears (e.g., fears of going out into public places such as streets, restaurants, open spaces), anticipatory anxiety, free-floating anxiety, and spontaneous panic attacks. While there may be restrictions in behavior only with respect to specific persons, places, situations, or objects, there may also be more generalized effects leading to a constricted life-style punctuated by distress and terror. Panic attacks are experienced as anxiety carried to its extreme, and they are more likely to occur when patients find themselves restricted in some way in their freedom of movement or in their access to help. This terror can be of such intensity that patients appear disorganized, disoriented, and depersonalized.

Anxiety responses, experienced as involuntary and irrational, lead to a variety of avoidance and escape behaviors. Rituals and various superstitious activities are common and may occur even though the patient is removed from the fear-producing stimulus. Excessive use of alcohol, stimulants, sedative-hypnotics, and anti-anxiety agents is common because these substances are of some value in reducing free-floating or anticipatory anxiety.

B. Treatment A comprehensive treatment plan is indicated for such patients and should include the following elements:

1. **An investigative-supportive relationship** A therapist can be of value in helping the patient to uncover the range of situations that cause the anxiety, and, subsequently, to identify the common aspects of these situations (e.g., fears of being unable to reach someone they depend on). In conjunction with eliciting the patient's history of anxiety and fears, efforts are made to relate any exacerbation or intensification of fears to contributing life events (e.g., the death of a loved one). Support is given to the patient as he confronts the fear-producing experiences or memories in a steady, progressive way.

2. **Antianxiety agents** Benzodiazepines are at present the agents of choice for the effective reduction of anticipatory and free-floating anxiety. Phenobarbital and amobarbital also may be employed, but they are not as consistently effective. (See Appendix II for dosages.)

3. **Antidepressants** Imipramine and phenelzine are beginning to achieve acceptance as effective agents for the treatment of panic attacks and phobic states. However, neither drug has been approved by the Food and Drug Administration for such use in the United States at the present time. In clinical-investigative work, these drugs have in several instances been dramatically helpful. Support for this application of these and related drugs can be found in the literature. Table 2-3 lists illustrative articles for the physician who seeks further information on this use of antidepressants.

   Imipramine dosage requirements are highly variable. It is best to start patients at low dosages and to titrate dosage until beneficial effects are observed or side effects are encountered. It is not uncommon for these patients (who are not primarily depressed) to be sensitive to low dosages of imipramine. Positive responses can occur with as little as 10 mg PO qhs. Side effects such as excessive stimulation or jitteriness can also be encountered at low dosages; tachycardia is not uncommon. When such side effects are encountered, the dosage may be reduced to a level at which side effects do not occur and the patient maintained at this level

Table 2-3.   Literature Supporting the Value of Antidepressants in the Treatment of Phobic-Anxiety and Spontaneous Panic Attacks

Geissmann, P., and Kammerer, T.   L'imipramine dans la nevrose obsessionnelle: Étude de 30 cas. *Encéphale* 53:369—382, 1964.

Gittelman-Klein, R., and Klein, D. F.   Controlled imipramine treatment of school phobia. *Arch. Gen. Psychiatry* 25:204—207, 1971.

Kelly, D., Guirguis, W., Frommer, E., Mitchell-Heggs, N., and Sargant, W.   Treatment of phobic states with antidepressants. *Br. J. Psychiatry* 116:387—398, 1970.

Klein, D. F.   Delineation of two drug-responsive anxiety syndromes. *Psychopharmacologia* 5:397—408, 1964.

Klein, D. F.   Importance of psychiatric diagnosis in prediction of clinical drug effects. *Arch. Gen. Psychiatry* 16:118—126, 1967.

Klein, D. F., and Fink, M.   Psychiatric reaction patterns to imipramine. *Am. J. Psychiatry* 119:432—438, 1962.

Lipsedge, M. S., Hajioff, J., Huggins, P., Napier, L., Pearce, J., Pike, D. J., and Rich, M.   The management of severe agoraphobia: A comparison of iproniazid and systematic desensitization. *Psychopharmacologia* 32:67—80, 1973.

Solyon, L., Heseltine, G. F. D., McClure, D. J., Solyon, C., Ledridge, B., and Steinberg, G.   Behavior therapy versus drug therapy in the treatment of phobic neurosis. *Can. Psychiatr. Assoc. J.* 18:25—31, 1973.

Tellenbach, H.   Über die Behandlung phobischer und anankasticher Zustände mit imipramin. *Nervenarzt* 34:133—138, 1963.

Tyrer, P., Candy, J., and Kelly, D.   A study of the clinical effects of phenelzine and placebo in the treatment of phobic anxiety. *Psychopharmacologia* 32:237—254, 19

Zitrin, C. M., Klein, D. F., Lindemann, C., Tobak, P., Rock, M., Kaplan, J. H., and Ganz, V. H.   Comparison of Short-Term Treatment Regimens in Phobic Patients: A Preliminary Report. In R. L. Spitzer and D. F. Klein (Eds.) *Evaluation of Psychological Therapies.* Baltimore: Johns Hopkins University Press (in press).

for several days before a dosage increment is again attempted. Most patients who are going to respond to this regimen can be treated with a single daily dose of up to 150 mg. Only rarely are higher dosages required. (See Chapters 1 and 3 for further information about imipramine.)

Phenelzine also has been found to be helpful to some patients, although its use is complicated by necessary dietary restrictions (see Chapter 19). Dosage increments should be titrated as described above for imipramine; side effects in the low dosage range are similar. A typical effective regimen might be 15 mg POtid.

With both of these drugs, relapses are common when the drug is discontinued. Any physician considering the potential value of antidepressants for a phobic-anxious patient with spontaneous panic attacks should be aware that this is not an FDA-approved indication for the use of these drugs. The physician should familiarize himself with the relevant literature so that the patient and physician will be informed about the potential risks and benefits. It is also advisable to seek consultation before embarking upon this approach and to have the results of this consultation documented in the patient's record.

3

The Classification and Treatment of Depressive Disorders*

Joseph J. Shildkraut
Donald F. Klein

In the original report in 1958 on the antidepressant action of imipramine (*Am. J. Psychiatry* 115:459–464, 1958), Kuhn noted the importance of differentiating among the various types of depressive disorders when prescribing treatment. Subsequently the differential treatment responses of various clinically defined types of depressions have been documented by other investigators, and there has been revival of interest in the phenomena and clinical classification of the depressive disorders.†

Much recent work has focused on refining the classic distinctions between endogenous (often equated with autonomous or vital) and nonendogenous (often equated with reactive or neurotic or chronic characterological) depressive syndromes on the basis of presenting signs, symptoms, and history. Although most investigators agree on the existence of a relatively homogeneous endogenous depressive syndrome, the precise definition and cardinal signs and symptoms of this syndrome still need clarification. Some investigators have focused on the absence of precipitants, but others have questioned the prognostic value and treatment relevance of this criterion. Instead, they have stressed the importance of various characteristics, such as pervasive inability to experience pleasure, loss of energy and vitality, psychic retardation, decreased interest or ambition, and decreased responsiveness to environmental events or interpersonal interactions. Although these characteristics often are present in apparently nonprecipitated depressions, they also frequently

*The authors wish to acknowledge the contribution of their colleagues to the system for classifying depressive disorders described in this chapter. They include Jon Gudeman, M.D., Jacov Avni, M.D., Barbara A. Keeler, M.S.W., Frederick Quitkin, M.D., Arthur Rifkin, M.D., and Rachel Gittelman-Klein, Ph.D. We also thank Mrs. Gladys Rege, who assisted in the preparation of this manuscript. This work was supported in part by USPHS Grant No. MH15413.
†The system for classifying depressive disorders embodied in the American Psychiatric Association's *Diagnostic and Statistical Manual of Mental Disorders,* 2nd ed. (APA DSM-II), provides little help in making rational and consistent treatment decisions. Most investigators in this field have abandoned the APA DSM-II system for classifying the depressive disorders, and a major revision of the APA system is expected in the near future.

are observed and are treatment-relevant in apparently precipitated depressions* (see J. J. Schildkraut, *Neuropsychopharmacology and the Affective Disorders,* Boston: Little, Brown, 1970).

The distinction between bipolar (manic-depressive) and unipolar depressive disorders also has been emphasized in recent years, and a number of biologic correlates of this clinical distinction have been reported. The diagnosis and classification of manic disorders as well as the differences and similarities between manic and schizophrenic disorders are currently undergoing a re-examination. These issues and related questions concerning the schizoaffective states reflect a longstanding problem in the history of psychiatric nosology.

The distinction between primary and secondary affective disorderst has been stressed by some investigators. Specific diagnostic criteria for identifying these disorders have been proposed by one group of investigators (*Arch. Gen. Psychiatry* 26:57–63, 1972), who have provided a preliminary validation of these criteria against followup data and family history. Further validation of these criteria against prediction of response to treatment or various biologic measures would be of particular interest. The distinction between primary and secondary depressive disorders (or dysphorias) is also a principal element in a recently proposed alternative, treatment-relevant diagnostic system (D. F. Klein, Differential Diagnosis and Treatment of the Dysphorias, in G. M. Simpson and D. M. Gallant [Eds.], *Tulane University International Symposium on Depression: Behavioral, Biochemical, Clinical and Treatment Concepts,* New York: Spectrum, in press).

Although the distinction between primary and secondary depressive disorder may be of some use clinically (and in research), when applied rigorously this distinction can sometimes lead to subcategorization with no evident prognostic or treatment-relevant implications. For example, the diagnosis of a bipolar manic-depressive patient with preexisting alcoholism or antisocial personality would have to be secondary rather than primary affective disorder, although prognosis and treatment of the affective disorder would remain the same.

Despite differences in approach, numerous studies have shown that the affective disorders can be separated into meaningful groupings on the basis of clinical signs, symptoms, and history. However, as in many other areas of medicine, disorders that appear clinically indistinguishable on the basis of

---

*Because many psychiatrists tend to equate the endogenous depressions with nonprecipitated depression, the term *endogenomorphic* has been suggested by one of us (D.F.K.) to stress the fact that both precipitated and nonprecipitated depression may share the salient characteristics of the endogenous state (*Arch. Gen. Psychiatry* 31:447–454, 1974). However, in this chapter we shall use the term *endogenous* to refer to such depressive disorders, defined largely on the basis of presenting signs and symptoms (as described here) irrespective of the presence or absence of precipitants. We hope this explicit definition will avoid both confusing terminology and neologism.

tPrimary affective disorders occur in individuals who have had no previous psychiatric disorders or else only episodes of depressions or manias. Secondary affective disorders occur in patients with a preexisting psychiatric illness other than depressions or manias (e.g., schizophrenia, anxiety neurosis, alcoholism, antisocial personality).

presenting signs and symptoms may nonetheless have different etiologies or underlying biochemical pathophysiologies. Conversely, some disorders with different clinical manifestations may nonetheless have similar biologic substrates. Thus, while various clinical criteria may be of value in determining the appropriate treatment for a patient with a depressive disorder, recent findings suggest that these clinical distinctions may soon be usefully augmented by various biologic criteria (*Psychopharmacol. Bull.* 10:5—25, 1974; or *Annu. Rev. Med.* 25:333—348, 1974).

I. **Classification of Depressive Disorders** The system for classifying the depressive disorders presented in this chapter represents an attempt to synthesize and refine two very similar systems developed independently by the authors and their respective colleagues over the past several years. Following the tradition of descriptive psychiatry, this system for classifying the depressive disorders relies on history as well as on the assessment of presenting signs and symptoms. In this system, depressions are classified as schizophrenia-related, bipolar manic-depressive, or unipolar largely on the basis of history. Specific depressive syndromes are defined largely on the basis of presenting signs and symptoms.

    An essential feature of this system is the separation of two discrete depressive syndromes, the endogenous depressions and the chronic characterological depressions (to which the term *neurotic depression* is often applied). These clinically defined syndromes appear to be separable entities in that few patients have been found to show both syndromes concurrently. Other specific syndromes, including agitated involutional depressive syndromes, are also identified. Some depressions, of course, fit no specific syndrome, and they are designated *nonspecific* in this system (Table 3-1).

Table 3-1. Proposed System for Classifying Depressive Disorders

Schizophrenia-related depressions

    Depressions in true or process schizophrenia
    Depressions in schizoid states (schizoid-affective depressions)
    Depressions in schizophreniform psychoses (schizoaffective depressions)

Bipolar manic-depressive depressions

Unipolar depressions

    Endogenous depressive syndromes
    Chronic characterological depressive syndromes
    Agitated involutional depressive syndromes
    Nonspecific depressive syndromes
        Situational depressions
        Other nonspecific depressive syndromes

A. **Proposed system for classifying depressive disorders** Depressive disorders, broadly defined, include patients with one or more complaints of depression, sadness, unhappiness, tearfulness, psychomotor retardation, apathy, anergy, or anhedonia. Since these symptoms may sometimes be manifestations of documented organic disease states (e.g. anemia, hypothyroidism, etc.) or drug-induced (e.g., by reserpine or oral contraceptives), it is important to rule this out by means of a careful history, physical examination, and laboratory investigation. *The following system for classifying depressive disorders assumes the prior exclusion of patients with depressive disorders that are drug-induced or that are manifestations of documented organic disease states.*

The modifier *psychotic* may be applied to any of the following diagnoses when formal psychotic elements are concurrently present (i.e., impaired reality testing, including delusions or hallucinations).

1. **Schizophrenia-related depressive disorders** From the group of depressive disorders we first separate patients with prior histories of schizophrenia, other schizophreniform psychoses or transient micropsychotic episodes* that are not affect-consonant (excluding those of toxic or documented organic etiologies), and schizoid disorders (characterized by chronic asocial behavior†). This group, termed schizophrenia-related depressive disorders, may be subdivided further on the basis of the history.

   a. The true or process **schizophrenic disorders** include those with well-documented schizophrenic psychoses that are characterized by thought disorders (e.g., communicative and inductive incompetence that is not due to the rate of thought and speech, a documented organic etiology, or sociocultural factors), delusions or hallucinations that are not consonant with concurrent depressive or manic affect,‡ and a history of chronic asocial behavior.

   b. The schizoid disorders include patients with histories of chronic asocial behavior but not of overt psychosis. These depressions may be termed **schizoid-affective disorders.**

*Transient micropsychotic episodes (clearcut, short-lived delusional or hallucinatory experiences) must be distinguished from malingering and vivid metaphorical communication (sometimes called hysterical).
†Chronic asocial behavior — which includes gradual deterioration in social functioning, extreme social isolation, or odd, bizarre, eccentric behavior of at least several years duration — is to be distinguished from antisocial, sociopathic, or psychopathic behavior.
‡Delusions or hallucinations consonant with depressive affect include those related to hopelessness, helplessness, worthlessness, guilt, impoverishment, decay of body, decay of possessions, and fearfulness, suspiciousness, and judgmental ideas of reference (including some persecutory delusions). Delusions or hallucinations consonant with manic affect include those related to euphoria, optimism, grandiosity, enhancement of power or wealth or possessions, and some persecutory delusions.

c. The schizophreniform disorders include patients with histories of psychotic manifestations (including transient micropsychotic episodes) that are not solely affect-consonant but that cannot be diagnosed as true or process schizophrenia, usually due to the absence of chronic asocial behavior. These depressions are termed **schizoaffective disorders** in this chapter. (See also Chapter 4, Section I.)

2. **Manic-depressive (bipolar) disorders** Of the patients remaining after removing the schizophrenia-related depressions, those with a prior history of mania or clear hypomania* are classified as bipolar manic-depressive. In clinical experience manic-depressive depressions generally present as endogenous depressive syndromes. (See also Chapter 5.)

3. **Unipolar depressive disorders** The remaining patients, the unipolar depressive disorders, are then separated into those with specific endogenous, chronic characterological, or agitated involutional depressive syndromes, and a residual group with *nonspecific* syndromes. This residual group will include most situational depressions, nonspecific depressive syndromes occurring in the context of other psychiatric disorders, and other depressive syndromes that cannot be classified more specifically.

B. **Criteria for differentiating among depressive syndromes** The specific depressive syndromes described below are defined mainly on the basis of presenting signs and symptoms, but elements of the history are also important in making these distinctions. Although this classification is mainly of value in differentiating among unipolar depressions, it is sometimes also useful to distinguish among these syndromes when evaluating patients with schizophrenia-related or bipolar manic-depressive depressions. Formal criteria for making these distinctions have been developed and are currently used in research studies (J. J. Schildkraut, J. Avni, B. A. Keeler, J. Gudeman, C. Neu, and R. D. Hunt, Clinical Inventory for the Diagnosis and Classification of the Affective Disorders [CIDCAD], unpublished). According to these criteria, a stipulated minimum number of core and supporting characteristics or combinations of characteristics are required for the diagnosis of each syndrome. This stringent requirement promotes diagnostic homogeneity at the cost of a certain number of false-negative misdiagnoses. However, in clinical practice

---

*Mania or hypomania as defined here include syndromes characterized by press of speech, euphoria, increased sense of vitality and well-being, flight of ideas, purposeful or quasi-purposeful hyperactivity, increased social activity, irritability, belligerence, decreased need for sleep, grandiosity, and spending sprees, occurring in the absence of psychotic elements that are not affect-consonant.

such formal criteria are rarely followed, since clinicians often must act on provisional diagnoses, thus accepting a proportion of false-positive misdiagnoses. Consequently, this chapter presents a list of the important characteristics of each syndrome rather than the more formal criteria devised for research use.

1. **Endogenous depressions** Endogenous depressive syndromes are characterized by psychic retardation (slowing and paucity of thought and speech with prolonged speech latencies, dull woolly-headed thinking, or decrease in decisiveness); anergy (loss of energy, impaired sense of vitality, or decrease in ambition or initiative); anhedonia or apathy (inability to attain usual satisfactions and pleasures customarily obtained from work and recreational activities or to maintain usual level of interest and emotional involvement in activities); decreased productivity; and diurnal variation (worse in mornings). Most important, endogenous depressions are further characterized by the autonomy of the depressive syndrome once it has been established, irrespective of whether or not the depression was initially precipitated by events in the patient's life. Thus, the patient's condition does not respond appreciably either to alterations in the environment or to social or therapeutic interpersonal interactions.

Agitation is a descriptor frequently used as a criterion for endogenous depressive syndromes. It refers to increased gross motor movements that appear expressive rather than instrumental in nature (e.g., hand wringing, pacing). These are often accompanied by vocal expressions apparently indicative of intense psychic pain (rapid, incessant, and often loud, vociferous supplication). Further, much of this activity seems directed toward producing somatic counterirritatant pain (hand wringing, hair pulling, head banging, cuticle picking). (Both authors agree that such behavior is a regular and distinctive concomitant of involutional depressions. D. F. K. believes that agitation is sufficiently distinctive that it should be made one of the core defining characteristics of endogenous depressions. J. J. S. believes that this descriptor, as a criterion, should be confined to the involutional depressive syndromes.)

Sadness of affect (depressive mood as a symptom) is often but not invariably present, and one must be prepared to make the diagnosis of an endogenous depressive syndrome even in the absence of the symptom of depressive mood. Other commonly occurring symptoms include sleep disturbances (insomnia or hypersomnia), anorexia (sometimes with appreciable weight loss), feelings of hopelessness, helplessness, worthlessness, guilt, and demoralization, and suicidal ruminations. However, these symptoms may also be seen in other types of depressions and are not among the core criteria to identify the endogenous depressive syndromes.

In the endogenous depressions, the depressive syndrome is often reported to be qualitatively different from those depressions of mood that the patient has experienced during the course of everyday life. Patients with endogenous depressions generally present histories of adequate premorbid social adjustments with a previous capacity to function well at work. Recovery from episodes of endogenous depressions usually occurs with complete clinical remission. Thus, the depressive episodes in such patients can be fairly well separated from both the premorbid and the postmorbid intervals.

The core criteria for identifying endogenous depressive syndromes differ markedly from the constellation of signs and symptoms of importance for the diagnosis of chronic characterological depressions (as outlined in Section I.B.2). It should be reemphasized that, in contrast to the chronic characterological depressions, the presence of depressive mood (feeling sad, unhappy, or blue) is not necessary for the diagnosis of endogenous depressive syndromes. The physician must be alert to this possibility since he may see patients who fulfill the criteria for an endogenous depressive syndrome but deny feelings of "depression" per se and who require treatment with antidepressant drugs or electroconvulsive therapy (see Section III. D. 1).

2. **Chronic characterological depressive syndromes** The syndromes designated chronic characterological depressions are typically (but not exclusively) seen in those patients whose depressions are an inherent part of a lifelong personality problem in which relatively minor stresses or changes in life pattern may precipitate symptomatology. Such patients frequently present longstanding histories of poor interpersonal and social adjustments, hence the term *chronic characterological* depressions. However, as in the endogenous depressions, in which the absence of precipitants is not essential for the diagnosis, in the chronic characterologic depressions, a specific type of character pathology is not essential, since the diagnosis is made largely on the basis of presenting signs and symptoms.

The signs and symptoms of importance for the diagnosis of chronic characterologic depressive syndromes include: unhappiness, dissatisfaction, weeping, preoccupation with losses or unpleasantnesses, feeling "shortchanged"; emotional lability, histrionic behavior, dramatic attention-seeking; blame avoidance; demandingness, complaining, clinging dependency; pessimism; irritability, anger; self-pity; anxiety; and hypochondriasis. (Other signs and symptoms often noted in these patients are marked secondary gain and frequent use of stimulants, sedatives, and alcohol. Manipulative suicidal threats occur, but so do actual suicides.) Patients with chronic characterological depressions generally are responsive to environmental events or interpersonal interactions, and they remain reactive to such external stimuli.

The chronic characterological depressive syndromes, as defined here, represent a heterogeneous collection of disorders that may include several, more specific clinical syndromes with specific responses to treatment. One of the authors (D. F. K.) has suggested two such syndromes, *hysteroid-dysphoric* and *phobic-anxious*. The detailed description of these syndromes and outlines for their specific treatment are contained elsewhere in this manual (see Chapters 2 and 17). It should also be noted that many of the patients with chronic characterological depressions, as defined here, may be classified as hysterical or borderline according to other diagnostic systems.

3. **Agitated involutional depressive syndromes** The diagnosis of an agitated involutional depressive syndrome may be made in conjunction with any depressive diagnosis. In practice this syndrome is usually observed as a subset of the unipolar endogenous depressions. The signs and symptoms of importance for the diagnosis of agitated involutional depressive syndromes include agitation (hand wringing or pacing), paranoid ideation or delusions, thoughts or delusions of bodily decay, and feelings or delusions of guilt. Most patients with such agitated depressive syndromes are over 45 years old (hence the term *involutional*), but this syndrome may be seen in younger people.

4. **Situational depressive syndromes** The situational depressions (sometimes called reactive depressions) are those depressive disorders that occur as a result of an overwhelming situational stress, such as the loss of a family member, job, fortune, or home. These depressions, which include grief reactions and mourning, are rather common. Symptomatology frequently includes tearfulness, brooding, preoccupation with the loss, feelings of tension, inability to shift attention focus from the inciting situation, loss of appetite, and insomnia. However, the patient maintains the reactive capacity for pleasure and interest and can be distracted from his brooding focus, as may be seen in a person at a wake.

Moreover, the affective state is not fixed, and a change in life circumstances may result in a prompt remission.

Situational depressions are usually self-limited disorders with remission generally occurring within a few months. Occasionally a situational depression may evolve into what appears to be an endogenous depressive syndrome in which the symptoms change their character and become autonomous of the initial precipitating stress or subsequent related life events. At that point the disorder should be regarded as a supervening endogenous depression and treated as such.

II. **Demoralization — A Difficulty in the Differential Diagnosis of Depressions** One poorly understood aspect of psychiatric illness is demoralization — the belief in one's ineffectiveness, engendered by a severe life defeat. It is a change in self-image (the complex of attitudes and evaluations toward the self) in the direction of helplessness. Although any life defeat may produce demoralization, it is quite common in depressions, since a feature of the pathological depressed state is the profound conviction of one's incompetence. This self-denigrating belief seems validated by the person's catastrophic life experience.

Demoralized patients are unable to engage spontaneously in even normal life tasks, since they view themselves as unequal to the effort involved. Therefore, they remain restricted in their activities, thus confirming their incapacity. Even after a depressive disorder has remitted, so that enjoyment is again possible, the ability to anticipate and plan competent activity may be severely diminished because of the persistent change in self-image. Demoralization is also a frequent consequence of other psychiatric disorders.

In contrast to many depressed patients, the demoralized person can enjoy himself in a setting in which no demands are made upon him. His appetites are not inhibited, and his sleep pattern is normal. Demoralization can be the secondary consequence of many different life defeats, and it will respond to a wide variety of encouraging measures. However, of practical importance is the fact that such a state of *attitudinal despair generally does not respond to antidepressant medication.*

A patient may present with a clear history of endogenous depression. This may have remitted, but the patient remains demoralized. The clinician may use an antidepressant, without benefit, and then embark on a prolonged search for the uniquely appropriate medication rather than providing the supportive, directive, remobilizing psychotherapy the patient requires.

III. **Treatment of Depressive Disorders**

A. **General considerations** This section provides an outline of recommendations for the treatment of the depressive syndromes described in Section I. It must be emphasized, however, that an appreciable number of patients will fall within the ill-defined areas between the diagnostic boundaries and will not be uniquely classified according to this system. Moreover, as with any nosologic approach based only on clinical signs and symptoms, the possibility of misdiagnosis must always be considered. The suggestions for treatment, therefore, are offered only as recommendations for the initial trial of therapy. Trial and error has not yet been obviated. If improvement does not occur after a suitable therapeutic trial of one treatment approach, the physician is advised to try alternative measures. Since depressions constitute a recurrent problem for many patients, clues to successful therapy may be found in the history of previous responses to one or another form of treatment. If a particular treatment has proved successful in previous episodes, the likelihood of its future success is enhanced.

Although the major aim of this chapter is to provide guidelines for the pharmacotherapy of depressive disorders, some comments on the role of psychotherapy are in order. As stressed here, decisions concerning the use and choice of antidepressant drugs are made on the basis of descriptive psychiatric criteria, namely clinical signs and symptoms and history. In contrast, decisions concerning the need for intensive psychotherapy and the specific nature of that psychotherapy are based on quite different criteria that include a dynamic assessment of the interpersonal and intrapsychic factors that may be related to the acute depressive episode and an assessment of the patient's level of social adjustment and functioning prior to the onset of the depressive episode. A final decision regarding the need for long-term intensive psychotherapy (in contrast to acute supportive, directive, or exploratory psychotherapy) is usually best deferred until after the resolution of the acute depressive episode. It must be cautioned that in acutely depressed patients, psychotherapy can sometimes foster a regressive dependency and demoralization by focusing the patient's attention and energies inward and onto their keenly felt deficits, thereby decreasing the patient's attempts at outwardly directed active coping behavior. Simple statements to such patients that depression represents their anger turned inward are not helpful and are potentially harmful. This may serve to intensify and prolong the depression or convert it into a demoralized state. According to a model proposed by one of us (J. J. S.), it is conceivable that inappropriately applied psychotherapy, by decreasing active coping behavior, could even counteract the specific neuropharmacologically induced revitalizing effects of antidepressant drugs (Schildkraut, *Neuropsychopharmacology and the Affective Disorders)*

Supportive or exploratory individual psychotherapy and family therapy may be of value in the treatment of some patients with acute depressive episodes. Patients whose depressions appear to have been precipitated by a recent loss or disappointment may be helped by having the opportunity to react affectively to these experiences. Involvement of key family members often is crucial in gathering objective information and ensuring treatment compliance. Milieu treatment directed toward social support, interaction, and distraction from brooding by concrete simple tasks that have the goal clearly in sight also may be helpful. Support of the patient's realistic attempts to maintain his activities during an acute depression is important to prevent further loss of self-esteem. However, excessive expectations for performance (whether coming from the patient or the family or the physician) should be avoided, since these may result in failure that will further decrease the patient's already impaired sense of self-esteem and increase his feelings of worthlessness. For patients who do not require hospitalization, remaining on their jobs may be helpful.

The decision to treat a depressed patient with psychotherapy does not preclude the use of antidepressant drugs any more than treatment with antidepressant drugs precludes psychotherapy. For many patients psychotherapy will help the patient to collaborate with pharmacotherapy. Each form of treatment has its own set of indications (as well as contraindications), and these are best considered independently of each other in determining the optimal therapeutic regimen for the individual.

It is important to emphasize the fact that the depressive disorders are, for the most part, treatable conditions. The eventual goal of treatment should be nothing less than complete restitution to the level of functioning maintained by the patient prior to the onset of the depression. All too often, clinicians and patients alike, impressed by the degree of improvement that has already occurred compared to the acute depressed state, settle for something less than total restitution. Although total restitution may not be attainable in every case, it is in most cases; the question of whether the patient has been restored to his or her usual self should be raised explicitly with the patient and with other people who knew the patient prior to the onset of the acute depressive episode.

All patients with depressive disorders, irrespective of diagnostic type, may be suicidal. The risk of suicide, therefore, must be recognized and evaluated in every depressed patient, and prevention of suicide must be assured as the first step in the treatment of patients with depressive disorders (see Chapter 20).

B. **Treatment of schizophrenia-related depressive disorders** Primary treatment of the schizophrenia-related depressive disorders should be directed toward the schizophrenic, schizophreniform, or other psychotic manifestations of these disorders as well as toward the schizoid or asocial behavior. This usually entails treatment with antipsychotic drugs as well as some form of interpersonal or social therapy. Group therapy focused on support and reality testing may be useful. These aspects of the treatment of schizophrenia and related disorders are considered in Chapter 4.

Depression sometimes constitutes the major manifestation of the schizophrenia-related disorder requiring treatment. This frequentl occurs after successful treatment of the psychotic manifestations with antipsychotic drugs or during the course of interpersonal therapy Following a period of treatment with antipsychotic medication, the patient may be improved but still show low spirits, inactivity, apathy, and lack of spontaneity. There is a difficult differential diagnosis here between a residual depression and the drug-induced conditions of overtranquilization or parkinsonian akinesia (even without manifes tremor or rigidity). Often this distinction is not possible on neurologic or behavioral phenomenological grounds. Although a reduction of dosage or discontinuation of the antipsychotic medication would demonstrate whether the condition was secondary to medication (i.e., overtranquilization or drug-induced extrapyramidal akinesia) or part of the course of the illness, this sometimes is not feasible for fear of relapse. If the patient is not receiving an antiparkinsonian agent, a short trial (several days) may show a sudden rise in spontaneity and participation, indicating that the problem was a drug-induced extrapyramidal akinesia. In contrast, some of the patients who do not respond to antiparkinsonian agents have drug-treatable depressions.

When the depression has the characteristics of an endogenous depressive syndrome, it should be treated with a tricyclic antidepressant (as described for unipolar endogenous depressions, Section **III. D**) except for the caution that antidepressant drugs may precipitate overt psychotic episodes in patients with schizophrenia-related depressions, particularly in those with true schizophrenias. (Should an overt psychosis be precipitated by an antidepressant drug, the antidepressant should be discontinued, and treatment with an antipsychotic agent such as chlorpromazine should be instituted immediately. Merely discontinuing the antidepressant is not sufficient.) When a schizophrenia-related depression does not have the characteristics of an endogenous depression, an attempt should be made to relate the syndrome to one of the other depressive syndrome described and treatment should proceed as outlined.

As indicated in Chapter 4 (Section I), it is sometimes difficult to separate schizoaffective disorders from manic-depressive disorders. This is particularly true in putative manic-depressive patients showing considerable psychotic disorganization (especially including paranoid belligerence) during manic episodes or, conversely, in putative schizoaffective patients when the psychosis is tinged with manic symptomatology (euphoria, grandiosity, press of speech, or flight of ideas) or depressive symptomatology (psychomotor retardation, anergy, or anhedonia). In fact, many investigators have questioned whether such distinctions are not rather arbitrary, and various biologic as well as clinical similarities in these groups have been observed. The use of lithium in the treatment of patients with schizoaffective disorders is currently undergoing experimental evaluation. Although conflicting findings have been reported, it does appear that lithium may be of value in the treatment of some patients with schizoaffective disorders. One may, of course, question whether such patients do not in fact have disorders that are manic-depressive variants, but in the absence of more definitive clinical or biologic criteria for making such diagnoses, this remains an empty, semantic issue.

C. **Treatment of manic-depressive (bipolar) disorders**   The depressive phase of manic-depressive disorders generally shows the characteristics of endogenous depressive syndromes. The acute depressive episode of manic-depressive disorders should be treated with imipramine according to the guidelines for unipolar endogenous depressions (Section III. D), even when a clearcut endogenous depressive syndrome is not apparent. As described in Chapter 5, lithium salts have been found to be effective agents for treating acute hypomanic or manic episodes and also for decreasing the frequency and intensity of both manic and depressive episodes in cycling manic-depressive patients. Moreover, lithium has been reported to be clinically effective in treating some patients with acute depressive episodes, particularly those occurring in the context of a manic-depressive disorder, although imipramine appears to be more broadly effective. The use of lithium for the treatment of acute depressive episodes is still undergoing experimental evaluation and cannot be recommended at the present time as a routine treatment.

When treating an acute depression in a manic-depressive patient undergoing prophylactic treatment with lithium, it is generally advisable to continue lithium at its usual maintenance level (particularly if the lithium has been found to exert some prophylactic benefit) and to add imipramine in usual therapeutic doses. Occasionally a monoamine oxidase inhibitor in conjunction with lithium may be particularly beneficial.

In some patients it may appear that lithium has contributed to the development of the depressive episode, particularly when this occurs shortly after initiating treatment with lithium; in such instances, it may be advisable to discontinue the lithium as the first step in the treatment of the depression.

Manic or hypomanic episodes may be precipitated by antidepressant drugs. This occurs much more frequently in patients with bipolar manic-depressive disorders than in patients with unipolar depressions. It is helpful to make members of the family of a patient with a manic-depressive depression aware of this possibility since these patients often fail to return for treatment once they become hypomanic or manic. Such drug-induced manic or hypomani episodes are treated by discontinuing the antidepressant drug and initiating treatment with lithium or an appropriate antipsychotic drug.

D. Treatment of unipolar depressive disorders

1. **Endogenous depressions**   An initial trial of treatment with a tricyclic antidepressant is usually warranted in this group of patients, provided there are no medical, particularly cardiovascular, contraindications. (Data concerning the cardiovascular toxicity of tricyclic antidepressants sufficiently firm to make definite risk-benefit analyses in individual patients unfortunately are lacking.) Differences in the effects of the various tricyclic antidepressants have not been conclusively demonstrated, although recent preliminary findings suggest that differential responses to amitriptyline versus imipramine or desipramine could be predicted on the basis of pretreatment biochemical data — i.e., the urinary excretion of 3-methoxy-4-hydroxyphenylglycol (MHPG), a metabolite of norepinephrine (*Am. J. Psychiatry* 130:695–699, 1973; *Arch. Gen. Psychiatry* 26:252–262, 1972). If clinical improvement is not obtained after an adequate trial of one tricyclic antidepressant, a trial of treatment with another tricyclic antidepressant or a monoamine oxidase inhibitor may be considered.

Some clinicians recommend the use of electroconvulsive therapy (ECT) in patients with endogenous depressions who fail to respond to treatment with a tricyclic antidepressant (see Chapter 6). Because of the delay in onset of the therapeutic effects of the tricyclic antidepressants, ECT may be selected as the initial form of treatment for some patients, particularly those judged to be highly suicidal; but this is subject to controversy.

A period of one to four weeks generally elapses from the time of initial administration of tricyclic antidepressants to the onset of definitive clinical improvement. Although the patient may appear to be relatively unresponsive to interpersonal interactions during this phase of treatment, a great deal of important interpersonal work nonetheless can occur as the physician offers support and optimism to both patient and family. Moreover, it is essential to provide all concerned with a realistic assessment of the patient's prognosis (which is very good in cases of endogenous depressions) in order to mitigate the patient's depressive sense of hopelessness and despair and the family's demoralization. The goals of the therapeutic work during this phase are to build a firm, trusting relationship with a patient and family (if available) and to keep the patient from acting on his suicidal impulses. Attempts to mobilize the patient into purposeful activity at this stage are often unsuccessful and may only reinforce the patient's sense of inadequacy, but support of the patient's realistic attempts to maintain his activities during this period is important. Vacations rarely are helpful, since they may simply give the patient more time to brood.

When a patient with an endogenous depression starts to improve on antidepressant drugs, the effect is often striking. The exact day of onset of clinical improvement can generally be defined, and the physician can usually ascertain this upon visual inspection. The patient's carriage may be more erect, his movements less restricted and more agile, and his face more expressive. The patient characteristically becomes more responsive to environmental stimuli at this time. During this phase of the treatment of patients with endogenous depressions, it may be of value to attempt to activate the patient through the use of various interpersonal techniques to promote both affective arousal and the resumption of purposeful activity. Timing is of critical importance here: the physician must be certain that the patient is no longer suicidal before attempting this.

It is generally recognized that decreasing environmental stimulation serves an important function in the management of the manic patient. The reversal of this technique may be of value in the treatment of the patient with an endogenous depression once clinical improvement has begun. Increasing the environmental input to promote affective arousal and a sense of initiative as well as purposeful action and active coping behavior may serve to hasten and perpetuate the improvement in affective state in patients recovering from endogenous depressions.*

*The possible role of noradrenergic and other monoaminergic neural systems in the regulation of affective states and levels of arousal as well as in the maintenance of a sense of initiative and a capacity to execute active coping behavior has been considered in relation to the effects of antidepressant drugs on monoaminergic neurons (Schildkraut, *Neuropsychopharmacology and the Affective Disorders*).

Intensive psychotherapy is not generally required or indicated for the treatment of endogenous depressive syndromes per se. However, some patients with endogenous depressions may demonstrate character pathology or problems in social adjustment and functioning that appear to warrant intensive psychotherapeutic intervention. As indicated earlier, a decision regarding the need for intensive psychotherapy is usually best deferred until after the resolution of the acute syndrome.

2. **Chronic characterological depressions**   Many patients with chronic characterological depressions show transient improvement with all forms of therapeutic intervention, including supportive interpersonal therapy or simply hospitalization. Many such patients are stuck in unrewarding life circumstances, and short-term psychotherapy may help them to make appropriate changes. However, sustained definitive clinical responses are not frequently observed, and intensive psychotherapy when available generally seems indicated for the long-term treatment of patients with chronic characterological depressions.

Although many of these patients are not particularly responsive to treatment with antidepressant drugs, some patients with chronic characterological syndromes do appear to improve during treatment with antidepressants. The authors of this chapter differ somewhat in their approaches to the treatment of these disorders. It must be stressed that these approaches are based on clinical experience and observations, and that differences in the effects of the various antidepressant drugs in specific clinical syndromes have not been conclusively demonstrated.

We recommend a trial (one to four weeks) of supportive psychotherapy (sometimes in conjunction with small doses of antianxiety agents) in all patients with chronic characterological depressions prior to considering the use of antidepressant drugs. If adequate improvement is not seen after this trial of psychotherapy, one of the authors (J. J. S.) recommends the use of a tricyclic antidepressant, usually amitriptyline, irrespective of the specific clinical characteristics of the presenting syndrome. The other author (D. F. K.) recommends treatment with one or another antidepressant drug, depending upon the presenting clinical syndrome. He recommends the use of monoamine oxidase inhibitors in patients with rejection-sensitive hysteroid-dysphorias who often manifest overeating and oversleeping (see Chapter 17), imipramine in patients with phobic anxiety syndromes (see Chapter 2), and amitriptyline or imipramine in patients with other types of chronic characterological depressive syndromes.

If the initially prescribed antidepressant drug does not cause remission of the acute symptoms, treatment with another tricyclic antidepressant or monoamine oxidase inhibitor may be considered. However, it should be noted that some patients with chronic characterological depressive syndromes may be very troubled by side effects and may do poorly on antidepressant drugs.

3. **Agitated involutional depressions**   Most agitated involutional depressive syndromes occur as a subset of endogenous depressions, and these syndromes, like other endogenous depressions, may be responsive to treatment with tricyclic antidepressants. The sedative properties of amitriptyline may be particularly helpful in agitated involutional depressive syndromes. Treatment with imipramine may be considered in patients who fail to respond to amitriptyline, and vice versa, although adequate data are not available to indicate the fraction of patients who will respond to one of these drugs after failing to respond to the other. Antipsychotic agents, such as chlorpromazine (up to 1200 mg/day), thioridazine (up to 800 mg/day), or perphenazine (up to 60 mg/day), may be particularly useful in the treatment of agitated involutional depressions with paranoid delusions or ideation. Antiparkinsonian medication may be required as an adjunct. After successful treatment of the agitation and the delusional component of the syndrome with an antipsychotic agent, the patient may show a lackluster akinesia and appear anergic; at this time one may want to gradually supplement, and eventually replace, the antipsychotic agent with imipramine. Many clinicians, though not all, regard ECT as the most effective treatment for agitated involutional depressions, and one may consider ECT when deciding on the initial treatment for these disorders. The use of ECT should always be considered in the treatment of agitated involutional depressions that fail to respond to pharmacotherapy (see Chapter 6).

4. **Situational depressions**   Situational depressions (which include grief reactions and mourning) are generally self-limiting conditions, and remissions usually occur within a few months. Some patients may require little more than the reassurance that they are experiencing a normal reaction to a loss, although others may benefit from psychotherapy directed toward helping the patient deal with the loss. Either of these approaches may be supplemented by symptomatically oriented pharmacotherapy to alleviate anxiety or sleep disturbance. Hypnotics (see Chapter 1) should be used sparingly and with caution. Antidepressant drugs

generally are not required unless there is an endogenous depression.

In determining the appropriate treatment for a patient with a situational depression, one must be aware of the possibility of contributing to the patient's impaired sense of self-esteem and endorsing the notion of patienthood in someone with an essentially normal response to loss that requires no specific treatment. However, even in clearcut cases, regular contacts for clinical reassessment (with experience some clinicians consider these contacts well handled by telephone) are important, since, as noted earlier, a situational depression occasionally evolves into a supervening endogenous depressive syndrome. This means a shift to symptoms that are autonomous from the initial precipitating stress or the subsequent related life events. Under such conditions, treatment of the disorder with antidepressant drugs or ECT should proceed as with any other endogenous depression.

5. **Other nonspecific syndromes** Treatment should be conducted in the spirit of clinical inquiry as one attempts to find an appropriate and effective form of treatment for each patient.

E. **Treatment of drug-induced depressions** The first step in evaluating and treating patients with drug-induced depressions is the identification and discontinuation (if medically feasible) of the drug responsible for the depressive syndrome (see Chapter 1). Many drug-induced depressions will undergo remission after discontinuation of the offending pharmacological agent. For those drug-induced depressions that persist, an attempt should be made to relate the disorder to one of the depressive syndromes described, and treatment should proceed as outlined in Section III. D.

F. **Antidepressant drugs**

1. **Doses** The approximate dose ranges listed in Table 3-2 are intended only as general guidelines for therapy. Recent studies have indicated that there is marked variation among individuals in the rates of metabolism of antidepressant drugs. The relationships between blood levels of these drugs and their therapeutic effects or side effects are currently under investigation. When prescribing an antidepressant, the physician must be familiar with the pharmacology of the particular drug and must, accordingly, take into account the specific clinical characteristics of the individual patient, including past responses to the drug. It is usually advisable to start medication at a fairly low dose and increase it gradually over a number of days to obtain a therapeutically effective dose.

Table 3-2. Approximate Daily Dose Ranges of Antidepressant Drugs

Drug	Approximate Dose Range[a] (mg/day)
Tricyclic antidepressants	
Imipramine	75 to 300
Amitriptyline	75 to 300
Desipramine	75 to 200
Nortriptyline	40 to 100
Protriptyline	30 to 60
Doxepin	75 to 300
Monoamine oxidase inhibitors	
Phenelzine	45 to 90[b]
Tranylcypromine	20 to 60[b]

[a]See Section **III. F. 1.**
[b]The upper limits that exceed manufacturers' recommended dose ranges are used routinely, when warranted, by one of the authors (D. F. K.).

Some clinicians feel that rapid increments shorten the time until clinical response, but this is not established. When the physician elects to discontinue an antidepressant, it is advisable to withdraw the drug gradually, since withdrawal symptoms (e.g., nausea, headache, malaise) may occur upon abrupt cessation.

The doses required for maintenance therapy with specific tricyclic or monoamine oxidase inhibitor antidepressants may fall below even the lower limit of the dose ranges suggested in Table 3-2 for active antidepressant treatment. Elderly patients generally tolerate these drugs less well, and lower doses are usually recommended for them (see Chapter 10). Because of the opportunity for closer clinical observation and the greater restriction of activity of patients in the hospital, the maximum doses that may be administered to hospitalized patients may exceed the maximum doses recommended by the pharmaceutical manufacturer for outpatients. We believe that the doses recommended by pharmaceutical manufacturers may not be sufficient for the treatment of many patients. The following section (III.F.2) outlines suggested schedules for the administration of two of the most commonly prescribed tricyclic antidepressants.

2. **Suggested schedules for the administration and withdrawal of imipramine or amitriptyline** Since imipramine and amitriptyline are the two most commonly prescribed tricyclic antidepressants, we have included suggested schedules for their administration and withdrawal. The two authors recommend somewhat different schedules. One (J. J. S.) recommends that imipramine or amitrip-

tyline be administered in an initial test dose of 25 mg. Blood pressure should be measured in lying and standing positions immediately prior to the administration of this test dose and 1 hour thereafter to determine whether the patient experiences severe hypotensive effects from the drug. If there are no untoward effects from this test dose, the patient should be instructed to take an additional 25 mg at bedtime. The dose of imipramine or amitriptyline is then increased by 25 mg/day up to a total dose of 150 mg/day. This should be given in divided doses (preferably on a three times a day schedule).

The other author (D. F. K.) questions the value of a test dose and blood pressure measurements and recommends that treatment with imipramine or amitriptyline be initiated at a dosage of 75 mg/day administered in a single dose at bedtime. The dose should then be increased by 25 mg every 2 days until the dosage is 150 mg/day by the end of the first week.

Some clinicians favor administering the tricyclic antidepressants in divided doses, while others recommend a single dose at bedtime. Each approach has its advantages and disadvantages. Administration of a single dose at bedtime may decrease the frequency and intensity of sedation and orthostatic hypotension during the day when the patient is active. However, administering the entire dose at bedtime may increase the likelihood of postural hypotension occurring at night if the patient gets out of bed (e.g., to urinate); and a large single dose could conceivably increase the incidence of cardiac arrhythmias (although this has not been established). As a compromise, some clinicians administer these drugs on a twice-daily schedule, with the larger fraction of the total daily dose administered at bedtime.

If the patient has not begun to show a clearcut clinical improvement after 2 weeks of imipramine or amitriptyline at a dosage of 150 mg/day, and there are no medical contraindications or manifestations of toxicity, the dosage may be gradually increased (at a maximum rate of 25 mg/day) to a maximum dose of 300 mg/day. Although recent studies have suggested that higher doses may be of value in the treatment of some patients (particularly when blood levels of the tricyclic antidepressant remain low even at a dose of 300 mg/day), doses in excess of 300 mg/day cannot be recommended for routine use at this time. If the patient shows a partial antidepressant response in the absence of serious toxicity, higher doses may be indicated.

After complete remission has been attained, the dose of antidepressant medication frequently may be reduced to a lower maintenance level (usually about one-half the therapeutic dose, although this may vary considerably in different situations). The dose should be reduced very gradually (imipramine or amitriptyline may be decreased by 25 mg every 7 to 14 days). When the appropriate maintenance dose level is reached, administration of the drug is generally continued for at least several months at this reduced dose. In general, the patients should be asymptomatic for at least six months before the medication is discontinued. In those patients for whom long-term maintenance therapy is not contemplated, the eventual discontinuation of the drug should proceed gradually. One of us (J. J. S.) recommends that the dose of imipramine or amitriptyline should be decreased by 25 mg every 7 to 14 days, whereas the other (D. F. K.) suggests a decrease of 25 to 50 mg per day. The physician must observe the patient carefully and often during this period, and he should be prepared to increase the drug dosage if depression recurs.

3. **Prophylactic treatment with antidepressant drugs**   The recognition that chronically administered lithium might prevent the occurrence of manic-depressive episodes, or at least decrease the frequency and intensity of such episodes, has led to an interest in exploring the possible prophylactic effects of the antidepressant drugs in patients with depressive disorders. Although this is still under investigation at the present time, recent findings do suggest that long-term administration of tricyclic antidepressants and lithium salts may be of value in preventing relapses in patients with unipolar depressive disorders. Tricyclic antidepressants do not appear to be as effective as lithium salts in the prophylactic treatment of patients with bipolar manic-depressive disorders because of the increased incidence of manic or hypomanic episodes during long-term administration of tricyclic antidepressants. The use of tricyclic antidepressants for the prophylactic treatment of recurrent unipolar depressive disorders is still under investigation and cannot be recommended as a routine form of treatment. However, if one is treating a patient with a severe, recurrent depression, the use of such a prophylactic regimen might be justified.

4. **Miscellaneous considerations**

   a. **Use of hypnotics in depressive disorders**   Prolonged administration of hypnotics is contraindicated in depressive disorders. An occasional hypnotic (for one night only) may be prescribed for some patients, particularly when the insomnia is associated with anxiety. In such instances, flurazepam or diazepam may be of value (see Chapter 1). Some hypnotic drugs (e.g., barbiturates) can stimulate liver microsomal drug-metabolizing enzymes and thereby increase the rate of metabolic degradation of the tricyclic antidepressant drugs (see Chapter 16). In most patients the insomnia associated with a depressive syndrome is best treated by treating the depressive disorder per se.

b. **Use of thyroid hormone in conjunction with tricyclic antidepressants**   Thyroid hormone administered in conjunction with tricyclic antidepressants has been found to speed the onset of antidepressant effects, particularly in women. Moreover, anecdotal reports suggest that some patients who are refractory to a tricyclic antidepressant may respond to the combination of a tricyclic antidepressant plus thyroid hormone. However, this combination may also lead to increased side effects. At the present time the combined use of tricyclic antidepressants and thyroid hormone is being investigated and cannot be recommended for routine clinical use.

c. **Combined use of monoamine oxidase inhibitors and tricyclic antidepressants**   The combined use of monoamine oxidase inhibitors and tricyclic antidepressants has been reported to be of value in patients refractory to treatment with either of these drugs alone. However, enhanced and severe toxicity, including hyperpyrexia and convulsive seizures, has been reported with this combination of drugs. Recent reviewers have suggested that the hazards of combined treatment with monoamine oxidase inhibitors and tricyclic antidepressants may be exaggerated. The routine clinical use of this combination of drugs is not recommended at this time. However, with a refractory patient, cautious clinical exploration with this regimen, under expert supervision, may be warranted.

5. **Brief summary of the contraindications, precautions, and side effects associated with the use of antidepressant drugs**   The cardiovascular complications associated with the use of antidepressant drugs probably constitute the most serious hazards. In the case of the tricyclic antidepressants, these include orthostatic (postural) hypotension, the precipitation of cardiac arrhythmias, and the exacerbation of preexisting arrhythmias or heart blocks. Sudden death has been reported in patients receiving tricyclic antidepressants; however, their specific role in such fatalities has been questioned in some recent studies. Considerable caution should be used when administering a tricyclic antidepressant to patients with preexisting cardiac disease. In the case

of monoamine oxidase inhibitors, the hypertensive crises, often induced by dietary substances (see Chapter 19) or other drugs, constitute a major hazard. Cerebrovascular bleeding has been reported in a small minority of such episodes. This has tended to decrease the use of these drugs as an initial approach to the treatment of patients with depressive disorders. D. F. K. advises his patients to carry with them 300 mg of chlorpromazine and to take it orally if they experience a sudden throbbing, radiating occipital headache; medical evaluation should be sought immediately thereafter. (The patient should be warned of possible sedation and orthostatic hypotension secondary to this dose of chlorpromazine.)

The tricyclic antidepressants also have significant anticholinergic properties accounting for complaints of dry mouth, constipation, and other atropine-like effects. These anticholinergic properties should be considered before prescribing tricyclic antidepressants to patients with prostatic hypertrophy, untreated glaucoma, or intestinal obstruction.

The physician must be alert to the possibility that a patient may present contraindications to the use of these drugs or side effects induced by these drugs that are not mentioned in this brief summary. The physician is advised to consult reference sources for up-to-date information prior to prescribing any antidepressant drug.

References

Feighner, J. P., Robins, E., Guze, S. R., Woodruff, R. A., Jr., Winokur, G., and Munoz, R. Diagnostic criteria for use in psychiatric research. *Arch. Gen. Psychiatry* 26:57–63, 1972.

Klein, D. E. Endogenomorphic depression: A conceptual and terminological revision. *Arch. Gen. Psychiatry* 31:447–454, 1974.

Klein, D. E. Differential Diagnosis and Treatment of the Dysphorias. In G. M. Simpson and D. M. Gallant (Eds.), *Tulane University International Symposium on Depression: Behavioral, Biochemical, Clinical and Treatment Concepts,* New York: Spectrum (in press).

Klein, D. E., and Davis, J. J. *Diagnosis and Drug Treatment of Psychiatric Disorders.* Baltimore: Williams & Wilkins, 1969.

Kuhn, R. Treatment of depressive states with G22355 (imipramine hydrochloride). *Am. J. Psychiatry* 115:459–464, 1958.

Maas, J. W., Fawcett, J. A., and Dekirmenjian, H. Catecholamine metabolism, depressive illness and drug response. *Arch. Gen. Psychiatry* 26:252–262, 1972.

Schildkraut, J. J. *Neuropsychopharmacology and the Affective Disorders.* Boston: Little, Brown, 1970.

Schildkraut, J. J. Norepinephrine metabolites as biochemical criteria for classifying depressive disorders and predicting responses to treatment: Preliminary findings. *Am. J. Psychiatry* 130:695–699, 1973.

Schildkraut, J. J. Biogenic amines and affective disorders. *Annu. Rev. Med.* 25:333–348, 1974.

Schildkraut, J. J. Biochemical criteria for classifying depressive disorders and predicting responses to pharmacotherapy: Preliminary findings from studies of norepinephrine metabolism. *Pharmakopsychiatrie-Neuropsychopharmakologie* 7:98–107, 1974.

Schildkraut, J. J. The current status of biological criteria for classifying the depressive disorders and predicting response to treatment. *Psychopharmacol. Bull.* 10:5–25, 1974

4

Approaches to Schizophrenia

Richard I. Shader
Anthony H. Jackson

Schizophrenia as a diagnosis is an elusive concept. Efforts over the past hundred years to define this illness or group of illnesses have been extensive. Yet there are no universally accepted criteria that have utility for planning treatment or establishing prognosis. Although for many patients clinicians would have little difficulty reaching diagnostic agreement, there are inevitably cases for whom consensus would be difficult and attempts futile. Such controversial patients are sometimes given other diagnostic labels, including borderline state (see Chapter 17), latent schizophrenia, pseudoneurotic or pseudopsychopathic schizophrenia, or psychotic depression. The tradition of categorizing the schizophrenias as functional has unfortunately contributed to the confusion of nosology. *Functional* suggests to some workers an exclusively interpersonal-social or intrapsychic origin for this group of disorders.

Although it is beyond the scope of this chapter to discuss the etiology of schizophrenia, currently available genetic data compel comment. Data from investigations of twins and of the children born to schizophrenic mothers but placed for adoption at birth argue for a major genetic factor in the etiology of the illness for some patients. There is reason to suspect that certain individuals inherit a susceptibility for the expression of schizophrenic disorganization. This susceptibility may lead to some early expression of symptoms, as in the schizophrenias of childhood and adolescence (see Chapter 8). Symptoms may otherwise appear later in life — perhaps when the stresses of separation from family or the requirements of living autonomously expose a schizophrenic vulnerability. An individual so burdened may be unable to bear the losses, disappointments, or defeats encountered throughout life.

I. **Symptoms and Diagnostic Considerations** In 1896 Kraepelin organized the observations of previous workers (Morel, Hecker, Kahlbaum) and developed the concept dementia praecox, which he saw as a peculiar pathologic condition of the internal connections of the personality resulting in a disturbed emotional and volitional life. E. Bleuler (1911) extended these efforts and offered the concept of a group of schizophrenias characterized by disturbances of thinking, feelings, and relation-

Table 4-1. Schneider's First-Rank Symptoms of Schizophrenia

Thought broadcasting — the sense that one's thoughts are escaping aloud from one's head.

Experiences of alienation — the sense that one's thoughts, impulses, and actions are not one's own but come from an external source.

Experiences of influence — the sense that one's thoughts, feelings, and actions are being imposed by some external force or agency to which one must passively submit.

Delusional perceptions — the organization of real perceptions in a private way, often leading to fixed beliefs that are in conflict with reality.

Auditory hallucinations — hearing clearly audible voices coming from outside one's head, commenting on one's actions or speaking one's thoughts. These voices must consist of more than one- or two-word phrases, unintelligible mumbling sounds, whispers, or the like.

ships to the external world. He isolated four fundamental diagnostic criteria — loosening of associations, inappropriate affects, autistic thoughts, and ambivalence. These criteria are commonly reported today, although some clinicians and researchers would emphasize an alteration in selective attention, information processing, or cue response (e.g., dog might be misheard as frog; green as an association would not be loose).

In the 1930s Schneider elaborated a phenomenological definition of the schizophrenias *(Die Schizophrenen Symptomverbande,* Berlin: Springer, 1942). He asserted the primacy of 11 empirically determined first rank symptoms, which he considered pathognomonic of schizophrenia. Later work has challenged their specificity to schizophrenia and thereby their value in prognosis *(Arch. Gen. Psychiatry* 28:847—852 1973). However, Schneider's work does usefully organize some of the disparate experiences patients report. In Table 4-1, Schneider's symptoms are grouped into five broad categories.

Conrad (described by Fish in *J. Ment. Sci.* 107:828—838, 1961) has delineated particular subtypes of schizophrenia. These derive from an awareness of the time course and differing stages of symptom appearance. Table 4-2 lists these progressive stages. Even though few patients may actually articulate such a progressive decompensation, we offer this conceptualization because it may help the clinician to appreciate the course of patients' experiences.

Table 4-2. Conrad's Progressive Stages of Schizophrenia

Trema
   Patients experience a loosening or lack of coherence between their sense of the inner and outer worlds; there is a feeling of loss of freedom, a sense that the environment has changed, or a feeling of inability to communicate.

Apophany
   The loosening and lack of coherence to the sense of the inner and outer worlds is so extensive that the inseparable can now seem separate, resulting in delusional and paranoid experiences.

Apocalypse
   There is complete breakdown of the sense of coherence and a fragmentation of psychic life.

Consolidating and Residual Stages

Table 4-3 lists the inclusion criteria developed by the World Health Organization (WHO) for their multinational studies of schizophrenia. Preliminary data from WHO for patients finally diagnosed as having schizophrenia suggest that schizophrenic patients as a group rate high on lack of insight, predelusional signs (e.g., ideas of reference, perplexity), auditory hallucinations, and experiences of external control (e.g., thought alienation, thoughts spoken aloud, delusions of control).

Table 4-3. World Health Organization Inclusion Criteria for Studies of Schizophrenia

Present	Present to a Severe Degree
Delusions	Social withdrawal
Definitely inappropriate and unusual behavior	Disorders of thinking other than delusions
Hallucinations	Overwhelming fear
Gross psychomotor disorder; overactivity or underactivity	Disorders of affect
	Depersonalization
	Self-neglect

From *The International Pilot Study of Schizophrenia,* Geneva: WHO, 1973.

Table 4-4 lists symptoms that a group of investigators at Yale have found correlate most strongly with the diagnosis of schizophrenia. It is of interest that this group reports observing depression as a symptom in 66 percent of patients diagnosed as schizophrenic.

Table 4-4. Symptoms that Correlated Most Strongly with the Diagnosis of Schizophrenia Developed by Astrachan and Co-workers

Delusions (unspecified as contrasted to depressive)	Blocking
Hallucinations, auditory	Inappropriate affect
Hallucinations, visual	Confusion
Bizarre thinking	Paranoid ideation
Looseness of associations	Excitement

From *Brit. J. Psychiatry* 121:529–539, 1972.

Biographic data from the patient's life may help in separating the schizophrenic psychoses from toxic or other causes of the symptoms of the syndrome and from other "functional" (primarily affective) psychoses. Life history criteria (see Table 4-5) are not expected to be diagnostic of a schizophrenic illness by themselves but are considered in conjunction with the symptoms described in the preceding paragraphs.

It should be apparent to the reader that the symptoms observed at any given point in time will depend on just when in the course of the illness the patient is seen, past and present treatments, and the type

Table 4-5. Criteria for Schizophrenia Developed by Feighner, Robins, and Guze

Chronic psychiatric symptoms lasting more than 6 months without remission.
Absence of a period of significant depressive or manic symptoms.
Poor premorbid history, including being unmarried and poor work history.
Family history of schizophrenia.
Absence of alcohol or drug abuse.
Onset of illness under age 40.

From *Arch. Gen. Psychiatry* 26:57–63, 1972.

and prognosis of the patient's illness. Diagnosis also must take into account whether or not the patient is psychotic at the time of observation; the presence of other etiological factors (e.g., the symptoms could result from toxic conditions such as from amphetamines); past history of alterations in mood, behavior, perceptions, and thought and present mental status; and social and cultural expectations (a belief in voodoo, for example, could significantly influence assessment).

A. Schizophrenia As a conclusion to this section we offer a **definition of schizophrenia** that draws on the American Psychiatric Association's *Diagnostic and Statistical Manual of Mental Disorders,* 2nd edition (APA/DSM-II) and the *British Glossary* to the *Eighth Revision of the International Classification of Diseases.* We define *schizophrenia* as a large group of disorders, usually psychotic in proportion. Schizophrenic patients show alterations in thoughts, percepts, mood, and behavior: subjective experiences of disordered thought are manifested in disturbances of concept formation, sometimes leading to misinterpretations of reality and at other times to delusions (particularly delusions of influence and ideas of reference) and hallucinations (particularly hallucinations of voices repeating the patient's thoughts or commenting on his thoughts and actions); mood changes include ambivalence, constriction, or inappropriateness of feeling, or loss of empathy with others; behavior may be withdrawn, regressive, or bizarre. Such alterations usually occur in a setting of clear consciousness, and disorientation and amnesia typically are absent.

Central to this characterization is the concept of a disorder of thought. This may be manifested in inappropriate rate, flow, or content of thinking. It may be evident in the supervening style of the thinking process and associated verbal productions. Typical **manifestations of disordered thought processes in schizophrenia** are:

1. Muteness.
2. Blocking, often associated with the subjective feeling of not being in control of one's own thoughts.

3. Neologisms, new personal language.
4. Verbigeration (the senseless repetition of words and phrases, seen particularly in chronic patients).
5. Private logic.
6. Thinking that is overly personalized and not abstract.
7. Difficulties in generalizing correctly and in seeing similarities and differences.
8. Things may be seen as identical because they share a common or similar property.
9. Difficulties in separating relevant from irrelevant and in screening out the irrelevant.
10. Overinclusive thinking in which usual conceptual boundaries are lost or blurred.

B. **Schizoaffective disorders** Clinicians often see psychotic patients who reveal delusions, hallucinations, and disordered thoughts but also appear elated or depressed. If the affective symptoms are pronounced, such patients are classified as **schizophrenia, schizoaffective type** (DSM-II). Patients with the "**excited**" **subtype** must be distinguished from patients in the psychotic phase of manic-depressive disease. In schizoaffective patients the disturbance in thinking is more typical of schizophrenia (e.g., blocking, illogical thinking, overinclusive thinking) rather than of mania (e.g., pressure to keep talking, racing thoughts). It also is typical for manic-depressive patients in an excited, psychotic episode to have an element of humor in their verbal productions (see Chapter 5). By contrast, schizoaffective patients are more likely to seem bizarre, and hebephrenic patients (who often are older and more chronically ill), to appear silly. Patients with the "**depressed**" **subtype** must be differentiated from patients with psychotic depressions, whose delusions usually involve guilt or bizarre somatic concerns ("my stomach is rotting away") or both. Also, patients with psychotic depressions are more often in the over 40 age group, while schizoaffective patients are typically younger. Schizoaffective patients usually have an episodic course with a good prognosis for a particular episode. They also are likely to have first-order relatives who carry a diagnosis of an affective disorder or alcoholism.

It is understandable that schizoaffective patients have been classified as atypical or as early forms of schizophrenia or manic-depressive disease. Leonhard, who would label many of these same patients cycloid psychoses, noted that their episodic course can become chronic with only partial remission from episodes once the illness pattern is well established. He considered these patients to have an independent endogenous psychosis that is neither schizophrenia nor manic-depressive disease (*J. Ment. Sci.* 107:633–648, 1961). One other alternative is to see these disorders as reflecting a genetic mixing of manic-depressive illness and schizophrenia. Careful observation of these patients suggests that they are in fact a very heterogeneous group.

C. **Depression symptoms in schizophrenic patients** In addition to patients who present acutely with schizoaffective symptoms, other schizophrenic patients may show depression or depression-like symptoms at some time in their course.

1. **Depressive position** Some patients appear to be in a depressive position or phase in the recovery from an acute episode of decompensation. Paranoid thinking or delusions and distortions, or both, are diminishing and are being replaced by depressive content ("they hate me" becomes "I hate myself").

2. **Depression per se** Clinical experience makes it clear that schizophrenic patients are not immune to depression. For example, a schizophrenic patient can experience and reveal dysphoric mood in connection with the loss of a significant person, yet not show any further worsening of schizophrenic symptoms that are already present. Antidepressant therapy added to their regimen of antipsychotic drugs may be of benefit to some of these patients. In other patients depression may appear before the onset of psychotic symptoms, in either a first episode or a reexacerbation of symptoms in a patient in remission. Although some may benefit from antidepressants alone, such patients are likely to become more overtly psychotic if antidepressants are prescribed in the absence of antipsychotic drugs.

3. **Neurasthenia** These patients appear "stuck." They may seem depressed, without the will to reengage with active life outside an institutional setting. In some patients this may be an iatrogenic condition, a result of prolonged hospitalization and inadequate rehabilitation and socialization. In others it may result when a therapist tries to get the patient to do what the therapist wants for the patient rather than to do what the patient wants for himself. The literature also contains the formulation that neurasthenia is a phase some patients must pass through as part of the reintegration process.

4. **Overtranquilized patients** Some schizophrenic patients who appear retarded and depressed may be simply overmedicated. Dosage reduction produces amelioration of the retarded-depressed presentation.

5. **Akinetic parkinsonism** Some patients may have neuroleptic-induced akinetic parkinsonism, which presents to the observer as depression and psychomotor retardation. A trial of anti-parkinsonian medication will identify this subgroup.

II. **Differentiating Schizophrenia from other Diseases that may Produce Similar Symptoms** The diagnosis of schizophrenia must be made in part by exclusion. Table 4-6 is a list of some disease states that can at times present with psychotic symptoms. Since many of the schizophrenic symptoms described here may be manifestations of a local or systemic process that alters CNS function, a complete discussion of these disorders is beyond the scope of this chapter.

Of primary importance in the differential diagnosis of these diseases is a careful personal and family history and physical examination, together with judicious use of the clinical laboratory. Of crucial interest may be a history of exposure to drugs or toxins, a family history of a

Table 4-6. Some Disease States that Can Manifest Schizophrenic-like Symptoms

Toxic and deficiency states
    Drug-induced psychoses (especially those induced by amphetamines, LSD, digitalis, steroids, disulfiram)
    Alcoholic hallucinosis
    Wernicke's encephalopathy
    Korsakoff's psychosis
    Bromism and other heavy metal intoxication
    Pellagra and other vitamin deficiencies
    Uremia and liver failure

Infections
    Syphilis
    Toxoplasmosis
    Viral encephalitis
    Brain abscess
    Schistosomiasis

Neurologic disease
    Seizure disorders
    Primary and metastatic neoplasms
    Early presenile and senile dementias
    Postencephalitic states

Cardiovascular
    Lowered cardiac output
    Hypertensive encephalopathy

Endocrine disorders
    Thyrotoxicosis
    Myxedema
    Adrenal hyperfunction

Genetic and metabolic disorders
    Acute porphyria
    Homocystinuria
    Niemann-Pick disease
    Electrolyte imbalances
    Diabetes mellitus

Collagen-vascular disease
    CNS lupus arteritis

genetic disease, the presence of neurologic deficits, or the stigmata of systemic disease.

III.   **Prognosis, Course, and Followup**   One of the crucial elements in Kraepelin's distinctions between manic-depressive psychosis and dementia praecox was the data generated by followup examination. Dementia praecox was seen as an illness from which recovery was not common. In the 1910 edition of his textbook, *Psychiatrie,* Kraepelin, although he acknowledged recovery in some 13 percent of patients, cited many contemporary investigations that emphasized deterioration and lack of recovery.

E. Bleuler's concept of a group of schizophrenias suggested the possibility of a broad spectrum of courses and outcomes. However, Bleuler emphasized that despite periods of arrest or reversal, patients would probably never be totally free of schizophrenia. Langfeldt has contributed extensively to a dichotomization of diagnoses based on outcome. Narrowly defined (nuclear) schizophrenic patients are predicted to have poor outcomes at followup. A subset of patients are seen to recover and are renamed schizophreniform, by virtue of both their recovery and the presence of certain features in the case material (e.g., acute rather than insidious onset, good premorbid adjustment, prominent depressive symptoms). Langfeldt, noting Sakel's observation that 88 percent of schizophrenic patients recovered, suggests that this was based on diagnostic error and that the patient population must have included many reaction types with a tendency to spontaneous recovery.

Several restatements of this same position by other authors are useful for emphasis: (1) ". . . apparent 'schizophrenia' with a good prognosis is not a mild form of schizophrenia, but is a different illness" (J. H. Stephens, Pg. 485); (2) "Schneider-positive patients with poor prognostic signs are probably suffering from Kraepelinean schizophrenia while Schneider-negative patients with good prognostic signs, although admitted as schizophrenic, are suffering from other non-schizophrenic illnesses" (M. A. Taylor, Pg. 67); (3) Discussing the 17- to 33-year followup of 33 adolescents hospitalized for schizophrenia, Roff also has delineated two groups. "One had a chronic schizophrenic course, the other had a psychotic episode with possible recurrence but a relative stable, neuroticlike adjustment at follow-up. The cases with relatively favorable outcome, although diagnosed schizophrenic, did not emerge as simply milder forms of process schizophrenia "Pg. 183. Roff's poor outcome cases were more likely to have relatives with chronic schizophrenia, a disturbed parent, below average IQ, hebephrenic subtype diagnosis, and distinctive developmental changes.

A vast number of followup studies have used a dichotomous concept of outcome — nonrecovered vs. recovered. This bimodal view is often related to dichotomous concepts of schizophrenia (e.g., nuclear schizophrenia vs. schizophreniform psychosis, process schizophrenia vs. reactive schizophrenia, good premorbid vs. poor premorbid schizophrenia). This use of followup data has had heuristic and theoretical rather than clinical significance to date.

The use of outcome as an element of diagnosis is complicated by intervening variables such as treatment, rehabilitation, and societal attitudes toward illness, to name only a few. More recent followup studies of schizophrenia have been extensively reviewed elsewhere. Poor outcome for schizophrenia, although still true for many patients, is by no means always found. A recent study in Poland reports an 88 percent discharge rate at nine months for 219 first-admission schizophrenics in 1956—1957. Forty-seven percent were never hospitalized again during a seven-year followup, and for those who were admitted again the average interval between first discharge and readmission was 1.9 years (± 1.5 years). At seven years, 35 percent showed an improvement in work performance, 10 percent had a decline in occupational status, and the remainder did not work. Russian statistics for 1413 schizophrenic patients reveal 16 percent still hospitalized at a two-year followup. Thirty-two percent were doing some form of skilled or intellectual-academic work. Ten percent of patients diagnosed as showing a malignant, continuous course were nevertheless able to do skilled or intellectual-academic work. A Canadian study of schizophrenic war veterans emphasizes that highly symptomatic individuals with many symptoms may be able to function outside institutional settings. Thirty percent of ambulatory outpatients showed the same level of pathology as 74 percent of a group who were still hospitalized after 10 to 15 years. Hospital versus nonhospital status appeared to depend on family emotional support and veterans' pensions and not on psychopathology alone.

A 12-year followup investigation in Mauritius reports 59 percent of patients showing a single episode with no further clear episodes of nonfunctioning. Sixty-four percent of the patients were living independently and with no symptoms. Limited data available from mainland China suggest that schizophrenia accounts for about 50 percent of all hospitalized psychiatric patients. One study of 2000 schizophrenic patients in Shanghai reports cure or notable improvement in 56 percent and moderate improvement in 15 percent, with 28 percent showing no improvement at all. Another investigation, which focuses on the use of chlorpromazine in the treatment of schizophrenia, reports that 30 percent were completely cured, while over 30 percent more showed notable improvement. The last-mentioned figures were obtained from a secondary source, and the time of outcome assessment and outcome criteria are not given.

Several important points can be made about followup and outcome. The timing of followup studies may be crucial. For example, in the Polish study 88 percent were discharged within nine months. A follow-up one year after discharge would not have revealed that a substantial part of this group was subsequently readmitted. Outcome must be considered not only in terms of manifest psychopathology but also in regard to adjustment or performance criteria as reflected by working capacity, interpersonal relationships, autonomy, or self-regard. Outcome can be seen as a process rather than as a dimension measured at a fixed point in time. M. Bleuler, for example, has outlined seven possible longitudinal patterns to describe the course and outcome of schizo-phrenia: (1) Acute onset leading to chronic severe psychosis, (2) insidious onset leading slowly to chronic severe psychosis, (3) acute onset leading to chronic mild psychosis, (4) insidious onset leading slowly to chronic mild psychosis, (5) several acute episodes leading to chronic severe psychosis, (6) several acute episodes leading to chronic mild psychosis, and (7) one or several acute episodes leading to recovery. The first four patterns show a rather continuous evolution, the latter three are phasic. Having followed the life experiences of a cohort of schizophrenic patients for 23 years, M. Bleuler feels that these patterns subsume the experiences of 90 percent of patients. Other patterns are certainly possible (e.g., insidious onset leading to recovery, chronic psychosis followed by acute episodes).

The Soviet classification of schizophrenia is dependent on the type and rate of the course of the illness as well as on symptomatology. Three basic forms are observed: (1) continuous, (2) periodic (recurrent), and (3) shift-like progressive (in the form of schubs). While the considerations presented by M. Bleuler emphasize the role of longitudinal course in considering outcome, the Soviet school makes course an integral part of diagnosis.

There are inherent problems in using course as an element in the diagnosis of disease. For example, the discovery of an effective treat-ment for a given disease could require a new diagnosis, at least for those who recover. Yet, the rate and degree of recovery can be highly variable, even for disease states with known pathology and specific treatments. The duration and degree of pathology before diagnosis and the institution of treatment can readily affect recovery, as can other variables within the patient and in the environment. Rarely does one disease have only one type of outcome, and commonly two or more diseases may show the same type of outcome.

It is clear that there exists a deep semantic and theoretical ambiguity in the use of the term *outcome.* Outcome may be used to describe the state at the end of a particular episode, the state at the end of a specific time period, or a summary statement about course. Can one be cured of or get over schizophrenia? Is remission merely a phase of arrest or reversal, as suggested by E. Bleuler? Does one remain predisposed to decompensations under the "right conditions"? If recovery is possible, is the illness still schizophrenia? An ulcer may heal, but a predisposition to hyperacidity may remain. Schizophrenia is not merely overt symptomatology; it is also the underlying condition. One does not get cured of diabetes, although the expression of and morbidity from the illness can often be greatly modified. At the moment there is no resolution of these conceptual difficulties, which are based on differing definitions among varied theoretical schools of thought. In the meantime further clarification could come from better definitions of concepts by the differing schools.

Despite their limitations, several studies do give a general picture of the course and outcome of cases diagnosed as schizophrenic. To return to Kraepelin, although he noted that about 13 percent of his cases recovered from the first attack, most of these relapsed in a few years, leaving only 2.6 percent with lasting recoveries. If those with mild residual defects were included, this percentage was increased slightly to 4.12 percent. Such figures are indeed forbidding. Followup studies of schizophrenia at that time were relatively simple since most patients remained hospitalized. Arnold, writing in the mid-1950s, reported on a sample of 500 schizophrenic patients followed for 3 to 30 years. His results revealed: (1) A phasic course of illness leading to complete cure in 15.6 percent, (2) a phasic course that became shift-like (new acute symptomatology followed by partial recovery) in 4 percent, (3) a phasic course leading to deterioration in 0.4 percent, (4) a phasic course that leads to deterioration punctuated by exacerbations of symptomatology in 3.4 percent, (5) a shift-like (some residual pathology) course in 9.6 percent, (6) a shift-like course leading to deterioration in 3.6 percent, (7) a shift-like course leading to deterioration punctuated by exacerbation in 14 percent, (8) a gradual deterioration in 7.2 percent, (9) a gradual deterioration punctuated by exacerbation in 38 percent, and (10) mixed psychotic courses in 6.6 percent. The important theme in these findings is that only about 16 percent recover, whereas 67 percent eventually deteriorate, again an ominous prognosis for those who receive the diagnosis of schizophrenia.

As noted earlier, M. Bleuler described seven patterns of evolution for schizophrenic patients that relate course and outcome. These patterns were generated from a study of over 500 patients seen by 1941. M. Bleuler began to accumulate a new cohort of over 200 schizophrenics starting in 1942. Writing in 1968 about a 23-year followup of these cases, he indicated that the pattern "acute psychosis leading to chronic severe psychosis" had almost disappeared. He further suggested that cases that evolve to a mild chronic psychosis had increased, while severe chronic psychoses had diminished. He cautions, however, that although the "most malignant *acute* schizophrenias are under control now, the most *chronic* schizophrenias are not. The percentage of chronic onset leading slowly to chronic severe psychosis has remained nearly the same within the last 25 years. . . . A further finding is also disappointing: it was not possible to increase the percentage of recoveries much over one-third of all cases."

Niskanen and Achté have examined the five-year outcomes of pati diagnosed as schizophrenic or paranoid psychosis. One hundred such patients were selected from each of the three years 1950, 1960, 1965 Several findings are notable. The average durations of first hospitaliza tion were 121.4, 147.7, and 72.0 days, respectively, for the three cohorts. Full recovery for the five years after the initial episode was observed for 30, 29, and 21 percent, respectively, showing a decreasir percentage of total recoveries. However, the second most frequent outcome, "apparent recovery from psychosis and ability to do the sar work," showed the opposite trend — 7, 11, and 21 percent, respectiv Thus 37, 40, and 42 percent, respectively, showed major, sustained recovery over the five-year followup intervals. Patients who remainec in the hospital decreased in number — 22, 14, and 10 percent, respectively. Average duration of total hospitalization also decreased — 335.0, 332.2, and 202.3 days, respectively. Although the authors note no changes in readmission frequency from the 1960 to the 1965 cohort, an examination of their data suggests a statistically significant and possibly important pattern of increasing readmissions over the three time samples. It does appear that patients now tend to spend le total time in the hospital, and this may be facilitated by an increased number of brief hospitalizations.

Three important aspects of such studies of course and outcome deserve further comment.

A. **Hospitalization as an outcome criterion** Many investigations use hospitalization as the single or major criterion of outcome. It is clear from the studies mentioned in this chapter that duration of hospitalization has changed over the years. Hospitalizations have become shorter, especially in the last two decades. At the present time, hospitalization practices in some countries are highly respons to the increasing costs of hospital care. The presence of communit and family support and the patient's role in the family have a majc effect on hospitalization practices. The presence of growing numb of alternatives to hospital care also contributes. Patients may resic in cooperative apartments with minimal supervision, boarding hom foster care placements, and the like. Thus, those who might have lived a semidependent status in the hospital can now do so outside the hospital.

It is also important to consider the mathematical handling of hospitalization as a dependent variable. Many studies simply look at a "yes" versus "no" dichotomy at a given point in time. An example of this is a prospective study of schizophrenic patients treated in Canada. The authors use "in" versus "discharged" at six months after admission. They are aware of the limitations of their choice and point out the trend toward increasing readmission rates. Wing has reported on a five-year followup in England of first-admission patients. Of interest in terms of the hospitalization variable is that 27 percent of patients were episodically disturbed, 11 percent were sick during the first half of followup but improved during the second half, and 35 percent were disturbed during the first year. One can readily see that this pattern would be missed by an "in" versus "out" variable. Also, patients in each of the three groups could in theory have the same duration of hospitalization (total number of days), which limits the usefulness of the hospitalization criterion. One could also question any use of hospitalization as a continuous variable, since there is an obvious discontinuity between being in the hospital and being out.

B. **Work as a criterion of outcome** The occupational performance of schizophrenic patients is an important dimension of outcome, especially where work has a societal importance. Just as hospitalization is a problematical variable, so is work. One can say whether or not a patient is working at arbitrary points in time. However, this ignores consideration of the quality of work, the relationship of the present level of work to premorbid functioning, the differing complexities of various jobs, and so on. One may question whether a negative finding reflects a true absence of work performance differences among subtypes of schizophrenic patients and whether the statistical model was the most appropriate.

Work status is highly influenced by other variables. Brown and collaborators point out that work success is dependent on past employment record, attitudes toward discharge, and the personality of the patient. The availability of work is also a crucial factor, particularly in countries with high levels of unemployment. A few studies that have focused specifically on work are of interest. Work as a predictor variable in a five-year followup was evaluated by Farina and colleagues, who noted that 98 percent of recovered males had worked prior to first admission, while only 80 percent of non-recovered males had worked. The corresponding figures for females were 70 and 87 percent, respectively. The work-recovery correlation for men was +.29 and for women −.20. Simon and co-workers conducted an eight- to nine-year followup of the performance of a group of schizophrenic patients whose performance had previously been evaluated in a one-year followup. Twenty percent showed further improvement in work performance, 50 percent were worse, and 30 percent were unchanged, again suggesting the need for longer evaluation periods. Cole and Shupe also followed a previously studied group. In their first study, schizophrenic male patients had lower work performance in comparison to controls matched for age, sex, specific job, and educational attainment. Problems arose for schizophrenic patients mainly in the areas of performance under pressure and interpersonal relationships. The schizophrenic patients were also rated lower on quality of work produced, judgment, and adjustment to new situations. Four years later these same two groups were again studied. Controls had more promotions − 47 percent as compared to 29 percent for schizophrenics. Of particular note was that controls had no medical retirements, while these were arranged for 15 percent of the schizophrenic cohort. Hall and co-workers examined the work experiences of the patients in the nine-hospital NIMH collaborative study of phenothiazines in acute schizophrenia (1961−1962). Job difficulties were experienced by 60 percent of these patients in the five-year period preceding their admissions. At followup one year after discharge, 72 percent were having difficulty, a figure mainly resulting from an increased number of unemployed. Of steady workers who had held a single job during the five years prior to admission 29.5 percent were unemployed one year after discharge.

Taken together, these findings support the use of work performance as a major variable for evaluating both the course and the outcome of schizophrenia. They also suggest, however, that work is a complex variable in terms of its dependency on variables not related to the patient's schizophrenia per se and that care must be taken in choosing and interpreting statistical procedures and results. In cross-cultural studies these difficulties are of course multiplied.

C. **Treatment as an intervening variable** In any study of outcome and course, a primary concern is the effect of any treatment intervention on the natural course of the illness. From many of the comments in preceding sections of this chapter, it is apparent that treatment is a meaningful variable in followup studies. Hospitalization as a treatment has its effects, usually positive in the short run but often negative when it is extended too long. Bhaskaran and colleagues in India, Wing in Great Britain, and Goffman in the United States have all described the harmful effects of institutionalization. Rehabilitation and socialization experiences and traditional inter-personal psychotherapies all make contributions and positively affect some patients. In general, however, as M. Bleuler's comments imply, the major changes have been with the middle range of patients. Chronicity and deterioration still occur, and the number of "cures" still remains about one-third.

Many patients are lost to followup. Are they treatment successes or failures? Some authors include them as successes in their analyses, some include them as failures in order to arrive at more conservative estimates, and some leave them out. Many patients in aftercare status do not follow their prescribed treatment regimen. They may pur-chase or pick up their pills, but do they swallow them? Reports from the United States and Sweden suggest that many chronic patients require at least two years of drug treatment before changes are seen but that these changes are often only in the direction of more integrated behavior in the hospital or in sheltered, structured living situations. Controlled studies do rather consistently show the benefits to both chronic and acute schizophrenic patients of the use of neuroleptic drugs during periods of hospitalization.

Aftercare effects have also been studied. The reports of Troshinsky and colleagues, Gross and colleagues, and Hogarty and colleagues support the value of neuroleptics (antipsychotic agents) in the after-care phase. These studies all employed random assignments and placebo controls, although they varied in their efforts to determine patients' drug-taking compliance. The Hogarty group, for example, noted a relapse rate of 31 percent for the drug group and 67 percent for the placebo group one year after discharge. Long-acting oral and injectible drugs, which require less patient cooperation, may alter this picture. Pharmacotherapy and other therapies do make a dif-ference, but at the present time there is no straightforward way to handle this variable in followup evaluations.

D. **Predictors of outcome in schizophrenia** Many authors have examined and reviewed prognostic features in schizophrenia. Table 4-7 sum-marizes some of the predictor variables that appear in these reviews. Robins and Guze have examined a number of predictor studies and conclude that the accuracy of prediction of poor outcome ranges from 55 to 91 percent and the corresponding range for good outcome is 36 to 83 percent. It would appear that one can predict more reliably those cases that will not do well than those cases that are likely to have a hopeful outcome. It is beyond the scope of this chapter to consider all the prognostic factors in detail. However, selected factors will be considered, particularly those that can be studied and expected to vary cross-culturally.

Table 4-7. Predictors of Outcome in Schizophrenia

Poor Prognosis	Good Prognosis
Insidious onset	Acute onset
Withdrawn behavior	Depressive symptoms
Emotional blunting	Good premorbid social and work history
Little overt hostility	Verbal aggression
Excessive persecutory delusions and paranoia	Concern with guilt and death
	Tension and anxiety
Schizoid or asocial premorbid personality	Clear precipitating factors
	Confusion
Hebephrenic clinical picture	No family history of schizophrenia
Clear sensorium	Family history of affective disorders
Family history of schizophrenia	
Single	Married
Absence of any affective symptoms	

1. **Heredity** Slater has extensively reviewed studies on the inheritance of schizophrenia. His summary suggests that schizophrenia can be found in 3.8, 8.7, and 12 percent of the parents, siblings, and children, respectively, of schizophrenic patients, regardless of outcome. M. Bleuler observed that 7 percent of his schizophrenic patients, regardless of outcome, had schizophrenic parents. Winokur and colleagues, studying the relatives of 200 carefully selected cases of schizophrenia, examined family histories and family member cases files and diagnosed schizophrenia in 5.5 percent of parents and siblings. A very conservative definition was used — the relative's illness had to begin before age 40 and go on either to chronic hospitalization or chronic social incapacity Vaillant, in a report on schizophrenic patients followed for varying amounts of time, noted no hereditary patterns among 44 patients who achieved a full remission, but a family history of schizophrenia was observed in 16 percent of 128 patients who showed an absence of full remission. McCabe and colleagues interviewed 144 of 263 living relatives of 28 good- and 25 poor-outcome schizophrenics. They observed an incidence of 3.3 percent definite cases of schizophrenia in the families of the good-outcome cases and an incidence of 11.6 percent for the poor-outcome cases. If suspected cases are added, these percentages increase to 5.5 and 15.1, respectively. It would appear from these studies that a family history of schizophrenia is associated with a diagnosis of schizophrenia that will more likely progress to chronicity. Waring and Ricks examined the records of mothers of 50 adult schizophrenics who had been seen with their mothers at a child guidance clinic before their adult diagnosis of schizophrenia. The adult schizophrenics were divided according to chronicity versus hospital dis-

charge. The records suggest that 16 percent of the mothers of the released group had received a diagnosis of psychotic, schizoid, or borderline type of character disorder as against 55 percent of the mothers of the children who later became chronic. This is reinforced by the finding that 20 percent of the parents of the chronic group had been diagnosed as psychotic as compared to 5 percent for the released group.

2. **Marital status** It would appear from the literature that unmarried schizophrenic patients have a less favorable prognosis than married schizophrenics. In an interesting study that exemplifies the complexity of statistical analysis of marriage data, Gittelman-Klein and Klein have shown that marital status, although a useful predictor, is highly dependent on premorbid asocial personality. Asocial people less often marry. The authors point out that asociality is associated with poor outcome, whereas nonasociality is associated with both good and poor outcomes. If linear partial correlation techniques are used to parcel out the effect of asociality on the relationship between marriage and outcome, a significant relationship still exists. However, if one properly considers the curvilinearity in the relationship between asociality and outcome and adopts nonlinear models, the relationship between marriage and outcome no longer appears independent of the premorbid asocial personality variable. Since marital patterns vary across cultures, cross-cultural studies are a fertile source of data for the investigation of marital status—outcome relationships.

3. **Premorbid asocial or schizoid personality** As suggested, asocial or schizoid personality is strongly linked to poor outcome and chronic course. In two other related studies, Gittelman and Klein and Rosen, Gittelman-Klein, and Klein observed that asociality was related to poor outcome for both sexes. Males, however, on average have greater asociality, so levels that are predictive of good outcomes for males are associated with poor outcomes for females. The greater asociality for males is observed in a higher degree of asociality before puberty; this high degree of asociality is not observed in women before puberty. This suggests that prepubertal boys who stay at home may be more likely to be labeled pathologic than girls who stay at home.

Longabaugh and Eldred factor analyzed a prognostic scale on a sample of schizophrenic patients and observed that the first factor was synonymous with the asocial, shut-in, schizoid personality dimension and the second factor was related to illness onset. The asocial factor was, in their sample, by far the more potent predictor of outcome; illness onset added very little predictive power. It is clear that illness onset is seen as less acute in patients who have had significant premorbid schizoid or asocial behavior. Watt and colleagues have provided an interesting confirmation of the role of premorbid personality. They studied the public school records of 30 children who as adults were hospitalized as schizophrenics. Ninety matched controls were also investigated. From these records it emerged that boys who later became schizophrenic appear to show a pattern of unsocialized aggression. They were more irritable, aggressive, negativistic, and defiant of authority. By contrast, the girls who later became schizophrenic showed more academic initiative and were more dependable, more calm, less nervous, and more insecure and emotionally immature. The girls participated less in groups, were more shy, sought less attention, and were less negativistic than their controls. These sex differences may be appropriately studied in the context of shifting child-rearing practices and attitudes toward sex roles.

IV. Treatment

A. **Hospitalization and milieu therapy** The onset of symptoms of schizophrenia is not in itself an indication for psychiatric hospitalization. If there is sufficient support in the community, and if the patient's illness does not constitute a threat to himself or others, outpatient treatment is often attempted. Such management at the very least may help preserve the matrix of social support that exists for the patient outside the hospital and may protect the patient from the unwanted effects of institutionalization. Recent studies of the process of psychiatric hospitalization suggest that many hospitalizations could have been avoided if more adequate family and community resources had been available.

If the patient is a threat to himself or others, hospitalization is indicated. Suicidal and homicidal ideation or gestures are especially serious in schizophrenic patients. They may lack the impulse control or judgment to modify such wishes, especially if voices are commanding them. They also may become panicked by delusional persecutory beliefs.

If a patient is confused, or so anxious that he cannot adequately care for himself, then hospitalization is also indicated. Although the sensorium is usually clear in schizophrenia, confusion with frank disorientation occasionally may occur. In assessing the patient's ability to care for himself outside the hospital, it is helpful to determine the patient's abilities to plan his daily activities and his capacity to get a full night's sleep.

Occasionally hospitalization of the schizophrenic patient may become temporarily necessary if those caring for the patient in the community become unable to do so or if interpersonal pressures on the patient become intolerable. Such occasions may include the illness of a parent or sibling or the birth of a child in the patient's family. The willingness of the hospital to help support a patient, and indirectly his family, often go far toward promoting the acceptance of the chronically disturbed patient within the community. Table 4-8 summarizes the major indications for hospitalization.

When the clinical decision to hospitalize the patient has been reached, the reasons for such action should be clear and should be explained to the patient in an unambiguous way. The patient's collaboration in such a plan should be obtained. Although patients may be too disturbed to participate in such a decision, often they will be able to respond in some positive way to the clinician's firm resolve that hospitalization will be temporarily helpful. Once hospitalized, the schizophrenic patient will soon experience the relief that follows from being in a place where he can feel relatively safe and where he can obtain help in controlling his impulses. The moratorium and distance from upsetting experiences may be beneficial.

Hospitalizing the acutely schizophrenic patient allows the physician a more complete opportunity for clinical evaluation and a more controlled setting for effectively titrating the patient's dosage of antipsychotic medication. It also presents the physician with the therapeutic challenge of helping the patient to use the ward milieu in a constructive manner.

In a large measure, our understanding of the therapeutic aspects of the milieu began with the observations of military psychiatrists during World War II of the power of peer group expectancies on patient's behavior. In the 1950s and '60s these observations were expanded and systematized by Jones, Stanton and Schwartz, Artiss, and others who developed therapeutic community programs or studied the therapeutic forces operating within the social organization of the hospital ward. In addition, the difficulties schizophrenics have with information processing were documented, thus adding a theoretical basis for some of the structure provided by the therapeutic milieu.

The frightening disruption in the continuity and quality of experience that occurs in an acute schizophrenic episode makes a structured environment one of the essentials of a therapeutic milieu. Such structure should provide the patient with a constant,

Table 4-8. The Purposes of Hospitalization

1. Protective-custodial
   a. Safeguarding the patient's life and reputation
   b. Safeguarding the community from the patient's behavior
   c. Removing the patient from a noxious environment
2. Diagnostic
   a. Closer observation
   b. Availability of specialized procedures
3. Therapeutic
   a. Motivation of the patient and family
      (1) to accept and support therapy
      (2) to make necessary life changes
   b. Pharmacotherapy
      (1) Administration of medication schedules too complex to be carried out at home
      (2) Rapid initiation of potentially toxic medication schedules that require careful observation
      (3) Assurance that confused or uncooperative patients take the prescribed medication
   c. Social-familial
      (1) Social rehabilitation, group therapy meetings, group living experience, exposure to therapeutic community, assumption of social responsibilities in hospital setting
      (2) Relief of family tensions so that exploration of critical relationships and issues can proceed without emergence of family crises
   d. Special therapy not possible outside the hospital (ECT or prolonged sleep treatments, or even concomitant observation and treatment of the patient and key relative or relatives)

From T. P. Detre and H. G. Jarecki, *Modern Psychiatric Treatment.* Philadelphia: Lippincott, 1971.

nonthreatening environment. If possible, another person, such as a nurse or attendant, should stay with the patient to help him maintain a reality orientation and tolerate his very powerful and disruptive feelings.

Communication with regressed patients should be clear, unambiguous, and brief. Studies of the failure of therapeutic communitie suggest that interpretive or oblique communications can increase patients' anxieties and disorganization.

Difficult management problems, such as acts of violence, inappropriate sexual behavior, and the refusal of food or medications, commonly occur. Because such activities can injure the patient or those around him, the clinician should act to prevent such behavior in a firm but nonpunitive way. Whatever the psychodynamic origins psychodynamic investigation before adequate controls are present is not in the patient's best interests. If clear verbal confrontation an exhortation will not deter the patient, then such behavior must be restrained with the least amount of coercion. Stimuli in the environment that promote violent or sexual acts should be minimized. If such behavior cannot be controlled by interpersonal intervention and placement in a quiet area, the use of a seclusion room may be temporarily indicated. Ideally, this need will be obviated by the patient's favorable response to treatment (e.g., antipsychotic drugs).

A patient's refusal of food or fluids should not be allowed to endanger his health. This contingency should be explained to the patient, and assisted feeding should be instituted if necessary. In such situations it is very important to pay close attention to the patient's overall fluid and electrolyte balance. Acutely regressed schizophrenic patients should not remain untreated when medications are clearly indicated. If patients refuse oral medications, intramuscular medications should be the alternative — patients usually will begin accepting oral medications. Such firmness in dealing with acutely regressed patients should not preclude the physician's trying to reach an empathic understanding of the feelings and wishes that the patient may be trying to express.

It is reasonable to assume that the potentially most useful therapeutic milieu will be one that provides the patient with the best opportunity for forming constructive human relationships. In order to maintain an atmosphere in which feelings of constancy, acceptance, and caring predominate, a good deal of attention must be paid to the functions of staff support, morale, and communications. When the patient has established some relationships, it is not uncommon to find elements of significant past relationships and conflicts expressed and reflected in his current ward situation. It is the task of the ward personnel to synthesize and communicate their impressions of the patient, understand these impressions in terms of the patient's past experiences, and construct an appropriately corrective therapeutic response. This process demands of the staff a willingness to interact on an affective level with the patient and an ability to share their impressions openly with one another so that a coherent image of the diverse aspects of the patient's personality may be obtained. Staff must also be able to tolerate the threats inherent in working with such patients and the frustrations that characterize social interactions with many of these patients.

In some settings, particularly with regressed, chronically ill patients, token economies and other social techniques based on behavior modification theory may be used to extinguish unacceptable behaviors and promote social adaptation. Such efforts have produced good results among some groups of chronically hospitalized patients. However, the generalization of such treatment effects to acute patients and to settings outside the hospital remains to be established. If such social systems are employed, they must remain sufficiently flexible to meet the various and changing needs of individual patients and of the same patient at different points in his course.

Table 4-9. Some Criteria for Patient Discharge

Does not constitute a danger to himself or others

Functions in an acceptable manner and is no longer harmful to himself or others

Behavior improvement is sufficiently strong to be maintained outside the hospital

Symptoms appear to be in stable remission

Has a stable living arrangement to return to

Assumes responsibility for his behavior

Suitable outpatient treatment is available

Has received maximum hospital benefits as an inpatient

Shows significant improvement in behaviors that precipitated hospitalization

Shows a reduction in deviant behavior that is incompatible with community adjustment

Able to continue in therapy on an outpatient basis

Has received maximum hospital benefits with no further improvement anticipated

In good contact with reality and capable of discussing his situation logically

Has increased socialization skills and is able to relate well to others

Capable of following prescribed medication regimen alone or with the help of a friend or relative

Social behavior and personal hygiene skills are acceptable

Capable of performing functional work independently

Has gained insight into his problem

Has adequate economic resources or a regular source of income

Has a good chance of obtaining immediate employment

Requests discharge against medical advice

Has a history of repeated elopements while hospitalized

Not involved in pending litigation

Adapted from R. C. Katz and F. R. Woolley, Criteria for releasing patients from psychiatric hospitals, *Hosp. Community Psychiatry* 26:33—36, 1975. Copyright 1975 by the American Psychiatric Association.

Discharge from the hospital-based phase of treatment to outpatient followup or community-based aftercare should be carefully planned. Premature discharge or discharge without adequate efforts to insure that the patient is entering an environment that can tolerate the patient's current level of functioning and psychopathology may make successful discharge and rehabilitation difficult if not impossible. These considerations are particularly relevant for chronically ill patients and those who may have become alienated from family and friends. Table 4-9 summarizes many factors that should be considered when evaluating the discharge readiness of patients.

B. **Pharmacotherapy** The efficacy of neuroleptic agents (antipsychotic drugs, major tranquilizers) in treating acute and chronic schizophrenic patients has been established by a vast number of adequately designed and controlled studies conducted over the past 20 years. These studies demonstrate the usefulness of neuroleptics in reducing disordered thinking, anxiety, delusions, hallucinations, social withdrawal, and other symptoms associated with schizophrenia. Although antipsychotic medications do not "cure" schizophrenia, they do

provide important symptomatic relief and can enhance the therapeutic effects of the ward milieu, of psychotherapeutic interventions,
or of social rehabilitation programs. See Chapter 1, Section I.D. and
Table 1-1 for a brief overview of the general pharmacologic properties
of neuroleptic drugs.

1. **Selection and specificity** Although there are numerous claims
   for differential therapeutic effects among the various antipsychotic
   medications, carefully controlled studies and attempted replica-
   tions thus far have failed to substantiate such differences. The
   choice of a particular antipsychotic medication rests primarily
   on consideration of the main and secondary pharmacologic properties, side effects, and toxicity associated with the medication, as
   well as attention to the patient's and the physician's past experience
   with the drug. Clinical experience might suggest that a given
   patient will respond better to one drug than to another; however,
   in the absence of history or pharmacogenetic data, drug selection
   is empirical. Appendix V presents the relative incidence of some
   common unwanted or adverse properties of various classes of
   antipsychotic medications Adrenergic antagonism, mentioned
   in Appendix V, is correlated with a drug's potential to produce
   orthostatic hypotension. In choosing an antipsychotic medication,
   the physician must anticipate the patient's probable overall
   reaction. For instance, an agitated or sleepless patient may
   benefit from the soporific effects of chlorpromazine, while an
   elderly or dehydrated patient might be harmed by the hypotensive
   effects of this drug.

   The patient's past experience with a particular medication also
   may partially determine the physician's choice. In addition to
   inquiring about a past history of drug allergy, the physician should
   try to ascertain which drugs the patient feels were of benefit to
   him and which drugs he feels were poorly tolerated because of
   particular unwanted effects. Such an investigation will not only
   supply the physician with needed clinical information, it will also
   promote the patient's cooperation with and participation in the
   treatment process.

   Finally, the physician should consider his own experience with a
   particular drug. Since there are many antipsychotic medications on
   the market today, extensive experience with all of them is unlikely.
   We recommend that the physician pick one or two representative
   drugs from each of the currently available classes (see Appendix III)
   and become thoroughly familiar with their clinical effects.

2. **Dosage adjustment** In titrating the dosage of a particular antipsychotic medication, the stage of the patient's decompensation

and his target symptoms, body size, weight, and known response to the drug or similar agents must be considered. Antipsychotic medications exert their therapeutic effects over a broad dosage range; particular patients who do not respond favorably to a drug at one dosage level may respond at a higher or lower dosage level.

When initiating the use of an antipsychotic medication, administration of a small test dose of the drug is recommended (25 to 50 mg PO or 25 mg IM of chlorpromazine or the equivalent dose of another antipsychotic drug). This will give the physician an opportunity to observe the patient for the development of orthostatic hypotension or other idiosyncratic effects. If such reactions do not occur within 2 hours of the administration of such a test dose, the physician may then begin titrating the drug dosage into an effective antipsychotic range.

Table 4-10 lists the approximate relative potencies of various antipsychotic medications by the oral route. These are at best rough approximations. For example, they may apply in the acute manage ment phase for a patient but not to maintenance. They are more accurate in the lower dosage ranges. Relative potencies of various drugs at high dosage ranges and for parenteral routes have not been studied adequately. Therefore, establishing the proper therapeutic dosage for a specific patient is largely an empirical process. Usual initial doses are given in Appendix III. These and other dosage recommendations that follow are meant as guidelines for the physic

Table 4-10.   Relative Potencies of Oral Forms of Currently Available Antipsychotic Agents (Reference: Chlorpromazine)

Generic Name[a]	Amounts (mg)
Chlorpromazine	**100**
Promazine	100 to 250
Triflupromazine	25 to 50
Mesoridazine	25 to 50
Piperacetazine	10
Thioridazine	60 to 100
Acetophenazine	20
Butaperazine	10
Carphenazine	25 to 50
Fluphenazine	1 to 4
Perphenazine	8 to 12
Prochlorperazine	15 to 50
Thiopropazate	10 to 15
Trifluoperazine	5 to 10
Haloperidol	1 to 5
Chlorprothixene	50 to 100
Thiothixene	2 to 10
Molindone	10 to 15
Loxapine	10 to 20

[a]See Appendix III for trade names and dose forms available.

as he adjusts the dosage of a particular antipsychotic medication to the needs of the individual patient.

The usual antipsychotic dosage range for acutely ill schizophrenic patients is 300 to 1800 mg daily of chlorpromazine or an equivalent amount of another drug computed from Table 4-10. Lower doses in such patients are not consistently effective, and higher doses, even if adequately tolerated, usually do not produce enhanced therapeutic effects. Although it is important to control a patient's agitated, destructive, or regressed behavior, "snowing" the patient with excessive doses of antipsychotic medication may only treat the staff's anxieties rather than the patient's symptoms. Furthermore, the clinician should remember that antipsychotic drugs often have a cumulative therapeutic effect. Such an effect usually begins within the first 48 hours of treatment, but it may require up to several weeks after beginning a drug. For younger patients who are acutely agitated and psychotic, it is reasonable to begin treatment with doses ranging from 600 to 1200 mg daily of chlorpromazine or equivalent (see Table 4-10). In patients over 40, or in those who have been psychotic for a long period of time, beginning doses of 300 to 600 mg daily of chlorpromazine or equivalent may be more appropriate. As a general rule we advise titration of dosage until an adequate therapeutic response is achieved or troublesome side effects are encountered.

Some authors advocate *rapid tranquilization* for acute schizophrenic patients. This may involve frequent intramuscular dosing (every 30 to 60 minutes) until improvement is observed. Haloperidol has received some acceptance for this procedure. Chlorpromazine has been used with some success, but it is associated with a higher incidence of serious hypotensive reactions. Rapid tranquilization with oral medication is also employed by some physicians. These methods emphasize the frequency of or time interval between dosage increments. Although these procedures may be of value to some patients, we do not feel that this approach has been adequately studied to date to determine fully its potential benefits and risks.

A related procedure (emphasizing amount of dosage) that is achieving some acceptance is the use of *early high oral or intramuscular doses* of drugs such as haloperidol, perphenazine, and fluphenazine. The recent increase in the upper dosage limit currently recommended for haloperidol to 100 mg has fostered this approach. Some clinicians and investigators feel that these high doses (e.g., 60 to 100 mg haloperidol per day) may place the drug in a clinically effective range that is no longer associated with the same intensity and frequency of unwanted extrapyramidal effects (the relationship between daily dose and extrapyramidal effects is postulated to be curvilinear). Although this approach may prove beneficial to some patients, it also has not been studied sufficiently to be generally recommended at this time. Long-term consequences have not been determined (e.g., will this approach increase or decrease the subsequent appearance of tardive dyskinesias?).

3. **Dosage schedules** After picking an antipsychotic medication and titrating its dose, the physician should carefully attend to rationalizing the patient's dosage schedule. After the first 48 to 72 hours of treatment, intensive administration of medication on a four or five times a day basis is usually unnecessary. However, frequent dosing may be indicated when the sedative properties of a drug (e.g., chlorpromazine) are desired during the daytime. Otherwise, antipsychotic agents have long half-lives in the body and are generally well tolerated in large oral doses. Reducing the number of daily doses (with appropriate increases in tablet or capsule strengths) to one (usually just before bedtime) or two a day will save important nursing time and costs and will reduce the cost per milligram of the medication and the inconvenience to the patient. Patient discomfort from many side effects also is minimized by single bedtime doses, since the patient is asleep during maximal anticholinergic or orthostatic hypotensive effects; this will be helpful unless the patient is not sedated.

4. **Maintenance and discontinuation of treatment** Once acute psychotic symptoms are controlled and the patient's condition is stabilized (usually 4 to 12 weeks), the daily dosage of medication may be gradually reduced. Often antipsychotic medications may be tapered over a period of weeks to a dosage range of 75 to 300 mg a day of chlorpromazine or equivalent.

For patients who are receiving or expected to receive antipsychotic medications for extended periods, the institution of drug-free "holidays" of one to three consecutive days a week may be accomplished in many patients without ill effects. Such drug-free intervals are advocated to reduce the total amount of drug ingested by the patient. This may lessen the likelihood of serious side effects associated with long-term use (e.g., tardive dyskinesias).

Other than serious unwanted effects, there are no clear guidelines that dictate the discontinuation of antipsychotic medications. Discontinuation of maintenance medications in chronic ambulatory schizophrenics often leads to relapse. In patients who have attained a complete remission for about six months or who have been chronically hospitalized and on very low doses of medication, it is reasonable to give the patient a trial with no antipsychotic medication. It must be remembered that neuroleptic drugs leave the body slowly; therefore drug-related relapse may not occur until weeks or months after discontinuing the drug. One possible approach to trial discontinuation in chronic patients is to decrease the maintenance dosage by about 30 percent. If no deterioration is seen in six weeks to two months, further decreases of 30 percent are attempted at similar intervals. If a patient's aftercare program provides for reasonably frequent visits, it should be possible for the physician to see whether a patient's clinical status is beginning to deteriorate. In most instances medication can be increased before frank relapse occurs.

5. **General comments**

  a. Oral dosage forms are usually effective. **Time-release** or **sustained-action forms** should not be necessary because of the long half-lives of these compounds. **Liquid forms** (see Appendix III) may be necessary for some patients, but they significantly increase the per milligram cost of most drugs.

  b. **Intramuscular forms** are available (see Appendix III) and may be necessary for some patients (e.g., for violence — see Chapter 7 — or for patients who appear not to absorb oral forms). Oral forms should be reinstituted as soon as possible.

  c. The use of **more than one neuroleptic at a time** is seldom indicated. There is little evidence to suggest that combining drugs is more useful than raising the dose of one drug or switching to another drug.

  d. **Long-acting neuroleptic agents** may be indicated for some schizophrenic patients who are unreliable drug-takers. Fluphenazine enanthate (usually effective for 10 to 14 days) and fluphenazine decanoate (usually effective for 14 to 21 days) are currently available intramuscular drugs. Dosage conversion is generally based on the assumption that 5 mg of oral fluphenazine daily equals 25 mg of either the enanthate or decanoate given every 10 or 14 days, respectively. Individual adjustment to a specific patient's needs is essential. Other long-acting drugs, including oral forms, are currently being investigated.

  e. The use of **electroconvulsive therapy** for schizophrenic patients is discussed in Chapter 6.

f. The use of **antidepressants** in schizophrenic patients is briefly discussed in Section I and in Chapter 3.

g. **Lithium carbonate,** when added to neuroleptic agents, such as chlorpromazine, haloperidol, or thioridazine, may be beneficial in some schizoaffective patients of the excited type who are not responding adequately to the antipsychotic medication alone. The use of lithium for patients not diagnosed as manic-depressive disease is not currently approved by the Food and Drug Administration. In many instances these patients actually may be atypical manic-depressive cases (in some, subsequent episodes clarify the diagnosis). Dosage of lithium should be monitored and kept as low as possible because reports in the literature suggest a lowered threshold to neurotoxicity from lithium when it is combined with major tranquilizers. For additional information, see Section I and Chapter 3 and 5.

6. **Side effects** Side effects and toxic reactions of antipsychotic drugs are varied and potentially very serious. They include neurologic and hepatic effects, hormonal alterations, blood dyscrasias, and pigmentary retinopathy (to avoid pigmentary retinopathy, an upper limit of 800 mg is placed on the use of thioridazine by the manufacturer). A full discussion of these reactions is beyond the scope of this chapter. The physician must thoroughly familiarize himself with these reactions before using antipsychotic drugs (see R. I. Shader, A. DiMascio, and associates, *Psychotropic Drug Side Effects,* Baltimore: Williams & Wilkins, 1970). Some side effects occur with sufficient frequency to merit brief review here.

a. **Nonspecific sedation** Agitation, hyperactivity, and disordered sleep are common manifestations of the syndrome of schizophrenia. Because major tranquilizers ameliorate the underlying thought disorder responsible for such manifestations, any drug of this type can have a calming effect and improve sleep in a psychotic patient. In nonpsychotic individuals major tranquilizers produce variable nonspecific sedation, depending on the particular drug and the patient's sensitivity to it. Phenothiazines and thioxanthenes with dimethylaminopropyl substitutions and, to a slightly lesser extent, piperidien phenothiaz have relatively strong sedative effects. Butyrophenones, dihydroindolones, and piperazine-substituted phenothiazines or thioxanthenes produce much less sedation. Dibenzoxazepines appear to be intermediate. Thus a drug such as haloperidol can appear to act differently depending on the type of patient who receives it. A healthy individual who is given haloperidol to treat nausea and vomiting may experience little or no drowsiness or sedation, but the same dose given to an agitated, sleepless schizophrenic patient can have a marked tranquilizing and soporific effect.

b. **Adrenergic antagonism**   Alpha-adrenergic blocking properties of major tranquilizers approximately parallel their nonspecific sedative effects. Dimethylaminopropyl derivatives of phenothiazines and thioxanthenes are potent alpha antagonists, whereas piperazine derivatives, butyrophenones, and dihydroindolones are weak. Dibenzoxazepines appear to be intermediate. Orthostatic (postural) hypotension is the most important consequence of this property, and this must be considered especially before chlorpromazine, promazine, or chlorprothixene is administered. In some cases, neuroleptic-induced hypotension has been serious or fatal, but it is not established exactly how frequently such events occur. As noted earlier, blood pressure measurements in supine and standing positions should be made before and after a test dose, particularly in the elderly. Orthostatic hypotension should not be treated with epinephrine, which is a stimulator of both alpha- and beta-adrenergic sites. Beta stimulators are contraindicated. Alpha stimulators, such as norepinephrine, are the treatment of choice. Serious hypotension and shock must be treated as a medical emergency (see Chapter 15, Section I.C.5).

A second consequence of alpha-adrenergic blockade is inhibition of ejaculation. For reasons that are not clear, this troublesome side effect is most commonly reported with the piperidien phenothiazines, thioridazine and mesoridazine.

c. **Extrapyramidal symptoms**   Major tranquilizers induce a variety of bizarre involuntary movements. Blockade of dopamine receptors in the basal ganglia is the postulated cause of these drug-related extrapyramidal movement disorders.

(1) **Acute dystonic reactions** are the most troublesome of the extrapyramidal symptoms. These acute spasms of nuchal, truncal, buccal, or oculomotor muscle groups can be frightening or disabling. Dystonic reactions usually are induced by piperazine derivatives (phenothiazine and thioxanthene) or butyrophenones, and they can occur in young, healthy individuals even after a single dose of one of these drugs. More chronic, insidiously developing extrapyramidal symptoms can occur with any of the major tranquilizers. These include a syndrome of motor rest-

Table 4-11. Antiparkinsonian Drugs in Current Use

Generic Name	Trade Name
Tropine derivatives	
benztropine	Cogentin
Piperidine compounds	
biperiden	Akineton
procyclidine	Kemadrin
trihexyphenidyl	Artane, Pipanol, Tremin
Ethanolamine antihistamines	
diphenhydramine	Benadryl
orphenadrine	Disipal

lessness or *akathisia* (usually experienced as an inability to sit still) and a triad of akinesia, rigidity, and resting tremor resembling *parkinsonism* (often associated with increased salivation). Middle-aged and elderly chronic schizophrenics taking major tranquilizers for weeks or months seem most susceptible to drug-induced akathisia or parkinsonism. For reasons that are not clear, piperidine phenothiazine derivatives uncommonly produce extrapyramidal reactions of any kind.

CNS cholinergic blockade effectively reverses movement disorders induced by major tranquilizers. Acute dystonic reactions may require parenteral treatment. Intravenous benztropine (0.5 to 2.0 mg) or diphenhydramine (25 to 50 mg) can provide dramatic reversal of such reactions. Akathisia or parkinsonism can be treated by antiparkinsonian drugs (e.g., benztropine or trihexyphenidyl in doses of 2 to 8 mg PO per day). Oral antiparkinsonian drugs (see Table 4-11) are effective in most patients when given on a once a day or twice a day basis. They do not compromise the antipsychotic efficacy of the major tranquilizers. Some authorities suggest that antiparkinsonian drugs should not be given prophylactically but only when extrapyramidal reactions appear. Once therapy is started, it need not be continued indefinitely. For some patients one to two weeks is adequate, and in most cases a three- to four-month trial need not be exceeded.

(2) **Tardive dyskinesias** (see Table 4-12) appear in an undetermined percentage of patients who have received long-term treatment with neuroleptic agents (they also may appear in patients who have never received these drugs). The symptoms of tardive dyskinesia usually

Table 4-12. Prominent Features of Tardive Dyskinesias

Lingual-facial hyperkinesias
  Chewing movements
  Smacking and licking of the lips
  Sucking movements
  Tongue movements within the oral cavity
  Tongue protrusion
  Tongue tremor with mouth open
  Myokemic movements (worm-like movement on the surface of the tongue)
  Blinking
  Grotesque grimaces and spastic facial distortions
Neck and trunk movements
  Spasmodic torticollis
  Retrocollis
  Torsion movements of the trunk
  Axial hyperkinesia (hip rocking)
Choreoathetoid movements of the extremities

appear with dosage reduction or discontinuation. In an occasional patient these symptoms appear to be related to the patient's becoming tolerant to a particular dosage level. Current hypotheses to explain tardive dyskinesias generally assume that the condition results from rebound sensitivity to dopamine in basal ganglion areas that have been subjected to the dopamine blocking properties of neuroleptic agents. An interaction between dopaminergic and cholinergic systems may be involved. The reinstitution of a dopamine blocking drug or an increase in dosage will usually mask symptoms. Antiparkinsonian drugs are most often of no benefit, and their use may exacerbate the symptoms of tardive dyskinesia. At the present time there is no accepted approach to the treatment of tardive dyskinesias. If symptoms are observed, it is advisable to try to discontinue the offending drug. If the patient's clinical condition requires continued use of neuroleptic agents, this benefit must be weighed (by both the physician and the patient) against the adverse implications of continued neuroleptic use. Reserpine (a dopamine-depleter), lithium carbonate, benzodiazepines, and other drugs have achieved some anecdotal support as potential sources of relief for the symptoms of tardive dyskinesia. However, their use has not been substantiated by adequate clinical study.

d. **Cardiac toxicity** The possible cardiotoxic effects of major tranquilizers have generated much concern. Reports of sudden unexplained deaths among previously healthy patients taking these drugs suggest that major tranquilizers may have the potential to precipitate fatal ventricular tachyarrhythmias. Although some experimental and pathologic studies are consistent with a cardiotoxic effect, it is not adequately established whether major tranquilizers do, in fact, have clinically important cardiac toxicity or cause fatal arrhythmias. In several reports thioridazine, in particular, has been implicated. Usual doses of thioridazine can produce electrocardiographic changes resembling hypokalemia that are reversible on administration of potassium. Such changes may be benign and unrelated to the presumed association with life-threatening arrhythmias.

e. **Cholinergic blocking**   Major tranquilizers have clinically important anticholinergic effects. Manifestations usually are limited to mild dryness of mouth or tachycardia. In predisposed individuals the drugs can exacerbate untreated glaucoma or precipitate urinary retention or intestinal obstruction. Major tranquilizers can potentiate toxicity due to other anticholinergic drugs and should never be used to treat delirium or hyperpyrexia due to cholinergic blocking drugs.

f. **Hepatic disturbances** have been reported with most major tranquilizers. The incidence of drug-induced jaundice appears to have diminished since the 1950s. Chlorpromazine has been more frequently implicated than other agents. Most cases develop during the third and fourth weeks of treatment. The clinical picture and time of onset suggest a sensitivity reaction — obstructive jaundice, fever, and eosinophilia are typical. Although clinical experience suggests that cross-tolerance is rare and that some patients can even be placed back on the same drug without a recurrence, conservative management should include switching to another class of antipsychotic drugs (e.g., from a phenothiazine to a butyrophenone or dihydroindolone), preferably after a drug-free interval.

g. **Leukopenia** and **agranulocytosis** rarely occur. Most cases appear during the interval between the end of the first month and the beginning of the fourth month. Elderly, debilitated women appear to be at greatest risk. However, careful clinical investigation should be made of all patients who develop pharyngitis or unexplained fevers. Discontinuation of the offending drug and the use of antibiotics may be indicated. Some clinicians are investigating the usefulness of prescribing lithium carbonate, which has been reported to increase white cell counts.

C. Psychotherapy Barring unforeseen development of new techniques, Freud discouraged psychotherapeutic work with schizophrenics because of his feeling that the withdrawal of libido from the object world prevents the formation of a transference. Subsequent therapists modified this view, and a large body of practical and theoretical work on the psychotherapy of schizophrenia has developed. Paul Federn, one of Freud's pupils, demonstrated that schizophrenics could form a transference, and he formulated the therapeutic task as that of helping the patient reestablish his faulty ego boundaries. Other specific approaches were developed by M. Klein, Schehaye, Rosen, Sullivan, Fromm-Reichmann, Bychowsky, Searles, and many others. A review of their work is beyond the scope of this discussion. This diversity of method has produced a variety of criteria by which to evaluate therapeutic efficacy. Well-designed, well-controlled studies have been rare. Only fragmented assessments have arisen from inconsistently researched data sources. A number of studies have nonetheless been carried out to evaluate psychopharmacologic treatment and individual and group psychotherapy in both chronic and acute patients. These studies suggest criteria we may employ to evaluate the effectiveness of psychotherapy. Some of the many variables that must be considered in evaluating psychotherapy with schizophrenics are listed in Table 4-13. Further work must focus on more limited objectives, including the clarification of patient, therapist, process, and outcome variables that may lead to specific psychotherapeutic results (see Section III).

Despite the uncertain state of our knowledge, some important conclusions are warranted: The majority of acute and chronic schizophrenic patients cannot be usefully treated by psychotherapy alone. From a public health point of view, the only useful single therapeutic intervention is antipsychotic medication, which is both the cheapest and most effective treatment of schizophrenic symptomatology. Preferable is a cogently designed multimodality treatment program that provides ample room for good psychotherapeutic management of schizophrenics or for the use of individual and group psychotherapy. The following discussion attempts to outline one useful psychotherapeutic approach.

In the early stages of psychotherapeutic contact with schizophrenic patients, the focus is on providing the essentials of a trusting relationship in which the therapist offers to the patient "lend-lease" ego strength. Establishing a stable, trusting human relationship is not an easy task for schizophrenic patients, in whom feelings such as fear, indifference, distrust, worthlessness, and hostility may predominate. In beginning such a relationship the psychotherapist

Table 4-13. Some Variables Involved in Defining the Efficacy of Psychotherapy for Schizophrenics

Patient variables
  Personality structure
  Age
  Socioeconomic background
  Expectations for treatment
Illness variables
  Schizophrenic subtype
    Paranoid
    Schizoaffective
    Simple
  Stage of illness
    Incipient psychosis
    Acute psychosis
    Partial remission
    Complete remission
    Chronic psychosis
  Prognostic indices (see Table 4-7)
    Genetic loading
    Clear precipitants
    Speed of onset of symptoms
    Presence of depression
Other treatments and supports
  Antipsychotic medications
  Hospitalization
  Community supports: family, job
	Therapist variables
	  Personality structure
	  Age and experience
	  Socioeconomic background
	  Expectations for treatment
	  Motivation
	  Comfort with frustration, strong
	    feelings, etc.
	Therapy variables
	  Patient-therapist fit
	  Frequency and duration of treat-
	    ment
	  Type of treatment
	    Supportive
	    Reality-defining
	    Interpretive—insight oriented
	Outcome measures
	  Baseline measurements
	  Duration of followup
	  Outcome goals
	    Length of outpatient stay
	    Ability to work
	    Interpersonal skills
	    Changes in psychopathology
	    Self-regard
	    Autonomy-dependency

often may be able to establish affective contact with his patient before gaining insight into specific conflicts. Since schizophrenic patients often are unable to communicate directly how they feel, it is important to pay close attention to their nonverbal communications, including facial expression, posture, and activity. Furthermore it is important to remember that words can take on peculiar and concrete meanings for these patients; the psychotherapist must speak to the patient in simple, direct, unambiguous terms. It is important for the psychotherapist to evidence constancy in his commitment to the patient, together with an ability to share some of his own human responses to the patient in an open, constructive way.

During the acute stages of a schizophrenic illness, it is best to avoid making interpretations concerning emotional conflicts that may have been associated in time with the patient's decompensation into psychosis. Instead, emphasis is placed on gathering a complete psychiatric history from the patient or the patient's relatives. Such an evaluation will give the psychotherapist an understanding of the early life experiences that may have contributed to the patient's later vulnerability to schizophrenia and an understanding of any events associated with the onset of decompensation. Equally important, the therapist must understand the areas of healthy personal and occupational functioning available to the patient.

In taking such a history the psychotherapist not only demonstrates a concrete interest in the patient and the facts of his life but also observes the patient's characteristic avoidances of unpleasant feelings and experiences. Such observations of the patient's patterns of denial, distortion, and projection may allow the psychotherapist to help the patient understand the areas of the patient's life that have been most painful.

It is crucial to bring the issue of medication into consideration and into the psychotherapeutic work. It is important to explore with the patient the feelings he has about taking medicine, and indeed about all other administrative issues, and to take them into account in planning treatment. The therapist also helps the patient to understand what is happening in the ward milieu.

As the acute psychotic process abates, and the schizophrenic patient begins the process of reintegration, many patients develop neurasthenic, hypochondriacal, obsessive-compulsive, and depressive symptoms. Suicide may become a serious risk in some. During this time as well, the patient may repeatedly test the therapist's interest in continuing the psychotherapeutic relationship. Appointments are often missed by the patient, and both patient and therapist may begin to feel that the focus of the therapy has become obscure. From time to time, however, patients are able to use the psychotherapeutic relationship at this stage to integrate some of the conflicts and sources of lowered self esteem that may have stressed them prior to their decompensation.

An empathic understanding with the patient of specific stresses and conflicts that may have led to the onset of the psychosis is seen as a means of helping the patient to anticipate future difficulties. The timing of such psychotherapeutic intervention is a crucial matter, usually dependent on the psychotherapist's judgment and intuition, and the patient's motivation and ability to undertake therapeutic tasks.

We assume that the patient's predisposition to disorganized thinking under stress leads the patient to have difficulties in adapting to and resolving problematical situations. This obviously affects the patient's self-image and his learning. The therapist tries to help the patient see what may evoke distortions of reality (e.g., not being able to "stand" feelings of loss, loneliness, helplessness, or rage) and what consequences these distortions may have. The therapist can try to help the patient tolerate uncertainty and ambiguity in his interpersonal relationships. Evaluation of family interactions may provide useful information for therapeutic work, and some patients are significantly helped by ongoing conjoint work with other family members.

D. Social rehabilitation and aftercare Following remission of the acute schizophrenic episode, it is not uncommon for patients to require many months to reach their premorbid levels of functioning. Furthermore, the patient's initial level of functioning may have been restricted by premorbid character traits or environmental hardships or both.

By rehabilitation we mean the process of helping the patient to learn or relearn those skills that could make him a productive member of the community. Such a process, while not necessarily associated with intrapsychic change, may be a major source of increased self-esteem, since it provides the patient with feelings of increased competence within his environment.

As mentioned in Section III, an individual's premorbid level of adult functioning is one of the better indices of his eventual ability to resume a socially productive life. Those patients who are married or who had a successful vocational adjustment prior to their illness have the best opportunity for a successful community adjustment upon recovery. The patient's ability to return to the community may depend as much on the social supports available there as on his level of psychopathology.

A number of clinical studies have demonstrated the usefulness of intermittent outpatient support facilities in maintaining patients outside a hospital. Such aftercare services usually involve a brief interview with a physician or other mental health professional and the prescription of an antipsychotic medication. The therapeutic factors within such aftercare programs remain obscure. In part, their usefulness may reflect the better organization or better motivation, or both, of the patients who choose to attend them. In part they may also reflect the combined benefit of antipsychotic medications and all available interpersonal opportunities. Although they help to maintain patients in the community, some aftercare programs can do little to improve the quality of his life there.

Some centers have utilized groups for the aftercare of chronically ill outpatients and report that the use of a group aftercare setting, although it does not affect rehospitalization rates, significantly improves the social skills of the patients involved. Such results await further clinical verification.

In addition to the deficits produced by the patient's environment, premorbid personality, and his illness, the side effects of institutionalization often become a stumbling block in the rehabilitation of the schizophrenic patient. This problem is particularly severe for those who have been hospitalized for two or more years. For chronically hospitalized patients, predischarge rehabilitation programs emphasizing vocational and interpersonal skills may be an important means of promoting their long-term community adjustment.

With the development of the open-door concept of psychiatric hospitalization and the large-scale use of antipsychotic medications, great numbers of patients are returning to live in the community. Leaving the hospital is, however, only a first step toward and one prerequisite for community adjustment. Active efforts by health care personnel are necessary to insure a patient's successful coping and productive reintegration.

References

Arnold, O. H. *Schizophrener Prozess und Schizophrene Symptomgesetze.* Vienna: Maudrich, 1955.

Artiss, K. L. *Milieu Therapy in Schizophrenia.* New York: Grune and Stratton, 1962.

Bleuler, M. A 23-year longitudinal study of 208 schizophrenics and impressions in regard to the nature of schizophrenia. In D. Rosenthal and S. Kety (Eds.). *Transmission of Schizophrenia.* Oxford: Pergamon, 1968. Pp. 3—12.

Brown, G. W., Bone, M., Dalizon, B., and Wing, J. K. *Schizophrenia and Social Care.* Maudsley Monograph No. 17. London: Oxford University Press, 1966.

Cole, N. J., and Shupe, D. C. A four-year follow-up of former psychiatric patients in industry. *Arch. Gen. Psychiatry* 22:222—229, 1970.

Farina, A., Garmezy, N., and Barry, N. III Relationship of marital status to incidence and prognosis of schizophrenia. *J. Abn. Soc. Psychol.* 67:624—630, 1963.

Federn, P. *Ego Psychology and the Psychoses.* New York: Basic Books, 1952.

Gittelman-Klein, R., and Klein, D. F. Marital status as a prognostic indicator in schizophrenia, *J. Nerv. Ment. Dis.* 147:289—296, 1968.

Gittelman-Klein, R. and Klein, D. F. Premorbid asocial adjustment and prognosis in schizophrenia. *J. Psychiatr. Res.* 7.35—53, 1969.

Goffman, E. *Asylums.* New York: Doubleday, 1961.

Gross, M. Hitchman, I. L., Reeves, W. P., Lawrence, J., and Newell, P. C. Discontinuation of treatment with ataractic drugs. *Recent Advances in Biological Psychiatry.* Vol. 3. New York: Grune & Stratton, 1961. Pp. 44—62.

Hall, J. D., Smith, K., and Shimkawas, A. Employment problems of schizophrenic patients. *Am. J. Psychiatry* 123:536—540, 1966.

Hogarty, G. E., Goldberg, S. C., and The Collaborative Study Group Drugs and sociotherapy in the aftercare of schizophrenic patients. *Arch. Gen. Psychiatry* 28:54—64, 1973.

Jones, M. *The Therapeutic Community.* New York: Basic Books, 1953

Langfeldt, G. The prognosis in schizophrenia. *Acta Psychiatr. Neurol. Scand.* (Suppl.) 110: 7—66, 1956.

Longabaugh, R., and Eldred, S. H. Premorbid adjustment, schizoid personality and onset of illness as predictors of post-hospital functioning. *J. Psychiatr. Res.* 10:19—29, 1973.

McCabe, M. S., Fowler, R. C., Cadoret, R. J., and Winokur, G. Familial differences in schizophrenia with good and poor prognoses. *Psychol. Med.* 1:326—332, 1971.

Niskanen, P., and Achté, K. A. A comparative follow-up study of first admissions for schizophrenic and paranoid psychoses in Helsinki in 1950 and 1965. *Psychiatria Fennica* 117—126, 1971.

Robins, E., and Guze, S. E. Establishment of diagnostic validity in psychiatric illness: Its application to schizophrenia. *Am. J. Psychiatry* 126:983—987, 1970.

Roff, J. D. Adolescent schizophrenia: Variables related to differences in long-term adult outcome. *J. Consult. Clin. Psychol.* 42:180—183, 1974.

Rosen, B., Klein, D. F., and Gittelman-Klein, R. Sex differences in the relationship between premorbid asociality and post-hospital outcome. *J. Nerv. Ment. Dis.* 149:415—420, 1969.

Simon, W., Wirt, A. L., Wirt, R. D., and Halloran, A. V. Long-term follow-up study of schizophrenic patients. *Arch. Gen. Psychiatry* 12:510—515, 1965.

Slater, E.: A review of earlier evidence on genetic factors in schizophrenia. In D. Rosenthal and S. Katy (Eds.). *Transmission of Schizophrenia.* Oxford: Pergamon, 1968. Pp. 15—26.

Stanton, A. H., and Schwartz, M. S. *The Mental Hospital.* New York: Basic Books, 1954.

Stephens, J. H. Long-term course and prognosis in schizophrenia. *Semin. Psychiatry* 2:464—485, 1970.

Taylor, M. A. Schneiderian first-rank symptoms and clinical prognostic features in schizophrenia. *Arch. Gen. Psychiatry* 26:64—67, 1972.

Troshinsky, C. H., Aaronson, H. G., and Stone, R. K. Maintenance phenothiazine in after-care of schizophrenic patients. *Pa. Psychiat. Quart.* 2:11—15, 1962.

Vaillant, G. E. Prospective prediction of schizophrenic remission. *Arch. Gen. Psychiatry* 11:509—518, 1964.

Waring, M., and Ricks, D. Family patterns of children who became adult schizophrenics. *J. Nerv. Ment. Dis.* 140:351—364, 1965.

Watt, N. F., Stolorow, R. D., Lubensky, A. W. and McClelland, D. C. School adjustment and behavior of children hospitalized for schizophrenia as adults. *Am. J. Orthopsychiatry* 40:637—657, 1970.

Wing, J. K. Institutionalism in mental hospitals. *Br. J. Soc. Clin. Psychol.* 1:38—51, 1962.

Wing, J. K. Five-year outcome in early schizophrenia. *Proc. R. Soc. Med.* 59:17—18, 1966.

5

The Treatment of Manic-Depressive States

Samuel Gershon

In the field of medicine, new treatments not only have important effects on theoretical concepts, they often raise new concepts in diagnosis and treatment as well. Within psychiatry such changes are currently taking place in the diagnosis and treatment of the affective disorders. In particular, the introduction of the lithium ion and its now established profile of action have necessitated a more careful consideration of diagnostic specificity. Thus, the label *mania* or *manic behavior* should no longer be broadly employed simply as a description of a behavior or a target symptom. Because diagnosis and treatment of such affective disorders are now more complex, they are now discussed in terms of diagnostic syndromes. As might be expected, these new patterns of description have resulted in marked discrepancies in incidence figures. Reviews of these current diagnostic descriptions are extensively presented in the literature.

Two of the factors that have been clearly established by diagnostic data are the relative infrequency of manic episodes and the high ratio of depression to mania. In addition, the clinical picture usually includes euphoria as well as irritability, hyperactivity of a motor or social or sexual nature, press of speech, flight of ideas, racing thoughts, grandiosity with delusional content, decreased sleep, distractibility, buying sprees, poor judgment, and social intrusiveness. The euphoria, joking, and jollity may be supplanted by anger and hostility if the patient is thwarted. Or, on occasion, the euphoria may give way momentarily to sadness and even tears when the patient is discussing a real life situation that may logically justify such a response.

For the diagnostician, however, the central problem is the considerable confusion that exists about the boundaries of the manic syndrome. There is uncertainty about how to regard these clinical variations, and some physicians think of them as atypical forms. In response to this problem, attempts have been made to develop inventories to record the behaviors characteristic of the disorder. In these efforts to establish specific diagnostic configurations, the most difficult problem is that presented by the schizoaffective states. This problem is important because of the hypothesis that these groups have a differential, adverse response to lithium. While the efficacy of lithium in the treatment of manic episodes has been established, the use of this drug with schizoaffective symptoms has produced less clearcut results. To further complicate matters, many naturalistic studies have reported anywhere from a 3 percent to an 82 percent change in clinical picture and diagnosis over time.

Some clinicians consider schizoaffective states to be a form of affective disorder, whereas others consider them to be a variant of schizophrenia; a third group views them as an intermediate stage between affective disorder and schizophrenia. Another important appraisal is a longitudinal view of the illness, which may include various phases such as delirious mania. Still another proposed approach is the unipolar-bipolar concept. Evidence has accumulated to indicate that manic-depressive disease is likely to be heterogeneous and that it contains at least two groups. In one of these groups, designated *bipolar* by most investigators, the patients exhibit both manic and depressive phases during the course of their illness. Patients in the other group experience only episodes of depression and are called the *unipolar* group. In addition to the qualitative and quantitative clinical distinctions given above, genetic and prognostic criteria developed in recent years suggest additional differences among depressive disorders (see Table 5-1).

Despite the apparent clinical polarity, the bipolar and unipolar patients share many common features, including inherent illness cyclicity and relapse potential. Aside from their subjective anguish, patients suffering from the bipolar and unipolar manifestations of affective illness frequently present with similar histories of family alienation, divorce, frequent hospitalization, an inability to hold gainful employment, and a tendency to get into difficulties with their co-workers or the law. The serious and almost tragic nature of manic-depressive disorder poses important and challenging therapeutic responsibilities, not only in treating the current episode of the disorder but also in attaining the goal of prophylaxis.

I. **Rauwolfia Alkaloids** Introduced in the early 1950s for the control of psychomotor overactivity of nonspecific type, the rauwolfia alkaloids are currently essentially discarded from routine psychiatric treatment use. Although some clinicians still consider reserpine to be one of the most effective psychopharmacologic preparations for the control of manic patients, a review of the literature offers no support for this. Instead the available reports suggest that the rauwolfias may in fact induce deleterious effects in manic individuals.

II. **Convulsive Therapy** ECT is still employed in treating manic patients, and its effects are reported to be almost immediate. Convulsive therapy does not prevent episodic recurrences of mania, and the duration of symptom-free intervals is not altered (see Chapter 6).

Flurothyl (hexafluorodiethyl ether) is a CNS stimulant that is used as a convulsive agent in therapy for mental disorders including mania,

Table 5-1.   Criteria for Behavioral-Chemical Differences between Bipolar and Unipolar Depressions

	Unipolar	Bipolar
Clinical features	Retardation-agitation Late age onset Greater tendency toward anger Physiologic complaints: anorexia	Retardation Early onset

Genetic		Transmitted on X chromosome:
		    Color blindness
		    Blood group XGA

Family history	Low incidence of mania	High incidence of mania Higher incidence of suicide
Biological features	"Reducer" on cortical evoked potential Normal or elevated 17-hydroxycorticosteroid excretion Plasma Mg^{++} is not changed during lithium therapy Lower CNS dopamine turnover RBC COMT markedly reduced	"Augmenter" on cortical evoked potential Low 17-hydroxycortico-steroid excretion Plasma Mg^{++} is elevated with lithium treatment RBC COMT slightly reduced
Response to psychoactive drugs	Antidepressant effect of Li_2CO_3 equivocal Antidepressant effect of tricyclics more marked No behavioral toxicity to L-dopa treatment	Antidepressant effect of Li_2CO_3 more marked Manic response to L-dopa treatment

and it is similar in safety and efficacy to ECT. The advantage claimed for flurothyl is that many patients prefer the drug to ECT, presumably because of the anesthesia-like state that precedes the convulsion. Commercially available under the name Indoklon, this agent, given by inhalation or parenterally, fails to demonstrate any clear advantages over ECT. In fact, any assessment of convulsive therapies for mania would be unlikely to demonstrate any superiority over pharmacotherapy.

The main disadvantage of convulsive treatment is the fact that frequent administrations are usually required; this may induce organic sequelae, albeit temporary, that include clouding, confusion, and memory impairment.

III.   **Effective Antimanic Drugs**

A. **Phenothiazine derivatives**

1. **Chlorpromazine**   Following the initial recognition of chlorpromazine's beneficial effects in controlling manic excitement and agitation, the drug became a standard treatment for these symptoms and at present is one of the most frequently used substances in

treating manic patients. Inasmuch as vigorous intervention is usually necessary in controlling the manic episode, intramuscular administration is often the preferred method of initiating treatment in the hospital; in less severe cases, liquid chlorpromazine may be given orally. Better still is the concomitant use of both oral liquid and intramuscular administrations. These routes offer the quickest effect and eliminate the possibility of the patient's "cheeking" and eventually disposing of the medication. When behavior has improved, intramuscular medication may be discontinued and capsules or tablets substituted for the liquid chlorpromazine.

Since underdosage is probably the most frequent mistake in treating this condition, care must be taken to insure that adequate doses are given. Dosage must be titrated individually, and progressive increments should be made until control of behavior and therapeutic response appear or side effects require intervention. Only if side effects of the extrapyramidal type occur should any antiparkinsonian medication be administered.

2. **Thioproperazine and thioridazine**   Many phenothiazine preparations are used in the therapy of manic patients. Favorable therapeutic results have been reported with discontinuous thioproperazine* treatment. Observers indicate that the dosage of thioproperazine should be raised swiftly.

Thioridazine has good neuroleptic potency and efficacy; its pharmacologic activity makes it a reasonable choice in the treatment of mania. In fact, a literature search indicates that there have been at least 50 publications dealing with the use of thioridazine in manic-depressive patients. Collectively, however, they contribute little if anything to defining the treatment efficacy of thioridazine in manic illness. Some authors suggest that the need for heavier sedation makes chlorpromazine the phenothiazine drug of choice. Some clinicians feel that thioridazine has a limited role since a toxic retinopathy can occur when thioridazine is used at sustained high dosage levels (greater than 800 mg per day) and no parenteral form is available.

B. **Butyrophenones**   Clinical trials with the butyrophenone haloperidol indicate its effectiveness in control or relief of psychomotor agitation, aggressiveness, assaultiveness, hostility, and other symptom parameters associated with acute or chronic psychoses. From available

---

*Editor's note: Thioproperazine is a piperazine phenothiazine that is widely used in Europe but not currently available in the United States.

open studies, it appears that behavioral and psychomotor activity in manic patients are brought under control within three days after initiating treatment with haloperidol and that, in a high percentage of cases, all symptoms are abolished in four or five days. These reports from open studies have not yet been fully supported by a recent controlled study.

In open studies that offer dosage information, the average maximum daily dose of haloperidol during the study periods is about 10 mg, ranging up to about 40 mg per day. Supplementation of the oral dose with an intramuscular dose was helpful in the more severe cases. Generally speaking, investigators give relatively low doses at the beginning of a research study, increase the dosage to achieve therapeutic effect, and then lower it to the minimum consistent with maintaining therapeutic effect. Thus, as shown by these figures, the effective doses of haloperidol for the treatment of manic patients tend to be small, considerably smaller than comparable doses of chlorpromazine or other potent phenothiazines. Of the currently available studies of lithium carbonate treatment in manic patients (see below), four have made comparisons of lithium with chlorpromazine. In light of the available information claiming efficacy for haloperidol in manic disorders, this compound *may* represent a more adequate reference drug than chlorpromazine. Ideally in such studies four drug groups should be used: lithium, chlorpromazine, haloperidol, and placebo. A recent study from our research group compares chlorpromazine, haloperidol, and lithium in the treatment of manic patients. It would appear from this double-blind controlled study that chlorpromazine and haloperidol are approximately equivalent in their antimanic activity, with haloperidol appearing superior in some respects.

C. **Lithium carbonate** The use of lithium salts for the treatment of mania was the first and only indication reported by Cade (*Med. J. Aust.* 36:349, 1949). Since that date, it is estimated that over 50 published reports have appeared on this subject, almost all of them supporting its efficacy. However, this literature includes trials not only in manic patients but in schizophrenic patients of various subtypes and in patients in several other diagnostic categories. Even in those studies in which the population is restricted to clearly defined and diagnostically typical manic cases, a number of factors make it difficult to assess the therapeutic efficacy of lithium: rating scales were not employed, other medications were used concomitantly, the drug washout period was inadequate, dosages of lithium varied widely, and plasma levels were not reported. In addition, diagnostic problems confuse this literature; large variation among reports as to the incidence of the disease seem to support the existence of a large variation in diagnostic criteria. Moreover, methodological problems are perhaps greater in the study of mania than in any other psychiatric condition, and these are complicated by additional problems arising from the management difficulties presented by these patients and the self-limiting and recurrent nature of their disease. All of these considerations are of great importance in evaluating published reports in this area and are discussed in more detail elsewhere (S. Gershon and B. Shopsin [Eds.]. *Lithium Ion: Its Role in Psychiatric Treatment and Research,* New York: Plenum, 1973).

The value of lithium in the treatment of mania is generally apparent from the numerous open studies: Although each of the five published controlled studies comparing lithium to placebo has its own methodological strengths and weaknesses, it is important to note that despite these differences the results are remarkably similar — lithium is clearly superior to placebo in the acute treatment of mania.

Even after more than 20 years of study, the conclusions that can be reached on the efficacy of lithium in acute mania are not absolutely resolved. Although it is probably safe to say that lithium is an effective agent in the treatment of mania and is superior in efficacy to placebo, its comparable efficacy over chlorpromazine for acute mania remains unclear (four studies). Controlled studies of small patient samples (12 to 28 cases) suggest its equivalence or superiority to chlorpromazine, whereas in a larger study of 250 cases the superiority of chlorpromazine over lithium during the acute stage is indicated.

Lithium's effect in mania differs distinctly from that of the neuroleptics (such as chlorpromazine and haloperidol) on three points. First, they have different time courses. Chlorpromazine and haloperidol usually act more rapidly than lithium, whose full effect cannot be expected till after 7 to 10 days of treatment. This is of considerable importance for the acute and unusually violent cases of mania, suggesting that the use of neuroleptics in such a treatment situation would be preferable. Second, while the sedative action of conventional neuroleptics is largely independent of the illness causing the agitation, lithium acts more specifically against mania, its best results being obtained in patients with clinical pictures dominated by mood elevation, irritability, restlessness, talkativeness, and jocularity. Third, and perhaps most important, the responses to lithium and neuroleptic treatments differ in quality. Neuroleptics, although they produce an effective suppression of the manic overactivity and restlessness, often are accompanied by a "drugged feeling" of sedation and drowsiness. Thus, the phenothiazines and butyrophenones merely "place a lid" over the manic state; the patients usually retain, below the surface, their characteristic symptoms of mania. Lithium, on the other hand, seems to remove the manic symptoms in a more specific manner, dissolving the elevated mood, hyperactivity, restlessness, talkativeness, and sleeplessness without sedation or the feeling of being drugged. The patient is "normalized," that is, he is brought into a state that cannot be distinguished subjectively or objectively from his normal, premorbid condition.

1. Therapeutic regimen

a. **Selection of patients** The treatment procedure must take into account both the patient and the physiologic or pharmacologic properties of the drug. It is important to clarify whether the treatment is for the control of a current manic episode or for maintenance and prophylaxis during an interphase, and to recognize that lithium is of most value for the specific diagnostic entity mania. The first issue, then, is whether the patient is one of those to whom lithium may be prescribed. The patient must be in reasonably good physical condition to handle the lithium ion upon its introduction into the body. Significant renal disorder, such that adequate elimination of the lithium ion in the urine might be impaired, is an absolute contraindication for lithium treatment. Other factors that mitigate against treating a patient with lithium include significant cardiac disease, organic brain damage, and regimens requiring restriction of dietary intake of salt (see Chapter 19).

b. **Stabilization** After selection of the patient for treatment, the therapeutic regimen may be considered in two phases, stabilization of the manic episode and maintenance. The initiation of lithium treatment in a manic patient needs to be considered as a matter similar to the institution of insulin in controlling a diabetic patient. The stabilization of a manic episode may take 5 to 10 days, and any lithium salt may be used for this purpose. The most readily available is lithium carbonate in tablets or capsules of 250 or 300 mg each, equivalent to 6.75 and 8.0 mEq, respectively, of elemental lithium (Table 5-2). The range of daily dosage during this phase may vary considerably (1 to 3 gm in divided doses over 24 hours). This initially higher dosage is given until the manic symptoms have abated. The size of the dose is determined by several factors,

Table 5-2.   Lithium Salts and Their Equivalencies

	LiCl	$Li_2SO_4H_2O$	Li_2CO_3	$Li_3C_6H_5O_7H_2O$
Molecular weight	42.4	127.96	73.89	279.96
10 milliequivalents	0.424 gm	0.37 gm	0.37 gm	0.93 gm
1 gram	23.6 mEq	15.6 mEq	27.0 mEq	10.75 mEq
10 grains (0.65 gram)	15.4 mEq	10.4 mEq	17.5 mEq	7.0 mEq

such as the severity of the clinical condition, body weight, age, physical condition, and rate of renal clearance of lithium. The steady state between intake and elimination is reached in 5 to 6 days; thereafter the serum lithium concentration in blood samples drawn approximately 12 hours after the last intake of lithium should be within the range of 0.8 to 1.8 mEq/L. Plasma levels of lithium should be determined approximately every 3 or 4 days during the stabilization phase. In addition to such chemical surveillance, careful clinical observation to record the appearance of any manifestations of toxicity is mandatory. If symptoms of toxicity appear or if the plasma lithium level approaches 2 mEq/L, the dose of lithium must be reduced or the regimen stopped.

When a patient's disruptive behavior becomes a significant management problem, the manic attack also can be treated with a combination of lithium and a neuroleptic such as chlorpromazine or haloperidol. The neuroleptic usually controls the more violent manifestations of the mania more rapidly, but when the effect of lithium becomes apparent, the neuroleptic can be discontinued gradually.

c. **Maintenance phase**   After the manic episode remits, the initially high dosage of lithium should be lowered and plasma levels continued until a stable plasma level is established. When the clinical condition is fully under control and a maintenance dose of lithium has been established, the patient can be safely managed with continued ingestion at that level, regular checks of plasma lithium levels, and clinical surveillance. During maintenance treatment, the intake of lithium must equal the elimination. Since lithium is excreted almost exclusively through the kidneys, it is primarily the renal lithium clearance that determines the maintenance dosage. The renal lithium clearance is usually a fixed proportion — about one-fifth — of the creatinine clearance. Like the latter, it varies a great deal among individuals and also falls with advancing years. Accordingly, the optimum maintenance dosage varies a good deal from person to person. In general, the maintenance level of plasma lithium is between 0.6 and 1.2 mEq/L, although maintenance dosage must be adjusted to each individual case in accordance with symptomatology and occurrence of adverse effects. Because of the usefulness of lithium medications as prophylactic agents in manic-depressive disease, it may be desirable to continue this medication for many years. As far as has been ascertained, other psychotropic drugs may be given in addition to lithium in the treatment of either the manic or the depressive phase without producing problems of drug interaction or increasing toxicity.

2. Toxicology

a. **The acute effects of excessive dosage** The most common features associated with mild toxicity and slightly elevated plasma lithium levels (usually over 1 mEq/L) are anorexia, gastric discomfort, diarrhea, vomiting, thirst, polyuria, and hand tremor (see Table 5-3). These often coincide with serum lithium peaks, and the effects may be related more to the steepness of the rise of the lithium level than to the height of the peak. Often they disappear or diminish without reduction of dose. However, some may persist, such as tremor (unresponsive to antiparkinsonian medication) and polyuria, which may give rise to a diabetes insipidus-like syndrome that usually clears upon withdrawal of medication.

Toxic effects seen at blood levels above 1.5 mEq/L are more serious and may include muscle fasciculation and twitching, hyperactive deep tendon reflexes, ataxia, somnolence, confusion, dysarthria, and, rarely, epileptiform seizures. These effects are often associated with reversible electroencephalographic alterations. A more reliable index of toxicity may be the intracellular lithium level rather than the plasma level. There is no specific antidote for severe lithium intoxication. From the studies carried out to date, treatment should consist of general measures to correct the effects induced on water and electrolyte balance (see Table 5-4). It has been suggested that forced diuresis should aid significantly in the elimination of lithium.

b. **Chronic effects** These effects, which have only recently been described, may be of considerable interest. Side effects appearing with chronic ingestion of lithium include a diabetes-insipidus-like syndrome, elevation of blood sugar, thyroid disturbances, and elevated white blood cell counts.

Table 5-3. Known Manifestations of Lithium Toxicity

Gastrointestinal symptoms
  Anorexia
  Nausea
  Vomiting
  Diarrhea
  Thirst
  Dryness of the mouth
  Weight loss

Neuromuscular symptoms and signs
  General muscle weakness
  Ataxia
  Tremor
  Muscle hyperirritability
    Fasciculation (increased by tapping muscle)
    Twitching (especially of facial muscles)
    Clonic movements of whole limbs
  Choreoathetoid movements
  Hyperactive deep tendon reflexes

Central nervous system
  Anesthesia of skin
  Incontinence of urine and feces
  Slurred speech
  Blurring of vision
  Dizziness
  Vertigo
  Epileptiform seizures

Mental symptoms
  Mental retardation
  Somnolence
  Confusion
  Restlessness and disturbed behavior
  Stupor
  Coma

Cardiovascular system
  Pulse irregularities
  Fall in blood pressure
  ECG changes
  Peripheral circulatory failure
  Circulatory collapse

Miscellaneous
  Polyuria
  Glycosuria
  General fatigue
  Lethargy and tendency to sleep
  Dehydration

The occurrence of **goiter** in patients on lithium was first
observed in 1970. In a study of 330 patients on maintenance
therapy for periods of five months to two years, 12 developed
diffuse, nontender thyroid enlargements while remaining
clinically euthyroid. Abnormal iodine metabolism was revealed
in several patients, as indicated by increased tracer uptake and
thyroid iodine clearance. Goiters usually disappear when
lithium is discontinued or when thyroid hormone is administere
concurrently with lithium medication, and their appearance

Table 5-4. Management of Severe Lithium Poisoning[a]

Clinical procedures recommended
1. Discontinue lithium.
2. Blood lithium level, stat; then daily or every two days as required.
3. Serum sodium and potassium estimations, stat; follow as required.
4. ECG, stat; periodically thereafter.
5. Temperature and blood pressure, every four hours.
6. Infection prophylaxis (e.g., rotate patient).
7. Optional: spinal tap, EEG.
8. If question of infection exists, blood culture and viral studies of blood and CSF are indicated.

Treatment methods recommended
1. Replace water and electrolytes (sodium, potassium, calcium, magnesium) as needed. Total daily fluid intake should be at least 5 to 6 liters per day. Do not oversalinize, and avoid abrupt changes in electrolyte intake. Monitor, if changes are made.
2. Forced lithium diuresis via urea, 20 gm IV 2 to 5 times daily (urea contraindicated if severe renal impairment antedates toxicity), or mannitol, 50 to 100 gm IV as total daily dose.
3. Increase lithium clearance with aminophylline (which also suppresses tubular reabsorption and increases blood flow), dosage 0.5 gm by slow IV (may cause sharp but transitory hypotension).
4. Alkalinization of urine with sodium lactate administered intravenously has been recommended as an adjunct.
5. If poisoning is severe, the patient should be dialyzed (peritoneal dialysis or artificial kidney).

[a]Primarily via Renal Excretion: 4/5 of filtered lithium is reabsorbed in the proximal tubule (normal half-life of lithium is 24 hours)

does not necessitate the permanent discontinuation of lithium medication. Hyperthyroidism, with enlargement of the thyroid, has also been reported.

Several reports, some at variance with one another, have discussed the modification of **carbohydrate metabolism** by lithium ingestion. Recent studies indicate that a reversible increase in blood glucose can result after lithium administration to patients in different diagnostic categories that will reach statistical significance at the 60 minute interval of the glucose tolerance test. The implications from these studies are that decreased glucose tolerance accompanying lithium administration is due to a physiologic effect of lithium ion and is not related to either psychiatric diagnosis or change in clinical state or duration of treatment with the drug.

A "consistent and striking" **elevation in white blood cell count** accompanying lithium administration was first reported in 1966. There have been three subsequent reports of similar findings. While the elevations in white blood cell count appear to be due to drug effect, they are not dose-related and are not dependent on the concentration of lithium found in the peripheral blood.

c. **Neurotoxicity** As early as 1950 sporadic reports of lithium-induced delirium began to appear. In 1970, in a series of controlled studies on lithium effects, it was found that most of the schizoaffective patients treated with lithium carbonate showed an overall worsening of their clinical status. A significant feature of this group was the appearance of symptoms of organicity, such as disorientation, confusion, and reduced comprehension. Along with these changes there was an increase in the severity of the basic psychopathology; thought disturbance often became more pronounced, as did psychomotor excitation, delusional thought, and hallucinations. These apparent drug effects occurred at blood levels not usually associated with severe toxic phenomena. In fact these central effects occurred in these cases without the usual lithium effects or toxic manifestations. The most consistent laboratory abnormalities involved changes in EEGs, including alterations in the alpha activity, diffuse slowing, accentuation of previous focal abnormalities, and the appearance of previously absent focal changes. The occurrence of neurotoxicity corresponds, therefore, to the presence and severity of EEG changes (see Figures 5-1 and 5-2). This drug-induced neurotoxicity will clear on cessation of lithium administration; plasma lithium level falls first, followed by changes in EEG and a related improvement in the clinical state.

It is also important to consider the possible **teratogenic effects of lithium if a pregnancy intervenes** in a patient being maintained on this medication. There is no ready way to calculate the true incidence of lithium-induced teratology from the available literature since no systematic randomized sample or even representative sample of births is available for analysis. While a large number of perfectly normal children have been born to mothers on lithium medication, some abnormalities have also been reported. Bearing in mind the possibility of potential risk, it might be wisest to suggest that women treated with lithium should not be routinely maintained on medication through a pregnancy. Furthermore, it appears even more important that *breast feeding* by lithium-treated women should *not* be permitted because lithium appears in the breast milk in concentrations approaching those in the mother's serum. Sodium depletion (from salt-restricted diets or diuretics) during pregnancy can also enhance lithium toxicity.

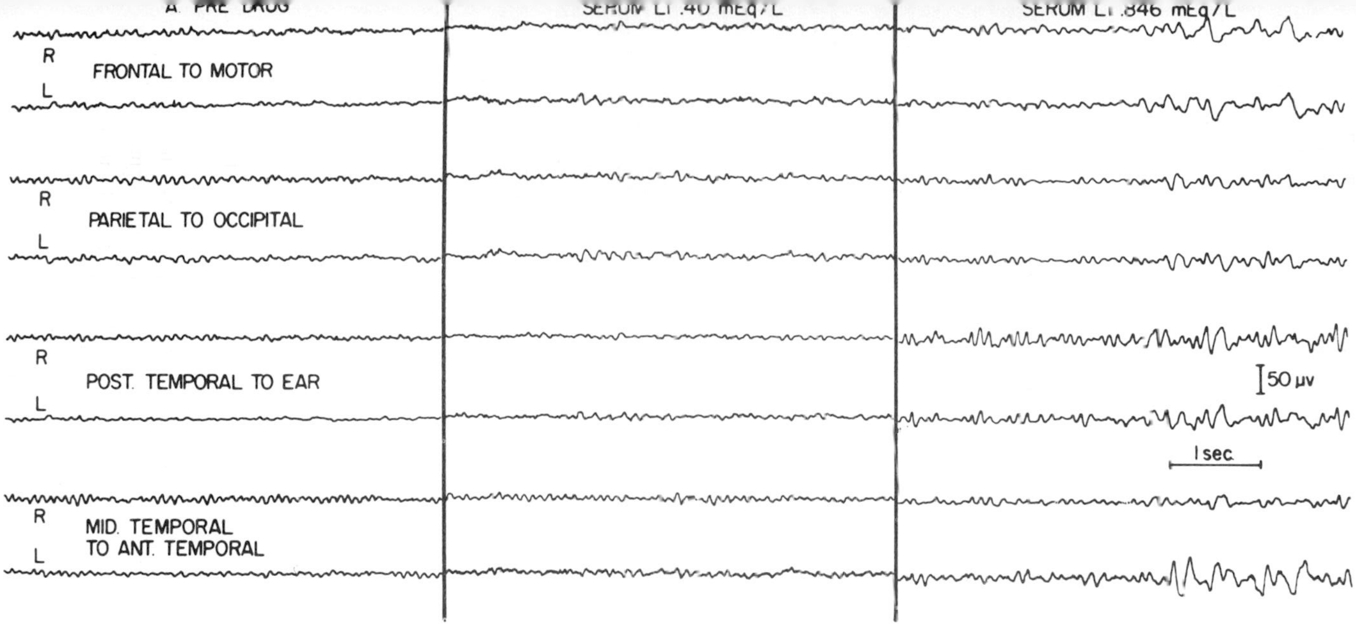

Figure 5-1. A. Predrug EEG (minimal asymmetry). B. EEG 2 hours after oral lithium, serum level 0.40 mEq/L (increased a pha amplitude, increased asymmetry). C. EEG during chronic lithium administration, serum level 0.846 mEq/L (moderate abnormalities — diffuse delta activity, increased alpha amplitude, and bursts). (From *J. Nerv. Ment. Dis.* 151:273, 1970.)

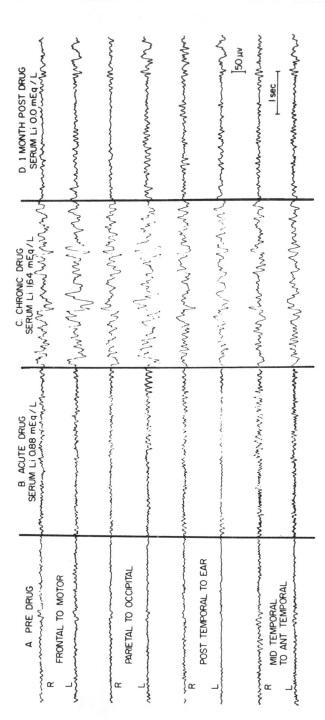

Figure 5-2. A. Predrug EEG (minimal asymmetry). B. EEG 2 hours after lithium ingestion, serum lithium 0.880 mEq/L (increased alpha amplitude, increased asymmetry). C. EEG during chronic lithium administration, serum lithium at 1.64 mEq/L (marked abnormalities — diffuse delta activity, increased asymmetry). D. EEG one month after lithium discontinued, serum level 0.00 mEq/L (persistence of left focal abnormality). (From *J. Nerv. Ment. Dis.* 151:273, 1970.)

6

Electroconvulsive Therapy

Carl Salzman

Electroconvulsive therapy (ECT) is an empirically derived treatment procedure developed in the 1930s. Since its introduction, this procedure has been the object of exaggerated praise as well as extreme vilification. In fact, ECT is neither a panacea nor a form of medieval torture. Its judicious administration is an important and sometimes life-saving psychiatric treatment that may offer substantial symptomatic relief, particularly for the severely ill. It is best employed as part of a general treatment program with other forms of therapy. For example, it may help a seriously disorganized patient to regain behavioral control prior to psychotropic medication's taking effect. In many cases, mute, severely retarded, or severely agitated patients who cannot or do not communicate verbally are able to enter into effective psychotherapy after some ECT. However, the physician never should use ECT out of frustration, as a punishment, or as retaliation against a difficult patient. And it should not be used as a way of controlling those expressions of anger that may be appropriate, therapeutic, and healthy. It should also be remembered that ECT does not ameliorate interpersonal events or psychological conflicts that may have contributed to or precipitated a patient's problems.

I. Indications

A. Affective illness

1. **Depression** Serious depression constitutes the outstanding indication for ECT. Recurrent unipolar depression, the depression of bipolar affective illness, involutional depression, postpartum depression, and severe depression of later life all respond well. Table 6-1 lists some of the symptoms of depressions that predict a good response to ECT. Agitated as well as retarded depressions respond to ECT, and suicidal preoccupation is often dramatically relieved. In considering this subject, it is well to remember that the term *depression* is ubiquitous; all patients who claim to be depressed may not be suffering from serious affective illness (see Chapter 3). Mild daily fluctuations in mood, for example, are not an indication for ECT.

Table 6-1. Symptoms that Predict a Good Response to ECT

Low self-esteem, feelings of worthlessness
A sense of helplessness and hopelessness
Anorexia
Weight loss
Constipation
Decreased sexual urges and functioning
Early morning awakening
Thoughts or acts of self-destruction

2. **Mania** ECT is useful in controlling or modifying hyperexcited and agitated behavior. Thus, it may often be helpful early in the treatment of mania before lithium carbonate becomes effective (see Chapter 5). However, there are no data to suggest that this regimen should be preferred to the use of neuroleptics such as chlorpromazine or haloperidol. Unless there is some contraindication to the use of lithium, the use of ECT in mania should be restricted to behavioral control problems that have not been successfully treated with psychotropic medication.

B. **Schizophrenia** There is general agreement in contemporary psychiat that catatonic stupors and catatonic excitements respond well to EC Considerable difference of opinion exists, however, regarding the efficacy of ECT for the general treatment of schizophrenic syndrom For example, ECT tends to have little effect on chronic schizophreni symptomatology. Recent research evidence suggests that phenothia-zines are the treatment of choice for most noncatatonic schizophren symptoms. ECT should be considered as an adjunct and limited to behavioral control.

C. **Miscellaneous clinical conditions for which ECT is useful** A variety of medical as well as psychiatric signs and symptoms are altered by ECT. Among these are akinesias that sometimes accompany pellagra psychotic symptoms that may be part of general paresis, thalamic pa and the severe pain of trigeminal neuralgia. In addition, anorexia nervosa has been relieved by ECT, but followup psychotherapy is a necessary part of the treatment program.

D. **Poor clinical indications for ECT** In general, ECT may offer some relief for severe depressive or agitated symptoms that accompany an psychiatric illness. There is little evidence, however, that ECT is use-ful in treating the primary symptoms of characterologic or psycho-neurotic illness. Table 6-2 lists the diagnostic categories that usually do not respond well to ECT.

II. **Contraindications and Risks** Modern, modified ECT is a safe procedur and can be administered to a wide variety of patients. There are always

Table 6-2. Poor Responders to ECT

Hysterical symptoms
Anxiety reactions
Obsessive-compulsive syndromes
Borderline character
Pseudoneurotic schizophrenia
Addictions
Sexual deviations, perversions
Sociopathic personality disorders

however, patients for whom such a procedure is contraindicated due to various physical factors. For example, increased **intracranial pressure** or any space-occupying lesion represents an absolute contraindication since ECT transiently elevates cerebrospinal fluid pressure with resulting tentorial herniation and death. Recent **myocardial infarction** represents another contraindication because arrythmias may possibly occur during the seizure. Once the electrocardiogram and cardiac enzymes have stabilized following a myocardial infarction, ECT may be used but with caution.

General anesthesia risks must also be kept in mind when using ECT. Thus, barbiturate allergy or personal or family history of acute intermittent porphyria precludes the use of barbiturate anesthesia. Intravenous diazepam may be substituted. Succinylcholine, used as a pretreatment muscle-relaxing agent to modify ECT, is hydrolyzed by serum pseudocholinesterase. Low or ineffective pseudocholinesterase from liver disease, malnutrition, congenital deficiency, or previous exposure to anticholinesterase agents (such as the organophosphorus inhibitor echothiophate, which is used to control glaucoma) predisposes the patient to prolonged apnea because of the absence or relative decrease of this enzyme. Healed vertebral fractures or vertebral osteoporosis are not an absolute contraindication to ECT, but particular care must be taken to insure adequate muscle relaxation so that the seizure will not exacerbate spinal pathology.

III. **Technique of Administration**   In addition to a careful diagnostic evaluation of psychiatric disorder, each patient should be medically cleared prior to administration of ECT. A complete physical examination with focus on cardiovascular and neurologic functioning is the first stage of this evaluation. Evidence of recent myocardial infarction or the presence of an arrhythmia should be noted and considered when determining whether or not a patient can undergo the ECT. Cardiovascular functioning must also be assessed by a pretreatment electrocardiogram. Evidence of neurologic dysfunction obtained by physical examination may be further assessed with an electroencephalogram, and particular attention should be paid to recent changes in neurologic status. Evidence of old spinal fractures (possibly from previous unmodified ECT) and degree of spinal osteoporosis may be assessed via x-ray of the dorsal thoracic and lumbar vertebrae. Degrees of cardiac, neurologic, or vertebral pathology that would contraindicate ECT are discussed in Section II.

Consistent with today's standards of psychiatric practice, all patients, prior to the first treatment, should be asked to sign a consent form that fully explains the nature and risks of ECT. When the patient is too sick to comprehend the nature of the consent form, a family member or guardian should sign the form.

A. **Preparation of the patient** In many institutions, ECT is administered in the early morning, and in such cases it is best to have the patient take nothing by mouth after the preceding midnight. If ECT is to be administered in the afternoon, an early, light breakfast may be taken. Prior to the treatment, the patient is given atropine (0.6 to 1.0 mg) to block the vagal stimulating effects of ECT as well as to decrease secretions. If atropine is given subcutaneously, it should be given about one hour prior to treatment, or, if administered intramuscularly, within 15 minutes of the ECT. In some institutions, atropine is given intravenously along with the anesthetic. Anxious or hyperactive patients may be helped by pretreatment administration of an antianxiety agent such as chlordiazepoxide (10 mg IM) or diazepam (5 mg IM) within an hour of the treatment.

Patients with loose teeth should have them extracted prior to an ECT series, since they may break and be aspirated during the seizure. Dentures must be removed before each treatment. Additionally, patients who are receiving ECT often are also taking antipsychotic or antidepressant medication. There is some evidence that these drugs may augment the hypotensive effect of general anesthesia. Therefore the dose prior to the treatment should be eliminated.

B. **General anesthesia** Prior to the induction of an ECT seizure, the patient is anesthetized with a short-acting barbiturate. In most cases, sodium methohexital (Brevital), 30 to 100 mg, given intravenously is preferred to sodium thiopental (Pentothal) because of the former's shorter duration of action (2 to 3 minutes). It also has been reported to produce less cardiac arrythmias and hypotension than sodium thiopental. When barbiturate anesthesia is contraindicated, diazepam (5 mg IV) may be substituted. It should not be given in the same syringe with atropine and succinylcholine because their aqueous diluents may cause the diazepam to precipitate out in the syringe. Anesthesia should be administered only by qualified, trained personnel. Emergency medications that should be available are listed in Table 6-3.

Table 6-3. Emergency Drugs for ECT

Aminophylline	550 mg
Calcium chloride	1000 mg
Chlorpromazine	25 mg/ml
Dexamethasone	4 mg/ml
Diazepam	5 mg/ml
Digoxin	0.5 mg/ml
Diphenhydramine (Benadryl)	50 mg/ml
Diphenylhydantoin (Dilantin)	250 mg/ml
Epinephrine	1:1000
Furosemide (Lasix)	10 mg/ml
Hydrocortisone	100 mg
Isoproterenol (Isuprel)	5 mg/ml
Levarterenol (Levophed)	0.2 %
Lidocaine	2 %
Naloxone (Narcan)	0.4 mg/ml
Neosynephrine	10 mg/ml
Phentolamine (Regitine)	5 mg (ampuls) (refrigerate)
Potassium chloride	40 mEq
Procaine amide	100 mg/ml (refrigerate)
Secobarbital	50 mg/ml
Sodium bicarbonate	44.6 mEq

C. **Modification of ECT: Muscle relaxation** The clinical efficacy of ECT is dependent only on central nervous system seizure stimulation and not on the production of peripheral seizure movements. For this reason, it is now standard procedure to modify the electrically induced seizure with the use of a neuromuscular depolarizing agent, succinylcholine (Anectine, Sucostrin). If facilities for EEG monitoring of the seizure are available, the peripheral seizure may be completely blocked with high doses of this drug (110 mg or more). More typically, one of two techniques is employed. An empirically determined dose of succinylcholine is chosen (30 to 80 mg) that will block the seizures so that only minimal clonic movements of the fingers and toes will be apparent. Alternatively, the circulation to one forearm is completely blocked by use of a tourniquet (blood pressure cuff inflated above mean arterial pressure). A dose of succinylcholine large enough to produce total blockade is then used, and seizure activity is observed only in the cuffed extremity.

D. **Technique of ECT administration** Safe, effective ECT requires adequate preoxygenation with 95 to 100% oxygen prior to the treatment. Adequate muscle relaxation is gauged by the presence of muscle fasciculations that begin at the head and move caudally. Only when the patient is fully relaxed may the treatment be given. Moistened soft electrodes are held firmly in place (see Figure 6-1), and the electric current is applied *in strict accordance with the directions for the particular machine being used.* For bilateral treatment, the electrodes are placed just above the bisection of a line that connects the outer corner of the eye and the beginning of the pinna

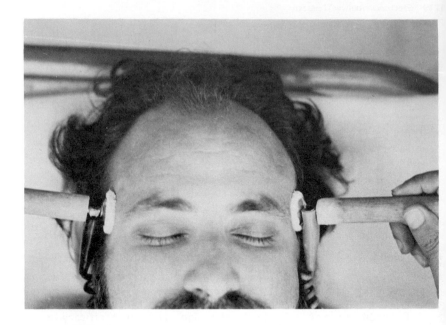

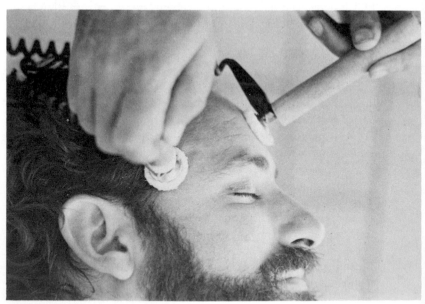

Figure 6-1. Placement of electrodes for bilateral (top photo) and unilateral (non-dominant lobe) ECT treatments.

of the ear. For unilateral treatment, the temporal electrode is placed in a similar position on the nondominant side (for about 95 percent of patients this will be on the right). The second electrode is held in the mid-forehead. To avoid superficial skin burns, the electrodes must be held firmly in place and must be moist; a dilute solution of sodium bicarbonate or saline may be used. A soft bite-block is inserted in the patient's mouth just prior to the induction of the seizure, and the jaw is held shut. Dentures must be removed, and loose teeth that were not removed prior to the treatment must be protected with gauze pads.

Immediately after electrical stimulation, a tonic seizure phase of 5 to 15 seconds ensues. The peripheral clonic movements then begin and last from 10 to 60 seconds. The first seizure of an ECT series is often the longest. Oxygen is provided to the patient during the clonic phase and then during the recovery period immediately following the induced seizure. The patient has no awareness of the seizure nor is any pain experienced. Succinylcholine is hydrolyzed within 1 to 3 minutes, and the sodium methohexital anesthetic is redistributed from the CNS in 2 to 4 minutes. Some patients awaken almost immediately after a treatment; older patients, with slower circulation times, may take a minute or two longer. Upon awakening there is a period of postictal confusion that is variable in length but usually lasts for about 15 minutes. During this recovery period careful supervision of the patient is mandatory, and monitoring of vital signs, maintenance of adequate respiration, and quiet reassurance are part of the care. Occasionally a patient will become very confused and agitated during this period; chlordiazepoxide (10 mg IM) or diazepam (5 mg IM) is helpful. There tends to be less postictal confusion and agitation following unilateral treatment to the nondominant hemisphere.

E. **Number of treatments** There is no absolute method for determining the number of treatments that should be used for an ECT series. As a general rule, treatments are given three days a week on alternate days at the beginning of a series and tapered to twice and then once a week near the conclusion of the series. Depressive reactions usually respond to 6 to 12 treatments. Early signs of response are improvement in sleep and in personal hygiene. Often, a patient will show signs of elation or euphoria as the treatment series progresses. It is best to suspend treatments at this juncture and continue if the depression returns.

Hyperexcitable states (catatonic excitement, mania, assaultiveness), as well as catatonic stupors, usually respond to 8 to 16 treatments, although a few more are occasionally needed. Behavior may then be brought under control, and pharmacotherapy and psychotherapy may be usefully employed. It is *sometimes* necessary to give more than one treatment on the same day to bring about behavioral contro in a seriously disordered, assaultive patient. The treatments may be given successively in such cases, allowing at least a one minute re-fractory period to pass between the end of the first clonic seizure movements and the induction of the second seizure.

Certain patients, particularly those with late life depressions, may reexperience depression after several weeks or months, even after a successful course of ECT. In these cases, it may be useful to continu with intermittent (maintenance) ECT, using one treatment every fou to six weeks.

A few authors recommend giving very large numbers of ECT treat ments (50 or more) to produce a regression in behavior (incontinence dementia, inability to care for self). Recovery from this state is said to be a successful treatment for very serious illness, particularly schizophrenia. Regressive ECT must be considered experimental at the present time.

F. **Outpatient ECT** ECT is frequently administered to nonhospitalized patients. In addition to the usual preparation of a patient, the close supervision of a responsible person, often a family member or friend, must be enlisted. This person assumes care for the outpatient ECT recipient in the following matters:

1. Ensuring nothing is taken by mouth for 12 hours before treatmen
2. Accompanying the patient from the treatment.
3. Close supervision of the patient for at least four hours following the treatment.

IV. **Effects of ECT**

A. **Side effects of ECT**

1. Prior to the use of muscle relaxants, the most frequent complicati of ECT was the development of **compression fractures,** frequently multiple, of the dorsal mid-thoracic spine between T4 and T8. This side effect has disappeared with the introduction of succinyl-choline modification.

2. **Memory loss** and confusion are now the two most common side effects of ECT. The memory loss is characterized by short-term decrease in ability to acquire new information (anterograde amnesia) as well as some amnesia for recent events (retrograde amnesia). Clinically, patients often complain of an inability to

Table 6-4. Physical Changes Resulting from ECT

Neurologic
Immediate loss of consciousness
Loss of superficial and deep tendon reflexes
Flattening of EEG activity followed by slow waves with a gradual return to normal; alpha waves reappear when consciousness is regained; in general, an approximately normal state is resumed within 5 to 30 minutes after the last seizure, with the frontal regions returning to their normal rhythm last.
Postictal automatisms and involuntary movements
No discernible correlation between clinical improvement, degree of mental confusion, and changes in brain metabolism or blood flow

Neuropathologic
Increase in blood-brain barrier permeability and capillary leakage in the CNS
Increases in spinal fluid nucleic acids, nucleases, and deaminases
Increased extracellular brain fluid, decreased electrolyte concentration, and cerebral edema with distention of perivascular space (all transitory)
No *proved* cell destruction
Cerebral oxygen drops moderately, and cerebral blood flow decreases very markedly immediately after ECT
Decrease in total brain norepinephrine but with an increase in neuronal discharge onto receptor sites; there is also an increased synthesis of norepinephrine and thus (presumably) increased utilization
Increased dopamine and serotonin turnover

Cardiovascular
Brief asystole with application of current
Bradycardia during the tonic phase, tachycardia in the clonic phase, and arrhythmias of several minutes' duration in the postconvulsive period; tachycardia runs 120 to 150/minute.
Blood pressure briefly decreases during the early tonic phase and then rises markedly (about 50 mg Hg) above the control level during the late tonic and throughout the clonic phase
Atropine *increases* the blood pressure rise
Blood pressure effects are independent of the peripheral convulsion and are centrally stimulated

Endocrine and autonomic nervous system
75% increase in plasma epinephrine levels immediately after the seizure, which subside in about 10 minutes; plasma norepinephrine concentration rises about 40%, with a slower decline to normal
With barbiturate and succinylcholine premedication, norepinephrine does not rise; it is concluded that the epinephrine rise is primarily due to stimulation of brain autonomic centers rather than secondarily due to the motor, cardiovascular, or anoxic components of unmodified ECT
Uniform rise in plasma 17-hydroxycorticosteroid levels and eosinopenia
Water retention
Menstrual cessation or irregularities
Transitory increases in plasma glucose, plasma protein, serum sodium, potassium, chloride, calcium and phosphorus, serum cholesterol and free fatty acids, BUN, NPN, blood carbon dioxide, serum uric acid, and lymphocytes and neutrophils

Sleep and REM time
REM sleep decreased but not completely absent
Decrease in the number of eye movements in REM sleep; this presumably indicates a change by ECT in the pontine reticular system

remember proper names. Memory loss usually does not appear until the fourth treatment and is proportional to the number of treatments received. Most lost memory returns within three to six weeks; the more treatments received, the longer it takes for memory to return.

Confusion from ECT appears as an acute organic syndrome with disorientation and impairment of social functioning. Like memory functioning, confusion increases with the number of treatments received. Elderly patients tend to become more confused following ECT than do younger patients.

In 1952 unilateral treatment to the nondominant hemisphere was begun in an effort to decrease the memory loss and confusion following ECT. Unilateral treatment is not quite as rapid as bilateral ECT. It does, however, decrease the amount of memory loss and confusion. More unilateral treatments may be required than bilateral to achieve the same clinical endpoint.

B. **Physical changes resulting from ECT**   A number of alterations in bodily functions occur during and after ECT. Most are only temporary, with return to normal occurring in minutes or hours after treatment. Table 6-4 lists some of these changes.

References

Fink, M. (Ed.)   Convulsive therapy. *Semin. Psychiatry* 4 (1): 1972.

Greenblatt, M., Grosser, G. H., and Wechsler, H.   Differential response of hospitalized depressed patients to somatic therapy. *Am. J. Psychiatry* 116:935—943, 1964.

Hoch, P. H., and Pennes, H. H.   Electric Convulsive Treatment and Its Modifications. In L. Bellak (Ed.) *Schizophrenia: A Review of the Syndrome.* New York: Logos, 1958. Pp. 423—455.

Holmberg, G.   Biological aspects of electroconvulsive therapy. *Int. Rev. Neurobiol.* 5:389—412, 1963.

Kalinowsky, L. B., and Hoch, P. H.   *Somatic Treatment in Psychiatry.* New York: Grune & Stratton, 1961.

Mendels, J.   Electroconvulsive therapy and depression. *Br. J. Psychiatry* 111:675—681, 1965.

Strain, J. J., Brunschwig, L., Duffy, J. P., Agle, D. P., Rosenbaum, A. L., and Bidder, T. G.   Comparison of therapeutic effects and memory changes with bilateral and unilateral ECT. *Am. J. Psychiatry* 125:50—60, 1968.

7

Management of Violent Patients

Joseph P. Tupin

I. **General** A person is violent when acting in a strong, rough, or harmful way toward something or someone. In this chapter consideration will be limited to harmful physical action between individuals, serious threats of such action, or recurrent fantasies of violence. This discussion will not deal with group violence such as wars, mobs, or sports activities whether legitimate or illegitimate. While this definition excludes much that is perceived as violent, it does draw the focus squarely to the individual and his immediate environment. Furthermore, physicians do not treat mobs or armies, but rather individuals and their families.

The President's Commission on the Causes and Prevention of Violence in 1969 drew a demographic portrait of the criminally violent individual: age under 25, social and economic deprivation, inner city residence, minority status, and male sex. Although it is statistically accurate, this profile hardly provides insight about a particular violent individual, but it does provide some insights regarding public policy, community mental health programs, and the effects of deprivation and discrimination.

II. **Clinical Assessment** Violent individuals may be self-referred or brought for examination and treatment by family, police, or others. The presenting complaint may be that the person fears acting in a violent way, plans to act in a violent way, is currently acting in a violent way, or has a history of violent actions. Each of these four circumstances suggests a different plan for evaluation and management.

A. **Diagnostic categories** There is no classification system or diagnostic label that is clinically useful in predicting violence, but a useful categorization is derived from Megargee's work (*Psychol. Monogr.* 80:1, 1966). He describes two types of individuals that commit violent acts, the *overcontrolled* and the *undercontrolled*. Studies of these two descriptive types have found that they differ on measures of personality traits and psychopathology. The overcontrolled individual tolerates a chronically frustrating situation, perhaps a destructive family relationship, quietly while resentment and rage grow. He is ostensibly cooperative and conforming, and is thought of by friends and neighbors as "good," only to suddenly erupt with bizarre and vicious violence, often directed toward those who have frustrated him and occasionally to strangers. By contrast, the under-controlled person is frequently violent, often from an early age, and is easily provoked by friends, family, or strangers. Thought of as having "a chip on his shoulder" or "a short fuse," he may be avoided by others, although he himself may seek confrontation.

In numerous clinical studies no single psychiatric diagnostic category seems to be invariably associated with violent behavior. Each diagnostic type suggests a different treatment approach. Paranoi states, psychosis, schizophrenia, and mania rarely are found in more than 20 percent of murderers. Personality disorder diagnoses are most common, but even so, numerous subtypes have been associated with violence, including sociopathic, antisocial, passive-dependent, explosive, and inadequate types. Serious or subtle brain injury with or without manifest seizures is also associated with violence. Also, depression, passivity, and homosexual panic have been associated with violence.

1. The suicidally **depressed** individual is often so pessimistic that he believes he must spare his family the agony of the future, so suicide becomes murder and suicide. Less extreme is the depressed individual who is agitated and irritable; this person may react under stress by becoming combative.
2. Occasionally, the **passive** individual or **mentally retarded** individual behaves violently when taunted excessively or when "going along with the gang" to gain acceptance.
3. Individuals who fear their **homosexual** tendencies may become panicked when such feelings emerge from the unconscious. Often this occurs with a general breakdown of psychological defenses, and violence may ensue. *Pseudohomosexual panic* is a term used to describe violence that erupts in an effort to reestablish self-esteem and masculinity in reaction to emerging dependency wishes that are symbolically expressed as homosexual fantasies (*Arch. Gen. Psychiatry* 27:255, 1972).

B. **Psychiatric examination** The psychiatric clinical assessment should explore fantasies, plans, explicit behavior, precipitating stimuli, frequency, nature and effectiveness of internal and external controls, intensity of behavior, guilt, age of onset, object of violence, and any association with particular conditions, such as drug or alcohol intake. Noting whether the behavior is ego-syntonic or ego-dystonic will be valuable in assessing motivation for treatment. The utility and re-liability of psychological tests have been reviewed by Megargee (*Curr. Top. Clin. Community Psychol.* 2:97, 1970).

1. The **Minnesota Multiphasic Personality Inventory (MMPI)** has received the most attention of those psychological tests found to be useful for assessing personality characteristics of violent individuals. It has been suggested recently that a 4-3 response pattern (peaks on the psychopathic deviation [Pd] and hysteria [Hy] scales on the nine-scale MMPI profile) is particularly characteristic of violent individuals (*J. Consult. Clin. Psychol.* 36:186, 1971). Other special scales have been developed that may, in the future, prove of clinical value (Foulds, G. A., *Manual of the Hostility and Direction of Hostility Questionnaire,* London: University of London Press, 1967; *J. Abnorm. Psychol.* 72:519, 1967).

2. Psychological tests that assess organicity may be the most effective way of determining subtle brain dysfunction. The Bender-Gestalt, *Wechsler-Bellevue Adult Intelligence Scale,* and the *Porteus Maze Test* are simple, widely used, reliable tests for screening for **subtle organic brain damage.**

3. **Projective tests**, particularly the more complex Rorschach, the Holtzman, and the *Thematic Apperception Test* (TAT), are useful in producing information about underlying aggressiveness, the quality of controls, and the capacity to correctly assess reality, all of which are important concerns in evaluating the risk of violent behavior. They are, however, difficult to standardize and poorly predict specific behavior. Other psychological tests await further study to determine their usefulness in assessing violence potential.

C. **Neurologic examination and history** are likewise important. There are well-known neurologic lesions that can promote violent behavior. Most often these lesions are located in the temporal or frontal lobes, particularly involving the limbic system in the area of the amygdala and hippocampus. A history of minimal brain damage or temporal lobe epilepsy may relate to violent behavior.

It seems unlikely, based on current evidence, that violence is a direct ictal phenomenon; rather, it may occur during an aura or in the postictal confusional state. Mark and others have described a behavior pattern characterized by periodic violence that they call the *episodic dyscontrol syndrome* (*Violence and the Brain,* New York: Harper & Row, 1970). Subcortical dysrhythmias or epileptogenic discharges have been noted in some cases. In other such individuals, past experience and psychological disorders seem prominent. The syndrome is characterized by the following:

1. A history of physical assault, especially wife-beating and child-beating.

2. The symptom of pathologic intoxication — that is, drinking even a small amount of alcohol triggers acts of senseless brutality.
3. Impulsive sexual behavior, at times including sexual assaults.
4. A history (in those who drive cars) of many traffic violations and serious automobile accidents. Violent tendencies may be expressed through the use of the automobile and through self-mutilation.

The neurologic evaluation should include careful neurologic and physical examinations, with attention to soft signs and an EEG with sleep, photic, and hyperventilation activation. Nasopharyngeal leads should be routinely used to identify anterior and medial temporal lobe abnormalities. A brain scan, echoencephalogram, arterio-encephalogram, or pneumoencephalogram is useful in verifying and localizing the lesions. Some studies have noted that the majority of the EEG abnormalities tend to be nonspecific and nonepileptiform. Minimal brain damage may persist into adulthood and then is more obscure than in the child, but mood lability, aggressiveness, difficulty with numbers or reading, and impulsiveness may persist. A history of childhood hyperactivity is sometimes noted (see Chapter 9).

III. **Other Elements in Evaluation** Since violence often results from the interaction of various factors, evaluation may involve considerable time, numerous tests, and specialists from several disciplines. Consideration usually must be given to each broad category mentioned in Table 7-1. Clearly there are exceptions to this statement both because of expedience and because occasionally, selected factors (e.g., manic psychosis) are preeminent.

Animal research and clinical studies have demonstrated a multiplicity of factors that relate to violent activity.[*] There is no reason to believe that these factors act independently to promote violence; rather, they more often act in concert in varying patterns. An evaluation ordinarily considers characteristics of the individual and of the victim, their inter-action, and the social setting.

A. **Childhood history** deserves special attention because of the apparent importance of family structure and dynamics and child-rearing practice in the production of violence. Impulsive, sociopathic behavior has been found in children from disorganized families and in families where there is an absent father, minimal expression of warmth, and rejection of the patient. These characteristics in themselves are not unique to the production of violence, but they are common in

---

[*]*Violence and the Struggle for Existence.* David N. Daniels, Marshall F. Gilula, and Frank M. Ochberg (Eds.). Boston: Little, Brown, 1970. P. 451.

Table 7-1. General Factors (with Examples) Related to Violence

Sociocultural
   Family stability
   Family closeness
   Social frustration (e.g., poverty, lack of jobs)
Selected legitimation of violence
   Romanticized violence (e.g., movies, TV)
   Models of violence
   Cultural model of manhood
Psychological
   Paranoia
   Impulsiveness
   Self-esteem
   Depression
Biologic
   Minimal brain damage
   Genetic defect (e.g., XYY)
   Hormone imbalance (e.g., altered testosterone level)
Inanimate
   Alcohol
   Availability of guns
   Drugs (e.g., amphetamines)

families of individuals with poor impulse control. Early violent behavior in one or both parents and toward the child may be an important model for later adult behavior. Physically abused children often become violent adults.

B. Another important consideration is the **sociocultural characteristics** of the patient. There may be sanctions for violent action from family, gangs, social groups, neighbors, or cultural ideals. What may be considered psychopathology in one setting may be acceptable behavior in another. "Defending one's honor" in one form or another is often associated with a concept of manliness and may lead to violence in some cultures. In this sense the violent act is customary, follows certain cultural rules, and does not necessarily arise from intrapsychic conflict; thus, strictly speaking, it is not psychopathology but culturally determined "deviant" behavior. Street gangs are another example. In cross-cultural studies, groups that emphasize child-rearing patterns that stress competitiveness, aggression, success orientation, and independence have been noted to have a high rate of violent crimes. These characteristics are widely valued in America. Social and educational discrimination and deprivation produce chronic frustration, which leads to violence.

C. **Interpersonal factors** are common precipitants of violent outbursts. Toch has described such processes and has emphasized the self-esteem enhancing and preserving aspects (*Violent Man: An Inquiry into the Psychology of Violence,* Chicago: Aldine, 1967). Violent individuals are often men described as *hypermasculine,* a term connoting a defensive exaggeration of masculine traits, fighting included, that masks underlying doubts about manhood. This circumstance leads to many "barroom brawls." Similar circumstances may be the basis for some marital fights. The violent individual may be provoked to action as much by the victim's needs as by the violent person's tendencies. Such provocation may be sudden and explicit — "You're too cowardly to shoot!" — or subtle and chronic. The latter pattern is noted in families in which an adolescent may be slowly repressed, abused, and rejected; the outcome may be a violent explosion.

D. **Genetic abnormalities,** specifically the XYY defect and altered testosterone levels, have been suggested as contributors to violent behavior. These conditions await further exploration and do not seem at the present time to merit inclusion in a routine clinical evaluation.

E. **Use of alcohol and amphetamines** has been implicated as facilitating violent behavior. Pathologic intoxication is a condition in which consumption of small amounts of alcohol leads to violence. In about 60 percent of the cases, victims and perpetrators of homicide are intoxicated with alcohol.

IV. **Management**

A. **Prevention** This approach is perhaps the most valuable from a social point of view; here, however, the individual practitioner has little expertise or opportunity to be effective. Perhaps in the future, identification and alteration of the family types that promote violence may be within reach of the practitioner, but it seems unlikely that most individual health professionals will be able to change poverty or discrimination. Perhaps through mass public education, strong programs in marital counseling, and other community health activities, they might influence basic family structure and social values. Before such programs of identification and intervention are mounted, a more precise description of those sociocultural conditions that allegedly contribute to violence is imperative. The physician must begin to act in the broader social setting to alter those social conditions that adversely affect health. There are a number of conditions that promote violence and hence should be the targets of prevention.

1. As mentioned above, **alcohol and drug abuse** play a role in the production of some violence. Consequently, efforts to reduce these problems may indirectly reduce violence. Particular attention should be given to the individual who after only a few drinks

"goes mad." This phenomenon of pathologic intoxication clearly warrants the attention of the mental health worker.

2. Community intervention programs aimed at diminishing **poverty** and **discrimination,** reducing **romanticization of violence** in movies and television, and limiting access to **handguns** and other weapons deserve careful review and support.

3. Factors such as **genetic defects, birth injury,** and **poor prenatal care** (e.g., untreated eclampsia), thought to contribute to brain dysfunction, which in turn may play a role in the development of violence, constitute another group of factors suitable for psychiatric-medical prevention programs.

B. **Early identification and intervention** This approach is particularly compatible with community mental health programs.

1. Further studies on the relationship between **childhood hyperkinesis** or **minimal brain damage** and adult violence may suggest some appropriate means of early intervention.

2. **Fire-setting, cruelty to animals,** and **enuresis,** a triad of childhood symptoms that have been linked to adult violence, could provide the basis for early identification and intervention programs.

3. Adults who were physically abused as children have an increased likelihood of behaving violently; consequently, **child abuse** victims are a high risk group suitable for early intervention.

4. New diagnostic techniques, including amniocentesis and karyotyping, may eventually provide the mechanism for another approach to early case identification.

5. Another avenue of early identification would be to utilize the **undercontrolled vs. overcontrolled typology** (see Section II.A). Since in undercontrolled individuals violent behavior is repetitive and often begins in childhood, early recognition and intervention is possible. Previous violent behavior appears to be the most accurate predictor of the risk of future violence. Early detection through school systems, public education, and social agencies may be particularly effective in identifying these undercontrolled high-risk youths.

   Little is yet known of the overcontrolled individual who explodes unexpectedly. By definition, he may appear to be one of the most law-abiding, compliant, and gentle of people. The overtly mild-mannered individual with brittle controls and repressed hostility should be taken seriously when he reports fantasies or plans of violence. Megargee suggests that these individuals are responsible for a disproportionate number of extremely violent assaults, supposedly because the instigation to aggression builds up over time and cannot be released through displacement or sublimation; thus, given appropriate stimulus conditions, all aggression is released in one extremely violent act.

C. **Treatment of the emergent condition** The last, and unfortunately the most common, circumstance is to begin treatment because violence has occurred. Intervention of this type can be conveniently divided into three levels on the basis of urgency: (1) *acute:* the combative, dangerous, actively violent individual; cooperation is not obtainable; (2) *subacute:* the severely agitated and threatening individual; violence has not yet occurred, but seems imminent; cooperation may or may not be obtained; (3) *chronic quiescent:* the recurrently violent person; currently in good control, he needs continuing care to prevent another act of violence; cooperation may or may not be obtained.

Control of the actively violent is an urgent matter, to avoid harm to others or to the person himself. Verbal intervention is hazardous and usually ineffective. Thus, physical restraint must be rapidly applied and followed, ordinarily, with appropriate medication. Acute and subacute situations may be managed as follows:

1. **Physical restraint** must be done by a number of individuals; a show of force may occasionally be adequate to gain some cooperation. If possible, the team that subdues the individual should be trained ahead of time and then briefed about the specific individual when action is required. A useful plan includes assigning one person to each of the violent individual's extremities. While the patient is engaged in some diverting activity, two or three members of the team may push him off balance and quickly gain control of the patient's extremities. This should be done in an area where there are few objects that could cause harm to the patient or staff.

   The combative individual must be controlled as quickly and humanely as possible. Prolonged fighting or physical restraint is neither humane nor good care; it only provides for increased risk of injury to patient or staff with subsequent anxiety or guilt. Rapid physical control by staff followed by intravenous medication is the desired procedure. Then the person can be placed in physical restraints.

2. The **medication** should be prepared, if possible, before the patient is restrained so it can be given as soon as possible, usually before placing the patient in four-point restraint. By giving the medication

slowly, intravenously, the level of sedation can be titrated, side effects minimized, and control gained quickly. Intramuscular or oral medication may take up to an hour to act, and even then control may be inadequate, requiring continued restraint of the patient and another dose. If absorption of the first intramuscular or oral dose was delayed, the second may be additive and may result in serious side effects. Medications that may be useful are:

a. **Barbiturates** — either the short- or intermediate-acting types may be administered intravenously or intramuscularly. Side effects include depressed respiration, laryngospasms, and transient hypotension; if the patient is underdosed, increased excitement may occur. Barbiturates may potentiate the effects of other CNS drugs, particularly depressants. Resuscitation and cardioversion equipment should be available. Sodium amobarbital is effective in doses of 200 to 500 mg. Intravenous administration of a 2.5 to 5% solution should be given at the rate of about 1 ml per minute. Barbiturates have the advantage of being widely available, commonly used, and effective in controlling seizures, should that be part of the behavior, and they are relatively safe if given slowly.

b. **Benzodiazepines** may be given either intramuscularly or intravenously, specifically to control patients who are agitated but not actively violent. These drugs have few side effects, although respiratory depression has been reported with larger doses given rapidly intravenously. Resuscitation equipment should be available. Enhancement of the depressant effect of alcohol, barbiturates, phenothiazines, monoamine oxidase inhibitors, and tricyclic antidepressants can occur. Diazepam, 5 to 10 mg given slowly intravenously, can be quite effective. Repeated use of diazepam is not recommended because of local venous reactions that may be due to the solvent system. It should not be mixed with water or placed in the same syringe with other medications.

c. **Phenothiazines and other antipsychotics** have been widely used for the control of agitation and combative behavior. These drugs are administered intramuscularly or orally and thus are slower to act. They potentiate CNS depressants, including narcotics, and also act additively with anticholinergics. Hypotension is the most serious acute side effect. Other acute side effects include tachycardia, laryngospasm, and extrapyramidal reactions. Numerous drugs of this type are available and effective; the choice should be based on the individual practitioner's experience. However, the high dose (low relative potency) type (e.g., chlorpromazine) has a higher incidence of hypotension. Large intramuscular doses of haloperidol (5 to 20 mg in a single dose, up to 100 mg/day) have been recommended for use in agitated and assaultive patients. Shader and Salzman and their colleagues have had success with a regimen that combines haloperidol (20 to 40 mg IM) and chlordiazepoxide (200 to 500 mg IM) given over 24 hours in divided doses.

3. **Verbal intervention** should help the patient recognize his angry feelings. This recognition must be accompanied by verbal reassurances that the staff will act in every way possible to prevent the individual from losing control of such feelings. Family member police, or other provocative people should be asked to leave. When homosexual panic contributes to the patient's turmoil and violence the patient's panic may be reduced by interacting with opposite-sex staff members. The person who is to work directly with the patien must be confident of his own skill and must avoid implying or exhibiting excessive anxiety, lest he confirm the patient's fear that he is dangerously out of control.

4. **Long-term control** of the potentially violent individual is a troublesome problem because of the multiple factors that may be causally involved and such individuals' often unstable, impulsive life-styles. Accurate assessment of the various factors contributing to the production of violence is essential. Obviously, the patient with a seizure syndrome or minimal brain damage will require a different treatment approach than the paranoid or psychopathic individual. Likewise, the psychotic must be managed quite differently from the individual with a personality disorder. It must also be remembered that some individuals are violent for cultural or ideological reasons and consequently may not be appropriate candidates for psychiatric intervention. Once an accurate assessment is made, treatment follows in the usual manner. Antipsychot are effective for those people with schizophrenic reactions or paranoid states. The various anticonvulsants are indicated for seizure states, and psychotherapy with antianxiety medications may be useful for the individual with a personality disorder or neurosis. Psychotherapy may also be useful to the borderline or frankly psychotic individual. Behavior therapy might be considered for some patients.

The patient with minimal brain damage may present an apparen personality disorder and may respond to CNS stimulants, anti-

convulsants, or one of the antipsychotics. Antipsychotics
(neuroleptics) that have been suggested as particularly useful for
control of aggression include haloperidol, thioridazine, chlorpromazine, and perphenazine; haloperidol has received the most
favorable comment. If the behavior arises from brain dysfunction
or seizures, phenothiazines and related compounds may be contraindicated since some of these drugs may reduce the seizure
threshold. One particular type of personality disorder, the
emotionally unstable character disorder as identified in adolescents
by Rifkin (*Biol. Psychiatry* 4:65, 1972), is thought to be closely
allied to affective illness because of the prominence of persistent,
transient, fluctuating symptoms of depression and hypomania and
the favorable response to chlorpromazine and lithium (see Chapter
17). These individuals have a marked mood lability consisting of
short periods of intense, empty unhappiness accompanied by
inactivity, withdrawal, depression, irritability, and sulking, alternating suddenly to periods of impulsiveness, frustration intolerance, rejection of rules, and shortsighted hedonism.

a. **Benzodiazepines** may be helpful on a long-term basis in some
   individuals with recurrent violent behavior. This regimen must
   be carefully evaluated, however, since some individuals instead
   may become disinhibited or have so-called paradoxical rages.

b. **Antiandrogen therapy** with cyproterone acetate or and progesterone has been suggested as a way of diminishing aggressive
   behavior associated with sexual activity.

c. **Lithium carbonate** has been reported as being effective in preventing the recurrence of violent behavior in some individuals.
   In one study (*Compr. Psychiatry* 14:311, 1973) the violent
   offenders shared some of the characteristics attributed by
   Rifkin to adolescents with emotionally unstable character
   disorders, that is, alternating mood states faintly reminiscent
   of hypomania and depression. Irritability, diminished tolerance
   to frustration, anxious depression, and a "short fuse" were
   particularly characteristic of this adult population. In addition,
   this group had a high frequency of abnormal EEGs, history of
   brain injury, or history of frank epilepsy. Behaviorally, the
   lithium responders all shared two characteristics: strikingly
   diminished capacity to delay violent reaction once provoked
   and a tendency to react maximally; in effect, these individuals
   "swing first and ask questions later." Lithium dosages averaged
   1800 mg a day to produce serum levels of 0.8 mEq/L. Side

effects included nausea, leukocytosis, activation of peptic ulcer disease, and apparent precipitation of psychosis in individuals with particularly brittle personality structure. With further study, lithium may offer a significant advance in the management of aggressive and violent behavior. Similar effec have been noted in animals and in various non-manic-depress conditions. The practicing clinician should note that this particular use of lithium in patients without manic-depressive illness is not yet approved by the Food and Drug Administra

5. **Psychosurgery** has been suggested by a number of authors for th control of aggressive behavior. Amygadolotomy is the procedur most often recommended. The serious ethical and medical consequences of this procedure, coupled with its permanency, indic extreme caution before use.

V. **Ethical Considerations**   Currently, violent behavior is seen by some individuals as legitimate and necessary to redress the grievances of the disadvantaged, poor, and exploited. Without question, these conditio do exist in our society, much to the detriment of the victims and of society as a whole. The debate as to what is a psychiatric or medical condition and what is a product of social or political discrimination rages continuously, and even in an individual case, the line of demarca tion is often obscure. Mental health workers in the employ of prisons and other agencies of criminal justice must be on constant guard lest they become captives of the system and act for the institution and its purposes rather than for the patient and his needs. Scrupulous assessr with determined review of social, cultural, psychological, and biologic factors must be the standard before the initiation of a treatment progi for individuals who commit violent acts. Errors are made when psychiatric and medical knowledge are used to subvert individual rights, maintain control, and inhibit legitimate social protests. Szasz (*The My of Mental Illness: Foundations of a Theory of Personal Conduct,* New Hoeber Med. Div., Harper & Row, 1961), has adequately delineated th risks of subverting civil rights through psychiatric procedures. The ris may be particularly grave when dealing with the individual exhibiting violent behavior.

8

Therapy of Psychiatric Disorders of Childhood

Magda Campbell
Theodore Shapiro

Most psychiatric disorders in childhood do not have clearly defined etiologies and are viewed as resulting from a convergence of genetic, acquired organic, and environmental factors. Therefore, definitive therapy based on etiologic certainty usually cannot be instituted.

The behavior repertoire of the young child is relatively limited, undifferentiated, and nonspecific. As he develops, he differentiates and integrates his various functions and exhibits progressively more complex behaviors. At an early stage he responds with the same symptoms and behavior to a variety of circumstances (e.g., his own slow maturation due to intrinsic factors, the frustration of being a late talker, a mother who is depressed and unstimulating or rejecting, gross neglect, central nervous system impairment, or any combination of these). Symptoms and behavior that can develop are hyperactivity, temper tantrums, withdrawal, delayed development, aggressiveness, or even self-mutilation. Moreover, a behavioral effect in any single sector of development may be secondary to a disruption of routines in another area.

I. **Diagnostic Process** The diagnostic process should include an adequate assessment of the child's (1) developmental status in regard to his motor, language, personal-social, and intrapsychic (libidinal and ego) landmarks, (2) his place in the family and social structure, and (3) the personality organization and psychopathology of his parents and their propensity to see psychopathology in their child. An evaluation should observe the following parameters: (1) chronological age, (2) developmental state (coping, ego landmarks, fantasy organization), (3) intellectual and perceptual functioning (clinical approximation or Gesell, WPPSI, WISC, or Stanford-Binet; Bender-Gestalt), (4) academic functioning (in relation to school and home standards; reading and language studies), (5) type of psychopathology (deviant behavior), (6) severity of psychopathology (ego-dystonic vs. ego-syntonic), (7) biologic studies (when indicated): EEG, neurologic examination, hearing and speech evaluation, metabolic and cytogenetic studies, (8) environment (family and social; peer and adult sectors).

A systems analysis including these sectors will help the diagnostician to make the proper plans for treatment. However, it is not always the child who requires treatment; it may be that the parents need counseling, reassurance, support, or therapy in order to tolerate and encourage the developmental process. Treatment of the child should be instituted only when symptoms persist or impede the developmental process.

The correct diagnosis is important both for the child's immediate treatment and for his future welfare. Finding a developmental, biologic basis for the child's problems or vulnerability may be therapeutic for the parents, relieving them of irrational guilt reinforced by vague diagnostic labels (e.g., "emotional disturbance") that carry a simplistic connotation of culpability. Early recognition of and intervention (including parental) in reactive psychopathologies may help to prevent the development of more crystallized neurotic behavior or personality disorders. It is therapeutic to help the parents see how recent changes in demand or structure can lead to symptoms in other sectors of behavior.

Symptoms can be used with benefit by parents as indicators of developmental process if they are viewed as temporary disturbances in achieving new landmarks (or functions) rather than as features of a disease process. For instance, transient zoophobia in a 3-year-old is so frequent in our culture as to be normal. Unless this phobia persists and pervades other behavior or inhibits the developmental flow, parents of such children should be reassured as to the transiency and normalcy of the phenomenon. Direct counseling, ego support, and desensitization frequently are helpful.

II. **Diagnostic Classification**   Some psychiatric disorders of childhood seem to have a clear biologic substrate underlying the disorder, even though reactive or situational factors may appear to be related to the onset of overt symptoms. In other disorders, environmental factors dominate, even though constitutional factors, such as temperament, are apparent, which suggests a biologic vulnerability. No single diagnostic classification system for disorders of childhood and adolescence has achieved unanimous acceptance. However, the system formulated by the Committee on Child Psychiatry of the Group for the Advancement of Psychiatry (GAP) (see *Psychopathological Disorders in Childhood: Theoretical Considerations and a Proposed Classification,* New York: G.A.P., 1966) is widely accepted and overlaps sufficiently with other nomenclatures to be broadly useful. Some of these disorders are elaborated below.

A. Healthy responses

   1. Developmental crisis.

   2. Situational crisis.

   3. Other responses.

This category subsumes a number of brief or transient alterations in the child's functioning as he or she develops and encounters stress in the course of day-to-day living. Separation anxiety in the preschool child and mourning (grief) following the death of a parent or grandparent or parental divorce are examples of this.

B. **Psychotic disorders**

1. **Psychoses of infancy and early childhood.**

   a. Early infantile autism.
   b. Interactional psychotic disorder.
   c. Other psychosis of infancy and early childhood.

2. **Psychoses of later childhood.**

   a. Schizophreniform psychotic disorder.
   b. Other psychosis of later childhood.

3. **Psychoses of adolescence.**

   a. Acute confusional state.
   b. Schizophrenic disorder, adult type.
   c. Other psychosis of adolescence.

Psychotic disorders can develop as early as the first two years of life and are characterized by withdrawal and overall retardation, particularly in the area of language and social behavior. If speech is present, it is predominantly noncommunicative and is characterized by echolalia, perseveration, and poor relevance to current context. Similarly, language comprehension is minimal, if it exists at all. Most investigators believe in a biologic basis for early infantile autism; while some would segregate it from childhood schizophrenia, others firmly believe it is the earliest expression of this more globally conceived disorder. Psychoses appearing after either normal or slightly abnormal development show less retardation. Latency-age childhood schizophrenics often present with introjected voices and bodies; only at prepuberty is the voice projected into hallucinations and external objects.

Generally speaking, manifestations of psychosis will be consonant with the developmental level of the child and therefore will take different forms at different stages of childhood. The earliest forms of psychosis are characterized by developmental arrests, in motor and physiologic sectors, while those with onset in later childhood are characterized by behavioral regression. As the child matures, other sectors will be influenced by the psychotic process. Poorly integrated speech and thought become evident as well as cognitive deficit and deviance. All these functions affect manifest behavior, so these children appear disorganized and bizarre, and they relate poorly to others. Psychoses can be primary, or secondary to toxic or metabolic aberrations and to mental retardation or brain damage. Manic-depressive psychosis is perhaps nonexistent under 10 to 12 years of age and is seen infrequently until the third decade.

C. **Psychophysiologic disorders** can occur in the first year of life due to lack of differentiation in emerging physiologic and psychological functions. Many have thought that autonomic responses during infancy provide the anlage for later short-circuiting of the affective responses in more differentiated psychological states.

D. **Developmental deviations** Some habit disturbances and lags in development are delays or distortions of development and maturation; they are seen more often in boys than in girls and are sometimes familial. Although these are listed as developmental, there may be a strong component of faulty training or interaction with parents. This category includes speech and language disorders and specific learn disorders that may manifest themselves as problems in reading, coding, or sequencing.

E. **Psychoneurotic disorders**

1. Anxiety type.
2. Phobic type.
3. Conversion type.
4. Dissociative type.
5. Obsessive-compulsive type.
6. Depressive type.
7. Other psychoneurotic disorder.

Psychoneurotic disorders in the first three to four years of life are usually seen only in the form of isolated neurotic symptoms. Most often, neurotic disorders in children are relatively less differentiated than those seen in adults. Single symptoms may appear that are typically ego-dystonic. Clinging to mother increases, and increased dependency is often the accompaniment.

F. **Personality disorders**

1. Compulsive personality.
2. Hysterical.
3. Anxious.
4. Overly dependent.
5. Oppositional.

6. Overly inhibited.
7. Overly independent.
8. Isolated.
9. Mistrustful.
10. Tension-discharge disorders.
    a. Impulse-ridden personality.
    b. Neurotic personality disorder.
11. Sociosyntonic personality disorder.
12. Sexual deviation.
13. Other personality disorder.

These disorders, like fixed neurotic disorders, are not seen in the earliest years of life, due to the immaturity of the child's psychic structure. However, early temperamental styles in interaction with specific family responses may fix a tendency toward a particular pattern. A child who is seen as willful in a punitive family may respond with withdrawal or paranoid-like symptoms. Also included in this category are children showing socially unacceptable behaviors that are partially internalized and crystallized. These symptom pictures must be distinguished from the developmental disorders, which carry a genetic or maturational component, and from the psychotic disorders. Children within this category who are *overly inhibited, isolated, mistrustful, or anxious* must be distinguished from children with psychoses of later childhood and adolescence. In the latter case, the responses are more chronic, less appropriate, and associated with more global personality disruption. Children with *oppositional, tension-discharge disorders,* or *sociosyntonic personalities* must be distinguished from those children with deviations in motor development who may be hyperactive and aggressive.

G. **Other disorders** The diagnosis of **minimal brain dysfunction** is one that is not included in the GAP classification. It may in fact overlap to some degree with other diagnostic categories (personality disorders, developmental deviations, and various organic brain syndromes) that describe children who are hyperactive and easily distractible and have a short attention span (see Chapter 9). The term *minimal brain dysfunction* is used to describe a group of children who have no known brain damage but whose signs and symptoms are similar to children with such damage.

Another psychiatric disorder that is not included in the GAP or standard nomenclature is **Gilles de la Tourette's syndrome** (maladie des tics). It is an uncommon condition, often aggravated by emotional tension, characterized by multiple tics, involuntary movements involving the whole body, inarticulate cries, echolalia, and coprolalia.

The etiology remains obscure, although subtle organic impairment has been implicated.

Chronological age and expectancy of developmental patterns will place a child in his normative framework. If he is not speaking in short sentences by age 3, he is relatively retarded in that function, but the same symptom at age 5 is more serious. Similarly, if a 2-year-old meets every frustration with a tantrum, we would assess the relationship of this symptom to his new toddling and getting into things vis-à-vis an anxious mother. If he were still having tantrums and head-banging episodes at 8, and in addition was withdrawn and without friends among his peers, we would think of a more malignant process, such as childhood schizophrenia.

Although in certain psychoses there may be no known brain tissue impairment, the prognosis for some of these subgroups (early infantile autism and childhood schizophrenia) may be as poor as that for children with gross brain damage resulting in mental retardation and psychosis. This is due to the fact that onset of illness in early life, when the organism and its functions are undifferentiated, affects the child more globally. Some authors assert that when communicative speech develops before the age of 5, there is a good prognosis in 50 percent of the cases for a marginally adaptive life. However, even those 50 percent frequently remain dependent.

In general, the prognosis of psychiatric disorders should be more favorable in childhood than it is in adulthood, given the assumption that children's symptoms are less crystallized. However, in the more severe forms of psychiatric disorders, treatments are often less effective in children because their total development is more globally affected (and arrested) by the illness.

Because all psychiatric symptoms and disorders in childhood interfere with development, intervention and treatment should be instituted early to encourage the process of maturation.

III. **Treatment Modalities**   In dealing with children, the process linking diagnosis with treatment is rarely a straightforward one. Treatment planning must give consideration to the child, his or her symptoms and level of maturation, the family (parents and siblings), the school, the neighborhood, and other factors. The following sections outline briefly certain of these considerations and appropriate treatment modalities. The interested reader will find another GAP report useful (see *From Diagnosis to Treatment: An Approach to Treatment Planning for the Emotionally Disturbed Child,* New York: G.A.P., 1973).

A. **Sectors of treatment**   Treatment may be directed toward the child, either or both of his parents, or the family as a unit. These treatment decisions are, of course, dependent upon the prior investigative process and the accuracy and precision of the physician's diagnostic skills.

1. **Treatment of the child**   A decision to treat the child should rest upon the discovery of maturational and developmental defects in the child that impair his progression to more mature forms of functioning. He should, in general, move from egocentricity to companionship, from lack of control over his body sphincters toward control, from playing with toys and his own body toward a proper balance of work and lesiure activities, and, finally, from a relatively autistic, need-satisfying world through a period of dependency to the ultimate attainment of self-reliance (A. Freud). Moreover, he should achieve the normative developmental landmarks in his motor, personal-social, language, and adaptive behavior. Interruptions in these paths require the direct application of techniques of treatment to the child himself. Any highly structuralized intrapsychic pathologic organization due to conflict may also be looked upon as reason for treating the child himself. This may include neurotic symptoms or perverse tendencies and may be temporary or chronic.

   a. **Educational and remedial techniques**   Tutoring or remedial techniques should be recommended if the child has a severe language disorder or reading difficulty or both. While there is a secondary overlay of psychological problems caused by feelings of inadequacy and the stigma of being "stupid," the educational techniques themselves will help the ego in its struggle for achievement and self-respect. Specific remedial techniques might include perceptual training, reading instruction, and math instruction. When a child's educational difficulties rest upon interpersonal problems, a tutor whose abilities include psychotherapeutic techniques may be very helpful.

   b. **Socialization groups,** such as therapeutic activity groups in a community center that are oriented toward rehabilitating delinquent or truant children, seem to provide significant role models and group peer relationships for socially deprived children.

   c. **Operant conditioning techniques** are used directly by parents as they unwittingly desensitize their children through gradual exposure to phobic objects. For example, when a child is fearful of a dog, the purchase of a puppy may be very helpful because the child may participate in caring for the animal in a nonthreatening circumstance. Professionals may be called upon for more systematic, specialized behavioristic techniques. A fixed schedule of conditioning, either desensitization or contingency pairing, may be utilized to initiate or discourage certain behaviors.

d. **Individual psychotherapy** may include a conjoint approach that utilizes simultaneous treatment of the mother and interview techniques with the child. Psychotherapy with children rests on bases similar to the treatment of adults. A therapeutic alliance is established in which child and therapist view the child's difficulties. The general problem is exposed through confrontation and clarification and is made ego-dystonic. At times interpretation is used to bring unconscious motivation to awareness. Play techniques seek to illuminate unconscious conflicts in young children (3 to 9 years) that underlie symptom and involve an interpretive approach based on the psycho-analytic model. These may be utilized in a limited way or extensively, depending on whether or not a transference as well as a realistic relationship to the therapist can be established

e. **Psychoanalytic techniques** include *play* and *interview therapy,* in which confrontation, clarification, interpretation, and possibly reconstructive techniques are all used. The trans-ference does not have as large a role in psychoanalytic thera-peutic techniques as it does in the treatment of adults. These techniques are applied generally to children who have a rather fixed internalized conflict and a character structure that is not amenable to other treatment and when the parents are not able to alter their behavior to help the child.

f. **Other psychotherapies** There are other psychotherapeutic techniques that involve the parent as well as the child. Some child therapists recommend joint treatment, in which the mother is an observing participant, in the treatment of psychotic children. Corrective object relations techniques are sometimes used in children who have severe difficulties with the develop-ment of their personal-social relations in regard to their parents or other adults. These techniques include some reeducation.

g. **Residential milieu treatment** A total treatment program requires the involvement and counseling of the parents or any adult caretaker, including teachers. The total treatment pro-gram, often referred to as milieu therapy, includes a well-structured clinical residential or day program with individual planning and therapeutic objectives for each child. Promotion of development is usually a multidisciplinary approach in the case of the psychotic child, particularly the younger child. It may include individual therapy, speech therapy, special education program, or remedial work or tutoring, or any combination of these. The patient may be hospitalized for diagnostic workup or as an intervention in crisis, but only as a temporary arrangement. Drug therapy has to be used in some cases as an adjunct.

h. **Group therapies: Therapeutic nursery school** Children selected for such programs are generally 2 1/2 to 6 years of age and require specialized attention, using specific educational techniques and interventions to support defective developmental lines. These nursery programs help a child adapt to acute stress, such as parental separation or loss. Teachers and other professionals under psychiatric guidance are sensitized to problems of children at risk.

2. **Treatment of the parent** The parent, on the other hand, must be looked at with regard to his specific role in relation to the child. This includes the assessment of the mother and father as models for identification, as well as the mother's specific role in care-taking, since our culture assigns a greater role to females in engendering the early development of young children. Among the areas to be considered as requiring clinical intervention with parents are: (1) role identification model distortions; (2) a tendency to treat a child as though he were a figure from the past, which leads to distortion of his status in reality; (3) use of a child for the parent's own psychotic or other purposes as an extension of the self; (4) a pathologic labeling of the child as "damaged" for personal and historical reasons; (5) traumatic symbiotic overconcern with separation from the parent or inappropriate permission for autonomous functioning when the child's developmental abilities do not warrant it; (6) overvaluation or undervaluation of the child; and (7) using the child as a foil in the parents' own struggle with each other. Once a proper assessment has been made considering all these relevant factors, an appropriate therapeutic modality may be chosen for the parents, either alone — without the child being treated — or paralleling and complementing the child's treatment.

a. Treatment of the parent may involve **counseling.** This is usually geared to the parent's needs in relation to the rearing of the child: the mother may need advice and education on child-rearing practices and childhood norms. She may need to reevaluate her assessment of the child.

b. At the earliest stages, such as infancy, teaching by **mirroring** and **identification with trained professionals** is most useful.

c. On the other hand, the mother may go into more intensive inquiry involving a **combination of counseling and individual psychotherapy** to explore her unconscious and conscious view of her child and the distortions she brings to her behavior with the child.

3. Treatment of the family The family itself may be the treatment object. Indications for treating a family include an improper labeling process in which the child is incorrectly looked upon as having the symptom. The family may be utilizing the child as a scapegoat for maladaptive group reasons; communication among and between the members of the family may not be adequate to support the developmental thrust. Finally, family therapy may be used as a precursor to individual therapy that can only come about after a sharing of mutual responsibilities among all the members of the family.

The group under treatment may include any responsible exter family member in what is called *family network treatment,* or it may pertain only to the immediate family grouping of elders and the index child, or it may be confined to all the family members who live under one roof. Such treatment is usually directed tow reassessment of the members' varied views of the actual situation and the investigation of the interrelations among the members of the family and how they operate as an organic whole. These con siderations may only incidentally touch upon the child. If the child himself needs some further help, he may be referred for additional individual therapy at a later time.

B. Psychiatric emergencies in children There are a few emergency circumstances in childhood that require rapid intervention. These include: acute school phobias, acute hallucinosis, acute homicidal and suicidal feelings, acute generalized anxiety, and agoraphobia. The general treatment procedure in these disorders is a rapid return to a normal social milieu, in accordance, of course, with the individual's capacity for adaptation and readaptation to the requiremen of his social environment. Too early a return from sheltered circum stances may lead to a sense of repeated failure. However, too permissive an attitude may lead to symptom "fixation."

1. **School phobias** are generally treated by immediate return to school, even though the child may not initially attend classes; this action is taken with the support of a parent or concerned school official. In many instances the young child's return to school can be facilitated by confronting and treating the parents' inability to allow the child to be separate or independent. Imipramine and related drugs have been reported to be very effective in the treatment of nonpsychotic school-phobic children. The child's returning to school per se is usually compatible with good prognosis. However, at times an assessment of the parental attitudes and other sectors may indicate more significant pathology; school phobia, especially in children over 12, may suggest graver diagnoses (e.g., childhood schizophrenia).

2. **Acute hallucinoses** usually mark the onset of acute psychotic episodes, frequently precipitated by traumatic events, and the child ought to be offered the possibility of talking about, exposing, and adapting to the traumatic experience. Differential diagnosis should consider ingestion of toxins, glue sniffing, and early meningitis or encephalitis, which can be confirmed by fever, confusional delirium with loss of orientation, and possibly stiff neck and petechiae.

3. **Phobic avoidances and agoraphobia** may be the end result of spreading single phobias. Management should include both psychological support and drugs to decrease acute anxiety, as in all the above-mentioned instances.

4. **Suicidal and homicidal gestures** Suicidal and homicidal thoughts are common in childhood, as are casual threats that may never be acted upon. During latency many children threaten to kill themselves or others in the midst of rages or temper outbursts. Usually remorse or even apology follows when the acute tantrum subsides. However, some children become morbidly preoccupied with vengeful feelings toward parents, or if this avenue of expression is blocked, toward themselves; this preoccupation may lead to actual attacks if impulse control is poor. Psychotic children and organically impaired children are most likely to exhibit such behavior during latency or preadolescence. When a child is actively and repeatedly suicidal or homicidal, prompt psychiatric evaluation is necessary, and the child may require protective hospitalization, tranquilizing drugs, and careful observation until the arousing circumstances have been ameliorated. Taunting siblings or excessively punitive parents may incite such dangerous behavior,

which in children with defective egos has been known to lead to death.

5. **Runaway children and fire-setting** Both of these behaviors are symptoms. Investigation should be carried out to discover the diagnostic category that underlies the emergent behavior. Running away is frequent and is benign if the child is in early latency and returns within hours. Precipitating causes, such as arguments, are easily discovered. Pathologic and repeated running away occurs in children with intolerable social and family conditions or in psychotic mentally deficient or severely neurotic children, whose ability to tolerate anger and frustration is limited. Evaluation of home and child, as indicated earlier, will determine the sector for treatment.

Fire-setting has its peak occurrence in boys in late adolescence but it can occur during the latency period. These children may use fire-setting for purposes of revenge, or they may have specific fascination with fire and fire rescue. For example, they may ascribe specific sexual or aggressive symbolization to fire, or may simply use fire as a means of covering another forbidden act, such as bed-wetting. Fire-setters must be evaluated with care to insure that no child will be incarcerated unfairly; but on the other hand firm measures must be taken to prevent a potential threat to the community from being realized. Constant care and supervision should be instituted.

IV. Drug Therapy

A. **Indications for drug therapy** Drug treatment may be a valuable addition to or an essential modality of the total treatment of both the psychotic and the moderately to severely disturbed child. In some instances drugs, correctly chosen, can make such children more amenable to educational and other therapies. However, with the exception of the "hyperkinetic" syndrome or minimal brain dysfunction, the effectiveness of pharmacotherapy in child psychiatry is yet to be established. Medication is helpful only when combined with other therapies or work with parents or both. Drugs themselves do not create normal adaptive or cognitive behavior, nor do they necessarily alter parental attitude, when administered to the child. In our present state of knowledge, there is no specific drug for any of the psychiatric diagnostic categories in childhood. Moreover, the severity of illness — even psychosis per se — is not always an absolute indicator for drug therapy. The very young, hypoactive, apathetic, psychotic child with no language or only sparse speech more often than not will fail to respond well or will even deteriorate when placed on a standard major neuroleptic such as chlorpromazine.

Currently available drugs are most effective in reducing target symptoms such as insomnia, hyperactivity, impulsiveness, irritability, excitability, disorganized behavior, psychotic thought disorder, and certain types of aggressive behavior. The hyperactive, distractible child may acquire some reading and writing skills when calmed down and able to focus his attention better. When the symptoms of an excessively aggressive, assaultive, or self-mutilating child are controlled by an effective drug, one hopes, he will develop positive and adaptive social interactions that in turn will improve learning. Experience suggests that such children fail to respond or respond only minimally to educational, remedial, and milieu therapies in the absence of drug treatment.

If apathy, hypoactivity, dreaminess, and withdrawal can in fact be affected by drugs, they are somewhat more susceptible to neuroleptics with "stimulating" properties (e.g., trifluoperazine and haloperidol) than to those with more sedative properties (e.g., chlorpromazine). However, some of these more "stimulating" psychoactive agents, although promising, are still under investigation (e.g., triiodothyronine).

B. General guidelines to drug therapy

1. Administration of psychopharmacologic agents is only part of the total treatment of a child.

2. The goal of all psychiatric treatments in childhood is to promote maturation and development (every psychiatric disturbance or symptom interferes with these trends, either individually or globally). Therefore, the purpose of drug treatment is not simply to alleviate certain symptoms but by doing so to make the child more amenable to other forms of therapy and to enable him to develop positive and adaptive social interactions that will improve learning of all types. Accordingly, if a drug or drug therapy interferes in any way with maturation, development, and learning, it should be discontinued.

3. We may influence not only immediate but also **long-term outcome** of the illness by drug treatment coordinated with a more global treatment plan. Although what a drug can do is limited, it is a misconception that a drug affects only symptom(s) and not the process of the illness.

4. Thorough acquaintance with the drug is essential. It is sufficient, however, to be familiar with one or two psychoactive agents from

each class of drugs. Additional research must be done to establish whether particular drugs affect specific symptoms or diagnostic categories. To be adequately informed about a drug one must be aware of the following:

a. **Therapeutic effects**

b. **Side effects and toxic reactions**

   (1) Specific for the particular drug or class of drugs (e.g., extrapyramidal, urinary, gastrointestinal, dermatologic).

   (2) Nonspecific; observed in most any drug or in all drugs at certain dose level (loss of weight or appetite, behavioral manifestations such as irritability, sleepiness, hypoactivity and hyperactivity).

   (3) Hypersensitivity reactions could occur with any drug in certain individuals. Drugs should not be given to a child with history of sensitivity to medications or general intolerance to medication. A history of allergy requires caution in the administration of neuroleptics.

   (4) *The usefulness of psychoactive drug combinations in children has not been demonstrated.*

5. **Fundamental differences between the child and adult**

   a. **Psychosocial** A child is dependent on an adult for the proper administration of a prescribed drug. The parent should be told about expected therapeutic effects, side effects, possible toxicity, and drug regulation. Major tranquilizers or potentially harmful drugs should be prescribed to a child on an outpatient basis only if the parents are cooperative and reliable.

   Parental attitude toward drug therapy may be positive or negative. In the latter instance, a parent may force the child to take medication as an expression of sadistic or controlling wishes or to align himself with the physician against the child. The parent may also fear drugs as a form of organic intrusion. On the positive side, a parent's need or wish for a quick cure or a physical solution to what is basically an interactional problem may cause him to be overly idealistic or hopeful about the effects of the medication.

   The child's interpretation of taking the drug may range from fear of loss of control, or fear of being poisoned or weakened, to a belief that he will feel stronger and better. Irrational beliefs, such as "the worse it tastes, the more effective the treatment," or "more medicine for increased symptoms," even after the dosage has been regulated, may confound therapeutic results. To some, a drug may represent a substitute for object need. A placebo effect should be looked for in a significant number of cases.

b. **Biologic action of the drug** There are not only quantitative but also qualitative differences to consider (including neurophysiologic central nervous system immaturities). We do not yet have answers to the sometimes paradoxical, contradictory, or inconsistent responses of the child to psychoactive drugs. For instance, while amphetamine is a stimulant and antidepressant in adults, in certain types of hyperactive children it is an effective agent in decreasing hyperactivity. Conversely, barbiturates are hypnotics in adults, whereas in young children the administration of members of this class of drug may result in insomnia and disorganization of behavior.

c. **Dosage** On the whole, children need or tolerate relatively higher doses of psychopharmacologic agents than do adults; therefore, dosages for children cannot simply be extrapolated from adult dosages. Weight and age are not always reliable guidelines. A more accurate way to determine the dosage for a child is by body surface. However, there still remain great individual differences in children as far as maximum tolerated or "optimal" dose is concerned, and this is often unrelated to either the individual child's weight and age or even the severity of his psychiatric illness. A frequent error is the maintenance of severely disturbed children on an excessively high dosage, the effect of which clearly interferes with functioning.

d. **Side effects and toxicity** Behavioral side effects in children may differ from those in adults. The younger the child, the more likely his expression of discomfort due to excess drug or drug side effect will be on an affectomotor level rather than on a verbal level. Since he is a relatively undifferentiated organism, the child's behavior repertoire is meager; he reacts to most anything by very nonspecific response, such as irritability, increased or decreased motor activity, or loss of appetite. Certain side effects, such as extrapyramidal signs, dystonic reactions, and tardive dyskinesia, are less frequently seen in children, particularly those under 6 years of age, than in young adults. Impaired liver function, drug-induced jaundice, and bone marrow damage also are seen less often in childhood.

However, children should still receive careful clinical and laboratory monitoring. It appears that the child's brain and whole organism are more "sturdy."

e. **Long-term effects**   Long-term pharmacotherapy may introduce some problems, including how such maintenance influences growth and certain endocrine systems or organs (including the reproductive system). Knowledge of these late effects is still limited. Only recently have there been a few reports regarding (1) the effects of drugs on offspring in experimental animals; (2) the effects of chlorpromazine, haloperidol, and lithium on the secretion of growth hormone in adults; and (3) the effects of methylphenidate and dextroamphetamine on growth in weight and height in children. There is some inconclusive evidence suggesting that neuroleptics, antidepressants (imipramine), and anxiolytics (chlordiazepoxide) may affect thyroid function; lithium has been found to have some antithyroid effect. In adults, elevated prolactin and galactorrhea have been observed with chlorpromazine, amitriptyline, perphenazine, imipramine, and chlordiazepoxide. The use of chlorpromazine in schizophrenic adults can be associated with ovulatory failure and increased pregnanediol excretion. In immature experimental animals, chlorpromazine was reported to inhibit luteinizing hormone (LH) secretion. The monoamine neurotransmitters (catecholamines and indoles) control the secretion of the hypothalamic neurohormones (releasing factors and inhibiting factors) that regulate the pituitary and other endocrine functions. These neurotransmitters are affected by various psychoactive agents. Since the hypothalamus is implicated in the initiation of puberty, drugs should be given with caution to prepubertal children.

All the foregoing must be viewed against the background that abnormal growth patterns and alterations in the onset of puberty are often seen in psychotic, retarded, and brain damaged children who have never received pharmacotherapy. Nonetheless, the possibility of late adverse effects of psychoactive drugs on a child cannot be dismissed. This is one of the reasons why the administration of psychoactive agents in general, and particularly over a prolonged period, should not be taken lightly; on the other hand, the long-term hazards of certain psychiatric conditions in childhood (particularly those of the severe behavior disorders or psychoses) have to be weighed against the possible adverse effects outlined. It is most important that the child calm down, concentrate, and remain in the classroom and in social situations to learn and to adapt to peer relationships.

Effects of drugs on learning and intelligence remain to be established. Some evidence suggests that the sedative type of neuroleptic drugs, such as chlorpromazine and thioridazine, decrease cognitive functions in psychotic and retarded children, while recent studies indicate that stimulants improve attention span and performance in general in hyperkinetic children of normal intelligence. The same drug may have different effects, depending on the child's IQ. More clinical evidence and research is necessary to clarify this important matter.

Addiction to or psychological dependence on drugs prescribed for specific behavioral or affective indications does not appear to pose a significant problem in the preadolescent child, although further confirmation of this is needed.

6. **Dose regulation** Stepwise progression is recommended, particularly with neuroleptics or certain antidepressants. The child is first placed on a low, usually therapeutically ineffective dose. Increments are gradual, at regular intervals (e.g., usually twice a week — Tuesday and Thursday), until therapeutic effects are obtained or untoward effects (e.g., behavioral, neurologic, excess sedation) are noted. The optimal dose is then determined, and the child is maintained on this dose. It is of paramount importance to explore the dose range fully, because maximum tolerated or "optimal" doses vary widely in children. A common error is to maintain the child on small ineffectual doses or on doses that are too high for him and produce negative effects (the same dosage might not even be sufficient for another patient). Some of these undesirable effects are actually exaggerated forms of the desired effects. For example, if the goal is to stimulate the child, excess dosage of a stimulant can result in irritability, excitement, or hyperactivity; on the other hand, if the drug is given to calm down the hyperactive, aggressive child, with too much drug he may become hypoactive or sleepy or might even fall asleep. Excess drug may be manifested as worsening of preexisting symptoms, including hyperactivity. This worsening should be distinguished from nonresponse due to an ineffective, low dosage. These phenomena of excess drug are transient and can be eliminated by decreasing the dosage. At times the drug may have to be discontinued for a day or two and then the dose lowered. However, even without lowering the dose, occasionally the child "gets used" (adapts) to the same dose, and the symptoms of excess dosage disappear. One should also be alert to another phenomenon: while the patient may not

show any untoward effects initially, such effects may eventually occur on the same dose due to drug accumulation. This should be distinguished from the patient's adapting to the positive, therapeu effects of the drug and exhibiting his baseline behavior.

7. **Observation of drug-induced behavioral changes** It is important that the child be observed daily to ascertain at what dosages positive and negative effects occur and thus determine the optima dose. This is readily done by the physician observing an inpatient Even then, however, and particularly in an outpatient setting, this has to be supplemented by reports from parents and teachers. While for the adult it is essential that he functions at work, it is equally important for the child to function well at play and in school. If the child is excessively sedated by a drug, this interferes with his functioning, and the dosage or even the drug must be changed.

   Two of the physician's major difficulties in drug therapy in children are the incidence of excessive sedation at dose levels that control certain undesirable behaviors or symptoms and obtaining the cooperation of a reliable parent or teacher.

8. **Failure of the child to respond to the given drug** should not be a reason to terminate drug therapy per se. If after one month of administration with adequate dose exploration, a drug yields no therapeutic response, other drug(s), either from the same class or with similar action or profile but from a different class, should be tried. Drug treatment is an essential part of the total treatmen of the psychotic preschool child. At a later age, or a later stage of illness, such a child may no longer be as responsive to drug therapy as he was in the first years of life. Nevertheless, one mus keep in mind that there may be children whose symptoms or illness are refractory to any kind of drug treatment, and therefore drug treatment may have to be superseded by other treatment modalities. Also, there are conditions, such as personality dis- orders, in which drug therapy may be of questionable or no value Polypharmacy, frequent changes of drugs, and unnecessary dosag escalation are usually ill advised in children.

9. **Duration of drug treatment** is an important issue for various reasons. In cases in which the child responds favorably to a psychoactive agent, he should be maintained on the medication for a fair amount of time, but certainly no longer than is necessar In some milder conditions, in which reactive elements are associa with some intrinsic factors, drug therapy may be needed only unt the vicious cycle is broken. In some acute psychotic episodes, on

month of drug therapy may be adequate. In more chronic cases, or where the pathology is entirely or predominantly intrinsic, the child will have to be kept on a drug for months or even several years. Due to possible hazards of prolonged pharmacotherapy (see Section IV.B.5), it is suggested that after each three to four months of administration, a drug be gradually decreased and discontinued for about a week (drug washout). This will allow assessment of how much of the newly acquired positive or more adaptive behavior and developmental gains are retained without the drug. If there is a recurrence of symptoms, drug treatment must be reinstituted. Careful clinical observation will determine the length of drug administration.

10. **Choice of drug** will depend on the child's age, the diagnosis, the severity of illness (with the same behavioral manifestations), and the duration of illness. The child's status — inpatient or outpatient — may be decisive in determining whether drug treatment is feasible or which drug should be used. Some medications require close behavioral or laboratory monitoring, and they should not be used for outpatients when parents are not reliable or cooperative, as discussed in Section IV.B.5.

C. Classification of drugs

1. **Neuroleptic drugs** (antipsychotic agents, major tranquilizers). See Appendix III for a comprehensive list of generic and trade names and dose forms.

   a. **Phenothiazines** The three subclasses of these antipsychotic agents differ in potency, side effects, and possibly other psychopharmacologic properties (see Chapter 1). The aliphatic subclass in general has more sedative-hypnotic action, while some of the piperazine drugs have stimulating properties; therefore, the former are presumably more effective in hyperactive, aggressive children and the latter in withdrawn, anergic, apathetic populations. Extrapyramidal signs occur more frequently with piperazine derivatives, particularly in older children. Baseline laboratory tests should be done in children who are placed on phenothiazines, as with all other neuroleptics, tricyclic antidepressants, and monoamine oxidase inhibitors. These should include a pretreatment complete blood count and differential, serum alkaline phosphatase, serum glutamic-pyruvic transaminase, serum glutamic-oxaloacetic transaminase, and urinalysis. If feasible, these blood and liver function studies should be repeated on a weekly basis during the first month of treatment, and thereafter once a month or as often as clinically indicated. Representative phenothiazines, their indications for use, daily dose range for children, therapeutic effects, side effects, and toxic reactions are given in Table 8-1. Further details on use of phenothiazines in children can be found in the literature (see B. Fish, Organic Therapies, in A. M. Freedman and H. I. Kaplan (Eds.), *Comprehensive Textbook of Psychiatry* Baltimore: Williams & Wilkins, 1967 Pp. 1468—1472).

b. **Butyrophenones and thioxanthenes** (haloperidol, thiothixene, and chlorprothixene) — see Appendix III. Although they are chemically unrelated, these two classes of neuroleptics are listed together because some clinical evidence indicates that along with their antipsychotic action, some members of the two classes may have similar stimulating properties (haloperidol and thiothixene). The combination of these two qualities may be desirable in chronic, apathetic, anergic schizophrenic and other young psychotic children, with or without brain damage. These children usually have some associated mental retardation and show little improvement even with the most intensive therapies available. Many of the preschool psychotics have never spoken. Functions such as language and adaptive skills must be *developed,* not merely returned to more normal levels, as in adults or other children in whom the psychotic process did not start in the first years of life. Sedation, so often produced in young children by the more sedative neuroleptics (e.g., chlorpromazine), can be associated with decreased functioning in speech and other areas, thus impairing learning. Some investigations suggest that haloperidol may be particularly helpful in Gilles de la Tourette's syndrome (*Arch. Gen. Psychiatry* 28:92, 1973). Haloperidol has a high incidence of extrapyramidal side effects in children, as does thiothixene, according to some reports. Clinical experience to date suggests that a lower incidence of sensitivity reactions (cutaneous, hepatic, and hematologic) occurs with these two classes of drugs. However, pretreatment and ongoing laboratory studies should be carried out, as indicated in the section on phenothiazines. Some drugs belonging to the above classes of neuroleptics are listed in Table 8-2, with daily dose range for children, indications for their use, therapeutic and side effects, and toxic reactions.

Table 8-1. Phenothiazines for Children

		Daily Dosage[a]	
Generic Name	Trade Name	Range (mg)	Number of Divided Doses
Chlorpromazine	Thorazine Chlor PZ	Oral: 9 to 200 IM (up to 5 years of age): max. 40 IM (5 to 12 years of age): max. 75	2 to 4
Triflupromazine	Vesprin	1 to 150	2 to 4
Trifluoperazine[b]	Stelazine	1 to 20	1 to 2
Thioridazine	Mellaril	10 to 200	2 to 4

Indications
  Psychoses, acute or chronic; mental retardation with behavior problems; moderate to severe behavior disorders; psychiatric emergencies; homicide and suicide attempts; and acute anxiety states

Clinical effects
  Antipsychotic effects; decrease of agitation, hyperkinesis, aggressiveness, excitability, irritability, anxiety, stereotypes, and insomnia

Side effects and toxicity[c]
  Acute dystonic reactions
    akathisia; parkinsonism; tardive dyskinesia; convulsive seizures; hypersensitivity reactions (cutaneous reactions, blood dyscrasias, hepatic findings); cutaneous disorders; lenticular and corneal opacities; and behavioral reactions

[a]Children 2 to 12 years of age. Dosage for adolescents is comparable to adult dosage. See Appendix III for available dose forms.
[b]For children over 6 years of age.　　　[c]See also Chapter 4.

2. Antidepressant drugs and psychomotor stimulants

a. **Tricyclic antidepressants** Imipramine is representative of this class of drugs. There have been few studies of their use in psychotic children, and those that exist are without controls and controversial. While the imipramine-like drugs are effective antidepressants in adults, particularly those with psychomotor retardation, their effects in "depressed" children cannot readily be evaluated. Childhood depressive states are not well-defined conditions, and manic-depressive illness is perhaps nonexistent in children under 10 to 12 years of age. The most extensive use of this class of drugs in the treatment of depressed children has occurred outside the United States. Reports from within this country support the effectiveness of imipramine as a nighttime medication for enuresis (*J. Pediatr.* 67:283, 1965), for hyperactive behavior disorders (*Am. J. Psychiatry* 128: 1425, 1972), and as a medication in school phobias in non-

Table 8-2. Butyrophenones and Thioxanthenes for Children

| | | Daily Dosage [a] | |
Generic Name	Trade Name	Range (mg)	Number of Divided Doses
Haloperidol	Haldol	2 to 16	1 to 2
Thiothixene	Navane	1 to 40	1 to 2
Chlorprothixene	Taractan	10 to 200	1 to 2

Indications
   Psychoses, particularly chronic, with apathy and anergy, with or without known
      impairment of brain tissue function
   Gilles de la Tourette's syndrome (haloperidol)
Clinical effects
   Antipsychotic effects; decrease of agitation, hyperkinesis, aggressiveness, excitability,
      irritability, and tics
Side effects and toxicity [b]
   Extrapyramidal symptoms; dystonic reactions; seizures; leukopenia, leukocytosis;
      impaired liver function, jaundice; dry mouth; blurred vision; insomnia, restlessness,
      worsening of psychotic symptoms; euphoria; behavioral reactions; pigmentary
      retinopathy and lenticular pigmentation (thiothixene)

[a]Except for chlorprothixene (approved for children over 6 years), none of the drugs in
these two classes of neuroleptics are approved by FDA for use in children under 12
years of age; literature is available on their use under 12. See Appendix III for available
dose forms.

[b]See also Chapter 4.

psychotic children (*Arch. Gen. Psychiatry* 25:204, 1971).
Table 8-3 summarizes the indications for use, therapeutic and
side effects, and toxic reactions of this class of drugs as well
as the daily dose ranges for children. The use of imipramine
for the treatment of enuresis has been approved by the Food
and Drug Administration. Its use in the treatment of hyperactivity (see Chapter 9) or phobias is still being investigated.

b. **Monoamine oxidase inhibitors**   Because of their toxicity, these
drugs should not be given to children.

c. **The use of psychomotor stimulants** in minimal brain dysfunctio
(hyperkinetic disorders) is discussed in Chapter 9. In psychotic
disorders, administration of amphetamine or methylphenidate
usually increases disorganization. Suicides and unsuccessful
attempts at suicide are reported with antidepressants, although
this mode of death is only rarely selected by adolescents.

3. **Antianxiety agents and sedative-hypnotics**   The value of antianxiety agents and sedative-hypnotics in children has not been

Table 8-3. Antidepressants and Psychomotor Stimulants for Children[a]

Generic Name	Trade Name	Daily Dosage[b]	
		Range (mg)	Number of Divided Doses
Imipramine	Tofranil Tofranil-PM Presamine SK-Pramine Imavate	6 to 225[c] (1 to 5 mg/kg/day)	1 to 2
Amitriptyline	Elavil	2 to 75	1 to 3
Nortriptyline	Aventyl	10 to 75	1 to 3
Amphetamine sulfate	Benzedrine		
Dextroamphetamine sulfate	Dexedrine		
Methylphenidate	Ritalin		

Indications
  Enuresis
  Depressive states
  School phobia (in nonpsychotics)
  Minimal brain dysfunction (hyperactive behavior disorders)
Clinical effects
  Alleviation of symptoms of depression and anxiety
Side effects and toxicity
  Restlessness; ataxia; tremors; seizures; extrapyramidal symptoms; bone marrow depression; jaundice; dry mouth; blurred vision; allergy; worsening of schizophrenic symptoms; insomnia; and behavioral effects

[a]Except for the use of imipramine for enuresis in children over 6 years of age, imipramine-like drugs currently are not recommended for children under 12. Literature is available on their use in the age group under 12. Psychomotor stimulants are discussed in Chapter 9.

[b]Children 2 to 12 years of age. Dosage for adolescents is comparable to adult dosage. See Table 1-2 for dose forms.

[c]Recommended dosage for enuresis: 25 to 50 mg, 1 hour before bedtime.

established with well-controlled studies, although they are in wide use in mild to moderately severe anxiety and neurotic states.

a. **Diphenhydramine** in effective doses is a safe therapeutic agent in these conditions (see Section **IV.C.5.a**).

b. **Chlordiazepoxide** may evoke rage reactions or worsening of preexisting aggressiveness in certain individuals, as well as florid psychosis in some borderline patients. This drug is not approved by the Food and Drug Administration for children under 6 years of age.

c. Antianxiety agents are ineffective in severely disturbed children. **Diazepam** appears to be of no value, and it has been reported to increase anxiety.

    d. **Barbiturates,** too, may worsen anxiety and disorganization in psychotic children.

    e. **Chloral hydrate** can be used as a nighttime sedative in insomnia, in doses ranging from 0.25 to 1 gm (up to 2 gm) (10 to 50 mg/k of body weight). Preparations: 250, 500 mg capsules; Noctec syrup, 100 mg/ml.

4. **Anticonvulsants** The usefulness of diphenylhydantoin in the treatment of behavioral disorders in childhood has not been demonstrated consistently.

5. **Miscellaneous**

    a. **Diphenhydramine** is a safe drug and effective in mild to moderately severe behavior and organic disorders associated with hyperactivity, and in anxious neurotic children. It can be used as a bedtime sedative. The effective dosage range is 25 to 600 mg per day in four divided doses. Among its untoward effects are skin rash, and dryness of the mouth and nose. Diphenhydramine, in doses of 25 to 50 mg IM, is also effective in relieving acute dystonic reactions caused by neuroleptics. Preparations: 25 mg, 50 mg capsules; 10 mg/ml elixir; 10 mg/ml 50 mg/ml IM.

    b. **Promethazine** The sedative effect of promethazine* can be utilized as a nighttime medication and antianxiety agent. Its toxicity is low. However, rare cases of leukopenia and agranulocytosis have been reported. Dosage: 12.5 to 25 mg hs (oral, rectal, or intramuscular). Preparations: 25 mg/ml; tablets 12.5 mg, 25 mg, 50 mg; expectorant, 6.25 mg/5 ml, 25 mg/5 ml rectal suppositories, 25 mg, 50 mg.

    c. **Lithium** In adults, the main indication for the use of lithium is in manic-depressive illness. The role of lithium ion in treatment of behavioral disorders of childhood is not yet established, and its use in children under 12 years of age is under investigation. There are some suggestions in the literature that this agent may have a mood stabilizing and normalizing action in children (as young as 3 years of age) and adolescents with undulating or periodic disturbances of behavior and mood. (Shader, R. I., Jackson, A. H., and Dodes, L. M., The antiaggressive effects of lithium in man. *Psychopharmacologia*

---

*Editor's note: Promethazine is actually a phenothiazine. The authors have elected to classify it here because its antihistaminic properties link it to diphenhydramine.

40:17–24, 1974; Campbell, M., Fish, B., Korein, J., Shapiro, T., Collins, P., and Koh, C., Lithium and chlorpromazine: A controlled crossover study of hyperactive severely disturbed young children. *J. Austism Child. Schizo.* 2:234–263, 1972.) While it appears that lithium has antiaggressive effects in severely disturbed children when aggressiveness (against self or others) is associated with excitability and explosiveness, its therapeutic usefulness in psychotic children with other types of behavioral profiles is only slight. There is some evidence that lithium is ineffective in hyperactive children.

Daily dose range of lithium in children over 3 years of age is 450 to 1800 mg per day. Starting dose should be 450 mg per day with weekly increments (steps: 450, 600, 900, 1350, 1800 mg/day). Dosage should be increased until therapeutic or untoward effects occur. Plasma levels of lithium should be monitored at regular intervals (twice a week during the drug regulation period and weekly during the period of optimal dose). Plasma lithium level should average 0.6 to 1.2 mEq/L and should not exceed 1.8 mEq/L. Laboratory studies before and during lithium maintenance include white blood count, differential cell count, hematocrit reading, BUN, urinalysis, thyroxine iodine level, free thyroxine level, and ECG. For side effects of lithium and toxicity, see Chapter 5 for details of lithium therapy in adults. Lithium carbonate is available in 300 mg capsules or tablets.

d. **Triiodothyronine** (T_3, liothyronine, Cytomel) There is some clinical evidence that T_3 has antipsychotic and stimulating effects in young children who are clinically euthyroid. It is currently viewed as an agent that is potentially effective in the treatment of childhood schizophrenia and autism (*J. Autism Child. Schizo.* 2:343, 1972; *Arch. Gen. Psychiatry* 29:602, 1973).

V. **Poisoning and Overdosage** For information on the management of poisoning and overdosage with psychotropic drugs see Chapter 15.

References

For additional information on the therapeutic and side effects of various psychotropic drugs, special problems in the use of these drugs in children, and a detailed bibliography, the following references are particularly recommended.

Campbell, M. Pharmacotherapy in early infantile autism. *Biol. Psychiat.* 10:399, 1975.
Conners, C. K. Pharmacotherapy of Psychopathology in Children. In H. C. Quay and J. S. Werry (Eds.), *Psychopathological Disorders of Childhood.* New York: Wiley, 1972.

Eisenberg, L., and Conners, C. K. Psychopharmacology in Childhood. In N. B. Talbot, J. Kagan, and L. Eisenberg (Eds.), *Behavioral Science in Pediatric Medicine.* Philadelphia: Saunders, 1971.

Fish, B. Problems of diagnosis and the definition of comparable groups: A neglected issue in drug research with children. *Am. J. Psychiatry* 125:900, 1969.

Lipman, R. S. Pharmacotherapy of children (bibliography). *Psychopharmacol. Bull.* 7:14, 1971.

Shader, R. I., DiMascio, A., and associates. *Psychotropic Drug Side Effects.* Baltimore: Williams & Wilkins, 1970.

9

Diagnosis and Management of Minimal Brain Dysfunction

Paul H. Wender

Minimal brain dysfunction (MBD) is probably the single most common behavioral deviation seen in the pediatric age group. Recognition of the syndrome is of practical importance because effective therapy is readily available, relatively inexpensive, and much less time-consuming than that of many other psychiatric syndromes. Synonyms for MBD, all of which emphasize differential attributes of the syndrome, are as follows: minimal brain damage, hyperkinesis, hyperactive child syndrome, minimal cerebral injury or damage. In addition, MBD overlaps that group of children designated as suffering from "specific learning difficulties."

I. Characteristics

A. **Attentional deficits** Teachers and parents report that the child has difficulty with stick-to-it-iveness both in play patterns and at school work, and he is frequently described as distractible or having a "short attention span." This symptom may be the sine qua non of the syndrome.

B. **Hyperactivity** Motor hyperactivity is seen in many but *not all* MBD children. For this reason, the phrase *hyperactive child syndrome* is inaccurate and at times misleading; some MBD children are normoactive or hypoactive. The hyperactivity, when present, is often a striking sign and one that is manifested from early childhood. The child is described by parents and teachers as never able to sit still, always on the go, driven like a motor. This hyperactivity diminishes with age and may be absent, although the other signs may still be present, after puberty.

C. **Coordination** Approximately half of MBD children show some abnormalities of coordination. These may be in the area of fine motor coordination, the children showing difficulty in learning to tie their shoelaces, in cutting with scissors, in coloring, and later, in handwriting. These difficulties may also be in the area of gross balance, so that the child has difficulty in learning to roller skate or ride a two-wheeled bicycle. Finally, they may be present in the area of hand-eye coordination, so that the child is inept in sports requiring the throwing, catching, and hitting of balls.

D. **Emotional behavior**   Many MBD children show abnormalities in that sphere of behavior loosely designated as "emotional." In general, MBD children show age-inappropriate characteristics of younger children, including affective lability, a short temper (or "short fuse"), and a low frustration tolerance.

E. **Interpersonal behavior**   MBD children typically show abnormalities in interpersonal behavior between themselves and their peers and between themselves and adults. With peers, the MBD child is characteristically immature, bossy, and dominating. As a result, he frequently has few friends. This sort of friendlessness should be differentiated from that of the schizoid child, whose isolation stems from social anxiety. The MBD child is typically outgoing and extraverted; he seeks friends but loses them. Because of his unpopularity and need to dominate, he may choose to associate with more compliant associates, with younger children, or, if a boy, with girls. With regard to adults, the MBD child is frequently refractory to social reinforcers. Parents and teachers report that discipline is ineffective in curbing the child's behavior, and this lack of social responsiveness, together with impulsiveness, forms a frequent basis for the child's referral to a clinic. Minimal brain dysfunction should always be considered in the child who is globally described as having "behavior problems."

F. **Impulsiveness**   The MBD child is very frequently impulsive. The sort of impulsive behavior that is socially offensive changes as a function of age. In toddler and preschool years, it may be his tendency to sphincter "accidents." In elementary school it may be his rushing off pursuing his own interests, irrespective of those of his teacher (which are, in fact, usually opposite in kind), and in preteen and adolescent years it may be acting out or antisocial behavior, including stealing, drug abuse, or sexual promiscuity.

G. **Perceptual and learning problems**   An appreciable fraction of MBD children show abnormalities of perceptual performance on certain psychological tests and impaired learning in school even in the presence of a normal intelligence quotient (IQ). In fact, academic underachievement is almost a hallmark of this syndrome. Even in the absence of perceptual problems, academic performance may be impaired by decreased attentiveness and low frustration tolerance. Thus, once sensory problems, psychosocial problems, low IQ, and teaching inadequacies are ruled out, MBD must be considered the most common cause of poor school performance. Because routine psychological examination often fails to discover the existence of this problem, it is desirable to have an evaluation done by an educational psychologist.

II. **Incidence** MBD, at least as currently defined, is more common in boys than girls, the sex ratio generally being at least 2 to 1. The prevalence in the population is hard to specify because differing diagnostic criteria have been employed. The order of magnitude would seem to be between 3 and 7 percent, making it a common psychiatric problem.

III. **Prognosis** MBD was formerly thought to be an age-limited problem that disappeared at adolescence. Followup and retrospective studies suggest that it is the motor hyperactivity that most commonly disappears at adolescence, while other problems frequently persist. In its more severe forms, MBD may be the forerunner of a number of personality problems, including sociopathy. Untreated, it is a frequent cause of school dropout.

IV. **Etiology** In the past MBD was thought to be a disorder secondary to intrauterine or postnatal brain damage. Recent evidence suggests that an appreciable fraction of individuals suffering from MBD develop the disorder on a genetic basis. Fetal maldevelopment *may* account for a certain fraction of cases.

V. **Diagnosis** The diagnosis of MBD can best be made on the basis of a careful review of the child's history. Adequate history-taking demands a broader knowledge of the signs and symptoms of the syndrome than is given above, and the reader is referred to the literature for more detailed information (*Pediatr. Clin. North Am.* 20:187, 1973). Informants should include all those who have lived with the child, including parents, parent surrogates, and teachers. Open-ended interviews often result in underestimation of symptoms; therefore, common areas of psychological malfunctioning should be directly investigated. It is important to emphasize that the syndrome is just that, and that all of the signs and symptoms do not necessarily or frequently occur in a single patient.

A. **Neurologic examination** is needed to investigate all possible etiologies of the child's behavior. However, approximately half of the children with the syndrome do not have neurologic signs. Some authors suggest the importance of less obvious findings (e.g., large head size, high palate, slightly misshapen ears). The electroencephalogram has no demonstrated diagnostic utility.

B. **Psychological testing** As noted earlier, an appreciable percentage of MBD children manifest no significant dysfunction on routine psychological testing (as opposed to educational testing).

C. **Chronic behavioral deviance**   It should be apparent that there are no absolute diagnostic criteria for minimal brain dysfunction. On the basis of history and psychological test performance indicators, the physician may suspect the existence of the syndrome. At a down-to-earth level this means that any child who has manifested chronic behavioral deviance either at home, with his peers, or in his school, or who is showing inadequate school performance despite the presence of normal intelligence, adequate teaching, and adequate nutrition, must be suspected of having MBD.

D. The existence of **problems in the home** should not be considered as ruling out MBD. These children often have alcoholic, sociopathic, or inadequate parents; this may simply be a reflection of the same biologic abnormality in the parents rather than evidence of the psychological forces that have produced a psychological syndrome in the child.

   Despite the best diagnostic workup, uncertainty will frequently remain. In such instances, the patient deserves a therapeutic trial.

VI. **Management**

A. **Education of the family and the child concerning the nature of the problem**   The single most important element of adequate management is an explanation of the problem to the child's parents and — with proper modifications — to the child himself. As a rule, most parents of MBD children are angry, confused, and guilty, believing that their child's problems are a reflection of their inadequacy as parents. Some believe that the child is willful and that he needs to have discipline "beaten into him." These parents should be helped to understand how physiologic abnormalities within the child may generate many of the problems the child presents. They should be helped to distinguish between the child's congenital temperamental problems and problems that have been generated by their management of him. The advantages of parent education are the same as for those of the parents of the retarded child. As part of the education of the family, techniques of child-rearing should be introduced and discussed, including both general techniques and more specific techniques such as behavior modification. The latter is currently being investigated and may show some utility with some MBD children.

B. When education problems exist, **proper educational placement** is mandatory. Many MBD children, either because of perceptual problems or because of a lack of the stick-to-it-iveness and attentiveness that are prerequisites for adequate school performance, are performing badly in school. No technique of management can succeed unless the child is given academic placement consistent with his needs. This may require special classes if perceptual problems exist or catch-up classes when the child is of adequate intelligence or has no perceptual problems but has fallen behind in school. Unfortunately, such desirable educational placements are frequently difficult to obtain in the community.

C. **Medication** is of benefit for approximately 75 to 80 percent of MBD children. Its effect, though often dramatic, is only suppressive, and this may necessitate medication being continued for several years until the child's signs and symptoms are reduced in intensity. In a few instances, the time course involved may be as many as 5 to 10 years.

1. The drugs of choice are the **stimulant drugs** — the amphetamines and methylphenidate. Overall, methylphenidate may be the more effective of the two, although an occasional child does better on amphetamines. An advantage of the amphetamines is that they are available in long-acting form, they are generically available, hence cheaper, and their absorption is not impaired by food. When maximally effective, the stimulant drugs do more than simply "calm" the child. They frequently reverse many of the psychological abnormalities described and promote "psychological growth" to an extent not seen before the drugs were administered. Many children will develop a longer attention span, increased frustration tolerance, greater emotional stability, increased social perceptiveness, and increased sensitivity to the requests and demands of peers and parents.

   Methylphenidate is administered in two (or three) daily divided doses — morning, noon, and possibly after school. It should be given at least one-half hour before meals. The amphetamines have a slightly longer duration of action and are usually given in morning and noon doses or in a once-daily long-acting dose. Total daily dose ranges for the drugs would be roughly: methylphenidate, 10 to 80 mg per day; d-amphetamine, 5 to 40 mg per day. The general procedure of administration is to begin the drugs at a low dose and increase the dose until the point of maximum therapeutic benefit or the presence of side effects is reached. Side effects include appetite loss, irritability, stomachaches, headaches, and insomnia if given too late in the day. Addiction to these drugs does not occur in childhood, and *in general* tolerance does not occur. Some children will do relatively well on a given dose for a period of one or two months and then backslide. In most such instances, increasing the dose does not result in further development of tolerance. In an occasional child, tolerance will develop to one of the stimulant drugs, and the general practice then is to switch to a member of the other class.

2. A number of **other drugs** have been used in the treatment of MBD children when the stimulant drugs have been ineffective. These include the major antipsychotic (neuroleptic) drugs and the major antidepressant drugs. Clinical consensus would seem to be as follows: The **antipsychotic drugs** (e.g., chlorpromazine, thioridazine) often will quiet a grossly hyperactive or aggressive child. However, these agents often decrease a child's attention span and hence further compromise the child in whom such a deficit already exists, thereby impairing academic performance. In most instances they do not have a beneficial effect on social refractoriness. These agents are more frequently associated with idiosyncratic reactions and other undesirable side effects. These unwanted effects do not constitute an absolute contraindication, but their use should be reserved for aggressive or unmanageable children who prove refractory to other agents.

More recently, the **tricyclic antidepressants** (e.g., imipramine) have been claimed to be of value in the management of some MBD children. Experience suggests that they are effective in larger doses than is claimed on the package inserts. Imipramine may be effective in small doses (e.g., 10 mg each morning), but some children show a positive dose-response curve to doses of up to 200 mg a day. Experience with other tricyclic antidepressants is more limited. Overall, they do not seem as effective as the stimulant drugs, and some children who respond initially become tolerant to their effects. A variety of other agents also have been used in the treatment of MBD children. These include anticonvulsant drugs, antihistamines such as diphenhydramine, and minor tranquilizers such as diazepam. In general, these agents have not proved to be consistently effective.

D. **Specific psychological therapies for the child and family** Psychotherapy, narrowly construed, has not been shown to be an effective agent in the treatment of MBD children. There is no doubt, even in the absence of controlled studies, that reduction of family tensions and structuring of the child's psychological environment are frequently of benefit. In those instances in which psychiatric pathology in the parent prevents him or her from modifying behavior toward the child, psychotherapy for the parents is useful when it is able to help the parents to change their behavior toward the child. Adequate psychological management of the child's problems includes an explanation to the child of the basis of his problems in terms that the child can understand. In an occasional older MBD child whose problems have received attention only after he has suffered the cumulative psychological effects of the syndrome for some years, psychotherapy may be of some benefit.

10

Psychopharmacology and the Geriatric Patient

Carl Salzman
Bessel van der Kolk
Richard I. Shader

Advanced age often presents a complex interaction of physical illness, reduced cognitive functioning, and psychopathology. In a society that is oriented toward the future and in which productivity and physical appearance are highly regarded virtues, the elderly may find themselves increasingly estranged and isolated. The psychiatrist is typically consulted when, as a result of these progressive multifaceted problems, family, friends, and other members of society or the other helping professions are unable to offer assistance. Characteristically, the elderly patient has now reached a level of disordered sleep, behavior, mood, or cognitive functioning that necessitates intervention with somatic therapy. Yet it is these special medical, cultural, social, and psychopathologic consequences of aging that demand particular thoughtfulness before appropriate and useful therapy can be effected. An appreciation of the many interactions between somatic therapy and altered biologic functioning, of the particular toxic consequences of somatic therapy in advanced age, and of the interaction between medical and psychiatric drug treatment is a prerequisite to effective psychiatric intervention.

I. **Etiology of Psychiatric Problems in the Elderly** Old age is characterized by the necessity of dealing with losses. Self-image and self-esteem wither as the external world, which once was the domain of the patient, gradually becomes less familiar through the loss of occupation, friends, social and cultural functions, and physical capacities.

   A. A psychiatric evaluation should include a careful **personal history** obtained from the patient and family or friends. Special emphasis should be placed on the following:

   1. Present as well as previous losses, including such catastrophic events as the loss of a spouse or close friend, or loss of a body function, or such seemingly minor deprivations as the loss of a pet, a hearing aid, dentures, or a familiar object in the environment.

   2. Responses to previous crises and losses and the means that the patient had at his disposal to deal with these crises. These involve both intrapsychic defenses and significant supportive persons in the patient's life.

3. The patient's attitude and adjustment to his present life circumstances, retirement, interests, and important persons in his life. It is helpful to get a picture of a typical day in the patient's life and of the highlights of the past few months.

4. Attitudes toward aging, its effects on self and spouse, and its effects on memory, sexual desires, and activity. Experiences with old age in parents and siblings.

5. A review of the patient's life, accomplishments, and disappointments; landmarks in the patient's life.

6. Attitudes toward religion, changes in church affiliation, if any; feelings about and preparations for death.

From this material the physician may derive an impression of the patient's prior adaptation, the quality of interpersonal relations, the prior existence of neuroses or psychoses, and the general level of mental and emotional strength.

B. A review of the patient's **present and past medical history,** as well as **thorough physical and neurologic examinations,** are part of every psychiatric evaluation. Four groups of physical disturbances may precipitate psychiatric symptoms in the elderly:

1. Bodily discomforts: e.g., pain, thirst, overheating, cold, or rectal and vesical distension.

2. Disturbed metabolism: e.g., fever, toxemia, electrolyte imbalance, hypovitaminosis, or defects in protein or carbohydrate metabolism.

3. Organic and functional states: e.g., cerebral anoxia, cerebral edema, meningitis, encephalitis, cerebrovascular accident, brain abscess, or brain tumor.

4. Pharmaceutical agents: Frequent offenders are bromides, opiates, and anticholinergic agents (those employed in the treatment of parkinsonism as well as those contained in over-the-counter preparations — see Appendix IV). Overmedication, especially with the psychotropic drugs, is a common problem in the elderly and frequently accounts for withdrawal, lethargy, and somnolence. Confusion and agitation in the evening are common, especially in patients on psychotropic drugs with hypotensive side effects. The natural drop in blood pressure toward evening combined with drug-induced hypotension may cause cerebral anoxia and its resultant psychiatric symptoms.

II. **General Principles of Pharmacology in the Aged** As the human organism ages there is a general trend for drugs to stay in the body longer, to have more prolonged biologic activity, and hence generally to have more powerful clinical and toxic effects on the organism.

Many psychoactive drugs are lipid-soluble. Because blood triglycerides increase with age, lipid-soluble drugs tend to be kept in the lipid compartment for a longer period of time. As the ratio of fat to parenchyma increases with age, lipid-soluble compounds are absorbed more easily and tend to accumulate in the fatty tissues. Some lipid-soluble compounds do not bind to plasma proteins but depend on other metabolic processes for elimination and secretion. Other compounds may be altered both by changes in the lipid compartment and by altered protein binding. A decrease in liver parenchyma causes a decrease in the metabolic enzymes needed for the rapid breakdown of psychoactive drugs. Hence, some metabolites may be formed more slowly in the aged, thereby prolonging drug activity. Protein fractions may also be reduced, which can have prominent effects on metabolism and binding.

Alterations in cardiac and renal functioning further contribute to extended biologic activity. A decrease in cardiac output and an increase in circulation time delay the circulation and distribution of drugs in the elderly. Renal blood flow, glomerular filtration rate, and tubular secretion diminish markedly with old age. The renal tubules reabsorb lipid-soluble compounds, so their duration of action is limited by their conversion to less lipid-soluble metabolites.

In the aged brain there is a gradual but dramatic loss of neurons, which are replaced by glial cells. The loss of functional neuronal tissue may be responsible for an increased sensitivity of the brain to the pharmacologic actions of drugs.

A. **Pretreatment evaluation** In addition to careful psychiatric evaluation, the medical condition of any elderly patient who is to receive somatic therapy must be accurately determined. Pretreatment assessment should include: blood pressure, erect and supine; complete blood count; total protein and albumin and globulin ratios; urinalysis; ECG; brief neurologic examination.

B. **Dosage** Intuitively, most physicians prescribe psychotropic drugs at lower dosages for elderly patients. As a general rule of thumb, starting doses and maintenance doses should be one-third to one-half those for younger adults. Increases in dosage should be gradual.

C. **Followup** Careful somatic therapy requires regular examination of a patient's physical health. For those who receive neuroleptic or antidepressant medication, biweekly checks of CBC and daily recordings of pulse and blood pressure are indicated during the first six weeks of treatment. A brief neurologic examination should be carried out at regular intervals in any patient receiving long-term neuroleptic or antidepressant treatment.

III. **Hazards and Precautions** All psychotropic drugs have some degree of toxicity. The elderly are more susceptible to all side effects because of their decreased ability to withstand stress, their already impaired organ systems, and their modified pharmacologic response to drugs.

A. **Cardiovascular side effects** The neuroleptics, particularly those phenothiazines having aliphatic (e.g., chlorpromazine) and piperidine (e.g., thioridazine) side chains, and the tricyclic antidepressants, which are structurally closely related, may produce serious orthostatic hypotension. Profound changes could expose the patient to cardiovascular or cerebrovascular insufficiency. Hypotension also can aggravate the symptoms of basilar artery insufficiency. A common complication of hypotension in the elderly is episodes of syncope that may lead to falls and resultant fractures, particularly of the hip. Epinephrine should not be used to counteract drug-induced hypotensi since it may cause a paradoxical lowering of the blood pressure.

Neuroleptics and antidepressants may cause tachycardia and arrhythmias. Sudden death, possibly secondary to arrhythmias, congestive heart failure, and sudden development of massive edema have been observed with both phenothiazines and tricyclic antidepressants. Such complications are rare, except for tachycardia and arrhythmias, but they do occur. They are not limited to the elderly, but their consequences obviously could be more profound in the elderly, particularly those with poor nutritional status.

Nonspecific ECG changes have been observed with neuroleptics and tricyclic antidepressants. They are most often manifested by a prolongation of the QT interval, a lowering and inversion of the T wave, and the appearance of either a bicuspid T wave or a U wave. These ECG changes are not correlated consistently with myocardial damage, and their clinical significance is largely unknown. At the present time, one working hypothesis is that these changes are a reflection of an efflux of cellular potassium.

B. **Neurologic side effects** Older people are generally more susceptible to the neurologic side effects of psychotropic drugs than are younger adults. **Extrapyramidal side effects** associated with neuroleptics are common in the elderly. Whereas the occurrence of dystonias diminishes with increasing age, the peak incidence of akathisia is between the ages of 40 and 50, and that of akinetic parkinsonian side effects is around 80 years. Akinetic parkinsonism usually starts 4 to 21 days after the onset of therapy and almost never arises de novo after three months. Antiparkinsonian agents are usually effective in keeping drug-induced parkinsonism under control, but they act additively with the anticholinergic effects of neuroleptics and antidepressants. Whenever possible, a decrease in the offending agent is the more advisable treatment approach. Since the incidence of extrapyramidal side effects is highest with neuroleptics having piperazine side chains and with haloperidol, these compounds should be used with caution in the elderly.

Tardive dyskinesia is a syndrome that includes disfiguring involuntary buccal and lingual masticatory movements. It occurs most typically in patients who have received high doses of neuroleptics for more than six months and is, at present, incurable. It is seen more in elderly females than in males. The physician may be able to reduce the risk of producing tardive dyskinesia by:

1. Minimizing the unnecessary use of neuroleptic medication (especially in high doses) in chronically ill patients. Many of the latter can be satisfactorily maintained for long periods without antipsychotic drugs. Drug-free holidays are advised in patients receiving long-term medication.

2. Discontinuing neuroleptics, if possible, at the first sign of abnormal oral or lingual movements or other possible manifestations of tardive dyskinesia.

Central nervous system symptoms, such as depression, paradoxical agitation, delirium, confusion, assaultiveness, delusions, and hallucinations, are found with increasing incidence and severity in the elderly in response to treatment with psychoactive drugs. Sedative-hypnotic agents, including the benzodiazepines, may cause fatigue, lethargy, and loss of ambition in the elderly. Lithium carbonate may cause generalized neuromuscular irritability and impairment of consciousness without focal neurologic signs.

C. **Side effects due to cholinergic blocking properties** The neuroleptics, the tricyclic antidepressants, and the antiparkinsonian agents all have marked cholinergic blocking properties that give rise to such symptoms as dryness of the mouth, loss of ocular accommodation, constipation (in rare instances leading to paralytic ileus), hypotension, incoordination, vertigo, sweating, urinary retention, atonic bladder, and increase in intraocular pressure (aggravating glaucoma). These anticholinergic effects are additive, thus making the use of antiparkinsonian agents in conjunction with neuroleptics potentially hazardous. Urinary retention may be of particular concern in men with prostatic hypertrophy.

Aggravation of glaucoma is of concern in the undiagnosed case
(the evaluation of elderly patients should include questions about
eye pain, seeing halos around lights, and the like). Systemic anticholinergic effects of psychotropic drugs rarely are strong enough to
override the treated glaucoma case. Anticholinergic effects also may
be of concern in patients with disturbances of cardiac rhythm.

D. **Allergic reactions** All allergic reactions to psychotropic drugs occur
with greater frequency among the geriatric population. Seventy
percent of all cases of agranulocytosis occur in patients between
the ages of 48 and 70. The phenothiazines are primarily responsible
for agranulocytosis and monocytosis in the elderly, although a few
rare cases of agranulocytosis due to tricyclic antidepressants and
meprobamate have been reported. Cholestatic jaundice has been
reported in up to 4 percent of all elderly patients on phenothiazines.
Dermatitis medicamentosa is found in up to 4 percent of geriatric
patients who receive phenothiazines. Sunlight aggravates drug-induced
dermatitis, and photosensitivity is high in geriatric patients. Chlorpromazine seems to cause more photosensitivity than do the other
phenothiazines. Pigmentary changes and cornea and lens deposits
occur in the elderly, as they do in the young. Retinal changes can
occur with thioridazine on doses exceeding 800 mg.

IV. **Somatic Treatment of Psychiatric Illness in the Elderly** Although advanced age is not a barrier to any form of psychiatric illness, most
problems requiring somatic treatment fall within one of four symptom
clusters: Behavioral disturbances, disorders of affect (depression and
anxiety), impaired cognitive functioning, and problems with sleep. Within
any category, there is a wide range of symptom severity; treatment
principles follow those established in younger populations. Thus, mild
disturbances require modest somatic treatment efforts with emphasis
placed on therapy for psychological and interpersonal problems. The
more severely disturbed elderly patient requires greater somatic therapy
intervention. Indeed, it is common to find that most nursing home
residents and elderly hospital inpatients with psychiatric problems are
receiving some form of somatic therapy.

A. **Treatment of behavioral disorders** Behavioral disturbances in the
elderly may result from psychotic, organic, or affective disorders.
Most schizophrenic and psychotic processes begin earlier and persist
into old age, when they may be accompanied by clear organic change
Psychosis that begins after 65 is almost always of the paranoid variety
(late paraphrenia) and is characterized by symptoms of agitation,
paranoid delusions, emotional distress, grandiosity, thought disorder,

and auditory hallucinations. So-called involutional psychotic reactions are characterized by depression (guilt, low self-esteem, self-deprecation, hypochondriasis), florid paranoid ideation, and agitated behavior. Late life depressions are often associated with severe agitation. The most frequent behavioral disturbances that accompany organic processes in the elderly include agitation, assaultiveness, noisiness, and wandering. The symptoms may fluctuate in intensity and often appear worse at night (sundowner's syndrome).

In geriatric patients, severe behavioral disturbances accompanying organic, psychotic, and affective illness provide a delicate treatment challenge for which a satisfactory solution cannot always be found. Neuroleptic agents are usually the treatment of choice. Most neuroleptics have a basically equivalent degree of usefulness in the geriatric patient population. Since these compounds do differ in the general pattern of side effects that are produced, selection of a particular drug depends more on these unwanted effects than on differential therapeutic efficacy. Representative compounds are presented in Table 10-1 (see Appendix III for a more complete list of available neuroleptics).

Aliphatic compounds such as chlorpromazine are high in sedative and hypotensive effects and thus have limited usefulness in patients who sleep during the day or who may seriously suffer from an orthostatic hypotensive episode. The sedative effects of chlorpromazine may be used to advantage at bedtime, however, or to help quiet an extremely agitated, uncontrolled patient. The piperazines and the butyrophenone, haloperidol, produce little hypotension and sedation but frequently cause extrapyramidal symptoms that may aggravate the discomfort of an elderly patient who already experiences difficulties in motor coordination. Among piperazine phenothiazine derivatives, acetophenazine produces the fewest extrapyramidal symptoms and is well tolerated by the elderly. Haloperidol, which produces significant extrapyramidal symptoms but minimal sedation or hypotension, can be considered for patients who have serious difficulties maintaining their blood pressure.

Acute agitation, severe psychotic outbursts, and crippling anxiety attacks often necessitate parenteral medication. Diazepam (5 mg IM) and mesoridazine or chlorpromazine (10 to 25 mg IM) have proved effective. Blood pressure should be monitored, and patients should be urged to lie down after intramuscular administration. Barbiturates generally should be avoided in the control of agitation and confusion in the elderly since cerebral anoxia secondary to depressed respiration may enhance the symptoms.

Table 10-1. Neuroleptics Recommended in the Elderly[a]

Generic Name	Trade Name	Usual Geriatric Dose (mg/day)	Relative Side Effects		
			Sedation	Hypotension	Extrapyramidal Symptoms
Chlorpromazine	Thorazine Chlor-PZ	50 to 300	Marked	Marked	Occasional
Thioridazine	Mellaril	50 to 300	Moderate	Moderate	Infrequent
Acetophenazine	Tindal	10 to 60	Mild	Mild	Occasional
Trifluoperazine	Stelazine	5 to 20	Minimal	Minimal	Frequent
Haloperidol	Haldol	1 to 6	Minimal	Minimal	Frequent

a .... with .... dibenzoxazepines in geriatric patients has not been as widely documented as the other drugs

Mania and hypomania occur with reduced frequency in old age. Symptoms include overactivity, poor judgment, hostility (verging on paranoia), and aggressiveness. Neuroleptics have proved useful. However, since extreme manic behavior is less common in the elderly, they have been largely supplanted by treatment with lithium carbonate. Cardiovascular, thyroid, and renal function must be carefully evaluated before commencement of lithium therapy (see Chapter 5). The incidence of lithium toxicity is higher among old people; the onset of coma may be quite sudden, without prodromal symptoms. Therapeutic and maintenance levels of lithium carbonate therefore must be carefully monitored and usually kept below levels recommended for younger adults.

Extrapyramidal symptoms that are produced by antipsychotic medication may be controlled with antiparkinsonian agents. These agents have strong anticholinergic properties that add to similar properties of the antipsychotic drugs. Thus, routine antiparkinsonian drug administration should be avoided; drug use should await the appearance of symptoms (see Section III.C).

B. **Treatment of depression** Depression of varying severity is common in advanced age. The development of symptoms may be insidious, with no clear precipitant, and increasing social isolation and deterioration of mental and physical capacities may aggravate the mood disturbance. Severe depression in the elderly often includes agitation or withdrawal and isolation, early morning insomnia, and severe anorexia. Somatic delusions, confusion, hostility, and increasing dementia may accompany depression and sometimes confuse the clinical picture. Depressed elderly patients, especially white males, may be high suicide risks; the only warning may be hypochondriasis of recent origin.

1. **Antidepressant medication** Tricyclic antidepressants are often effective in the treatment of mild to moderately severe late life depressions (see Table 1-2). In the healthy patient under 60 years of age,* these compounds may be used as they would in younger adults. The starting oral dose is usually 25 mg bid or tid, with dosage increments of 25 mg, leading to a therapeutic dose range of 150 to 250 mg/day. It is generally advisable to give a test dose of 10 to 25 mg and after 30 to 45 minutes examine the patient sitting and standing to check for orthostatic hypotension. Because of the potentially serious complications of a hypotensive episode, blood pressure should be checked prior to the onset of medication and then followed at weekly intervals until a stable dose level is achieved. In patients who are over age 60,* or who have unstable

---

*Editor's note: The choice of age 60 is arbitrary. It is meant merely to call attention to the issue of advancing age as a factor in patients' susceptibility to drug effects.

cardiovascular function, the side effects of tricyclics are likely to be more hazardous. Starting doses should be no more than 40 mg/day, with weekly increments of no more than 25 mg/week, leading to a therapeutic dose range of 75 to 150 mg/day. Blood pressure and cardiac rhythm must be checked repeatedly.

Amitriptyline may be somewhat more effective than imipramine in women. Imipramine has some activating properties that may lead to increased agitation and restlessness in anxious patients, while amitriptyline has more sedative effects, especially when first used. The new tricyclic antidepressants, such as desipramine, nortriptyline, and protriptyline, all are effective antidepressants that hold no particular advantage over the older tricyclics. The activating properties of both protriptyline and nortriptyline may be useful in anergic and apathetic states but make these drugs unsuitable for patients with a large anxiety component to their depression. Doxepin may have some benefit when depression is mild and accompanied by manifest anxiety (see Chapter 1, Section II.C.2). Neuroleptics may have a significant role in the treatment of some depressions. Thioridazine, for example, has been shown in some studies to be more effective than imipramine in the treatment of agitated and anxious depressions.

Precautions: *The tricyclic antidepressants may activate psychotic or manic symptoms in patients with underlying schizophrenic, schizoaffective, or manic-depressive illness.* Tricyclic antidepressants also may produce toxic confusional states in the elderly with visual hallucinations, disorientation, delusions, anxiety, agitation, insomnia, and nightmares.

The monoamine oxidase inhibitors adversely interact with many medical drugs and may cause such serious side effects so as to make their routine use in the elderly too hazardous when weighed against their potential benefits. Psychomotor stimulants such as the amphetamines or methylphenidate may cause increased agitation, confusion, and disorientation and should not be used to treat depression in the elderly. In low doses, they may have some positive effect on mild states of apathy and anergy.

2. **Electroconvulsive therapy** As mentioned earlier, serious depression in the elderly has lethal potential, either resulting from suicide or as a consequence of severe anorexia and insomnia leading to inanition and exhaustion. For these reasons, rapid treatment of severe depression may be a life-saving procedure. Since tricyclic medication may require several weeks to produce clinical relief of depression, a faster-acting alternative treatment is often needed — electroconvulsive therapy. This treatment procedure, when

Table 10-2. Summary of ECT Problems in the Elderly

Problem	Considerations
Increase in confusion; acute organic brain syndrome	Use unilateral treatment to the nondominant hemisphere
	Use fewer treatments than for younger adults; 2 to 6 treatments will usually suffice
	Space treatments to avoid compounding of the confusion following each treatment; use at least an alternate-day treatment schedule
Cardiac arrhythmias	Get a pretreatment ECG, and then follow cardiac rhythm during treatment with a cardiac monitor or ECG
	Use of pretreatment atropine may protect patient against poststimulus arrhythmias; may need higher doses of atropine in elderly patients
	In patients with recent history of infarctions and arrhythmias, pretreatment with lidocaine may be indicated; a cardiologist or internist should attend the treatment of elderly patients with serious cardiac pathology; hyperoxygenate just prior to treatment
Augmentation of hypertension	Consider elimination of or reduction in dose of pretreatment atropine
	Pretreatment with 5 mg of diazepam IM may protect against a large increase in blood pressure
Increased susceptibility to fractures	Requires careful determination of adequate dose of succinylcholine to achieve complete muscle relaxation
Prolonged sleep	May require lower dose of barbiturate anesthesia
Prolonged apnea	Serum pseudocholinesterase may be reduced or absent due to hydrolysis by another medication, such as echothiophate treatment for glaucoma

properly administered, is safe, rapid, and remarkably effective in alleviating the symptoms of severe depression. The reader is asked to refer to Chapter 6, which describes more specifically the use of ECT. A summary of the problems with ECT that have particular relevance to the elderly is presented in Table 10-2.

C. Treatment of anxiety Neurotic disturbances in the elderly typically arise at a younger age. Loss of important people, feelings of uselessness, and the experience of physical and intellectual deterioration may serve to aggravate preexisting neurotic conditions. A heightening of old neurotic defenses is a common response to the onset of an organic brain syndrome. Neurotic symptoms in the elderly usually take the form of anxiety, depression, and obsessive-compulsive behavior. Hypochondriasis, lethargy, or restlessness and agitation are often accompanying symptoms. Psychotherapy with the patient, as well as intervention in his social environment and in his family, is of prime importance in the treatment of neurotic symptoms in the elderly. Within the past 15 years, the traditional use of low doses of barbiturates (e.g., phenobarbital) has been replaced by other, less toxic antianxiety agents. Antianxiety agents may be of considerable assistance in managing anxiety and agitation in the elderly (see Appendix II). Side effects of antianxiety agents include drowsiness, often even at lower doses than those used in younger adults, particularly with drugs having long half-lives. Diazepam, for example, tends to accumulate in the blood, and a useful clinical regimen might be to omit one dose every other day. Ataxia and incoordination may occur and may result in falls and fractures. See also Chapter 2.

D. **Treatment of cognitive disorders: organic brain syndrome** Organic brain syndrome is defined as any mental disorder caused by or associated with diffuse impairment of brain tissue function. At least 50 percent of the geriatric population in mental hospitals and nursing homes suffer from this syndrome. In addition, a sizable number of noninstitutionalized elderly (with estimates up to 30 percent) have such symptoms.

1. **Acute organic brain syndrome** Acute organic brain syndrome is defined as reversible impairment of brain tissue function. The onset is usually sudden, and an underlying organic cause can be found. Precipitants include (1) bodily discomforts, (2) disturbance in metabolism, (3) organic and functional states, and (4) pharmacologic agents, toxins, and alcohol. The symptoms of acute organic brain syndrome include: sudden restlessness, confusion, disorientation, disordered behavior, incontinence, and hallucinosis. Treatment consists of diagnosis and remedying the underlying cause of the syndrome. Agitation and uncontrolled behavior can be controlled by use of phenothiazines and related compounds (see Section **IV.A**).

2. **Chronic organic brain syndrome** The symptoms and signs of chronic organic brain syndrome include impairment of recent and remote memory, deficit in immediate recall, disorientation, lack of attention and concentration, fluctuation of state of consciousness, and impairment of judgment and social functioning. The patient's symptoms may get worse when he is removed from familiar surroundings and at night. An acute organic brain syndrome may be superimposed upon an already existing chronic condition.

   The patient's response to his mental impairment is largely a function of his remaining cortical functioning, his premorbid personality, and his present life circumstances: changes in mood and behavior frequently accompany the development of chronic organic brain syndrome. One may see such diverse symptoms as anxiety, agitation, depression, apathy, withdrawal, paranoid ideation, delusions, and hallucinations. Supportive individual, group, milieu, and family therapy may be of great value to patients who are mildly or moderately impaired by chronic organic brain syndrome. Physical and mental stimulation as well as meaningful interpersonal interactions are essential to keep the patient from further deterioration.

Cerebral vasodilators have been claimed by some to increase the blood flow to ischemic areas in arteriosclerotic brains. Controlled studies have yielded inconsistent results. Positive findings tend to be in the area of improved socialization and behavior rather than in consistently improved intellectual functioning. Cerebral vasodilators are not specific for the brain, hence they may produce hypotension. The best-studied vasodilators are cyclandelate given in doses of 800 to 1200 mg per day and papaverine given in doses of 150 mg every 12 hours.

Dihydrogenated ergot alkaloids (e.g., Hydergine) have been shown to act on the metabolism of brain cells. Most studies done with Hydergine have demonstrated modest improvement in social functioning and mood, but there has not been consistent improvement of intellectual functioning. Hydergine does not cause hypotension, and no significant side effects have been noted with the usual dose of 4 to 6 sublingual tablets per day.

Pentylenetetrazol (Metrazol), anticoagulants, RNA and RNA precursors, procaine, glutamic acid, vitamin B, pipradol, and hyperbaric oxygen therapy all have been proposed for the treatment of organic brain syndrome with incomplete or ambiguous results.

Depression, which frequently accompanies progressive organic brain syndrome, may further compromise intellectual functioning. Following successful alleviation of the depression there may be a demonstrable improvement in memory. Clinically, many cases of early senile deterioration are actually depressive equivalents in which the symptoms result from a withdrawal of interest in daily functions. Psychotherapy that helps the patient to put his life in perspective can be helpful. Antidepressants also may help in some cases.

E. **Treatment of disorders of sleep**   Insomnia, a frequent complaint of the elderly, usually can be categorized as difficulty in falling asleep or early morning awakening. Mild difficulties in falling asleep are very common in the elderly and may be attributed to daytime napping, anxiety about the future, or physical distress (see Chapter 1 for a discussion of hypnotic agents). Confusional states and paradoxical agitation following barbiturate ingestion are well known in the elderly. Chloral hydrate, 250 to 1000 mg given at bedtime, is a drug of time-proved effectiveness. Although it rarely causes paradoxical excitement the treating physician should be alert for this unwanted effect. As noted in Chapter 1, flurazepam has the least effect on suppression of REM sleep. Mild insomnia may also be safely treated with occasional evening or bedtime doses of antianxiety agents or chlorpromazine (25 to 50 mg) without significant suppression of REM sleep.

Early morning awakening is also common in advanced age. Mild disruptions of sleep may be due to physical discomfort. More severe awakening and inability to return to sleep are often symptoms of late life depression. Treatment of the affective disorder often alleviate early morning awakening.

Precautions: One of more frequent toxic consequences of nocturna sedation occurs when old people awaken at night to use the bathroom Falls due to confusion and unsteadiness are a constant danger. Since nocturnal sedation greatly increases the incidence of such falls, the lowest possible dosage should be used at all times. In some instances side rails for the bed may be essential.

11

Bad Trips

David J. Greenblatt
Richard I. Shader

"Bad trip" refers to an adverse drug reaction following the use of a pharmacologic agent for purposes of pleasure. Since self-harm is not the intent of drug use, bad trips usually do not involve overdosage of the drug in question. Patients with acute poisoning from psychotropic drugs (see Chapter 15) present with various degrees of central nervous system depression. "Trippers," however, are awake and usually responsive, manifesting any of a variety of possible symptoms, signs, and alterations of mental status. Bad trips occur when actual drug effects deviate from the desired ones. Manifestations can be the actual pharmacologic effects (e.g., unwanted hallucinations, distorted perceptions, dysphoric affect, delirium) or the patient's emotional reaction to them (e.g., depression, despair, fear, panic). It is not always possible to distinguish drug-induced changes in mental status, mood, and affect from the patient's response to the experience.

Many drugs produce bad trips. Most notable are the illicit hallucinogens (LSD, mescaline, psilocybin, marijuana), which have no established therapeutic use and are exclusively drugs of abuse. A number of legitimate therapeutic agents also are used for consciousness-altering purposes. These include amphetamines, anticholinergics, antihistamines, and certain sedative-hypnotics (barbiturates, glutethimide, methaqualone). The hallucinogenic properties of scopolamine-containing proprietary hypnotics have recently been exploited on a large scale. Obviously, bad trips can also follow alcohol ingestion or abuse of other CNS depressants.

I. **Epidemiologic Determinants of Bad Trips** Why, how often, and in whom bad trips occur are questions for which there are no adequate answers. Many investigators and experienced drug-takers express the impression that a number of nondrug factors may be powerful determinants of the response to agents deliberately used for hallucinogenic or consciousness-altering purposes. The following factors are frequently mentioned in the literature. It should be emphasized again that this list has been generated by clinical impression and intuition rather than controlled study.

   A. **The setting** Bad trips often occur when subjects are in an unfamiliar place, alone, or with unfamiliar people. Conversely, intimate sympathetic groups and familiar surroundings are conducive to favorable drug experiences. An experienced, knowledgeable drug-taker who serves as group leader (guru) can do much to guide the novice and prevent unwanted drug reactions.

B. **The subject**

1. **Prior drug experience**   Bad trips appear to be less common in experienced drug-users, particularly when their previous drug experiences have been favorable.

2. **Expectation**   Subjects who do not anticipate characteristic drug-induced changes in perception, mood, and mental status can be surprised, frightened, or even panic-stricken when they occur. On the other hand, those who expect orgasmic, "mind-blowing" drug effects can become despondent or profoundly depressed if they do not occur. Many individuals having unfavorable drug experience report grandiose revelations on the state of humanity or the universe that are extremely depressing or anxiety-provoking.

3. **Emotional state**   This is a controversial and complex determinant of the subjective response to pleasure-giving drugs. Many clinicians feel that individuals who are emotionally stable and well-adjusted benefit most or are harmed least by drugs of abuse, while those who are labile of affect and who have difficulty coping with ambiguity, uncertainty, dysphoric sensations, or distorted perceptions are more likely to experience adverse drug reactions. From the same line of reasoning comes the concept that drug-related psychoses merely represent an unmasking of prepsychotic tendencies already present, thus hastening a psychotic episode that would have occurred eventually. These conceptual links between drug response and premorbid personality make intuitive sense, but their validity has not yet been conclusively demonstrated.

II.   **Classification of Bad Trips**   Adverse reactions to drugs of abuse can be divided into three categories depending on when they take place relative to drug use.

A. **Acute reactions** occur shortly after the drug is ingested. The causal relationship to drug-taking is usually obvious.

1. **Apprehension, fear, and panic** are common sequelae of hallucinogenic drug abuse. They occur when distortions in perception or affect are anxiety-provoking rather than pleasurable. Subjects who experience hallucinations may find them ego-dystonic and intrusive. Some individuals are simply afraid that they are "losing their minds."

2. **Psychotic-like reactions** (including hallucinations, lability of affect, and delusions) can follow abuse of amphetamines or hallucinogens. In some patients, these manifestations are ego-dystonic and can be attenuated or terminated by reality testing. In others, psychosis can merge with disorientation and delirium. Occasionally subjects cause harm to themselves or others during such drug-induced psychoses.

3. **Delirium** is said to occur when orientation is lost and cognition is significantly impaired. Drug-induced delirium is usually accompanied by hyperactivity or combativeness. Psychosis frequently merges with delirium in bad trips due to hallucinogens, anticholinergics, or antihistamines. In amphetamine abuse, however, delirium is usually absent.

4. **"Crash"** refers to an episode of depression of mood, which characteristically follows termination of a "speed" (amphetamine) trip. This depression can be profound and can even precipitate suicide attempts.

5. **Adrenergic crisis** can accompany the psychosis of acute amphetamine intoxication and sometimes constitutes a medical emergency. Possible manifestations include diaphoresis, mydriasis, tachycardia, hypertension, hyperpyrexia, cardiac arrhythmias, and seizures. Adrenergic hyperactivity also may accompany hallucinogen abuse, but then it is usually less severe.

6. **Anticholinergic crisis** follows ingestion of atropine-like drugs or antihistamines. Tachycardia, mydriasis (unresponsive to light), absent sweating, dry skin and mucous membranes, paralytic ileus, urinary retention, and hyperpyrexia are common manifestations.

7. **Obtundation** and **coma** due to drug ingestion are discussed in Chapter 15.

B. **Delayed reactions** can occur anywhere from days to months following drug ingestion. There are two important varieties.

1. **Amphetamine psychosis** can develop insidiously with prolonged amphetamine abuse. The reaction occurs with continued, prolonged exposure to the drug.

2. **Prolonged hallucinogen-induced psychosis** refers to a psychotic state following use of a hallucinogen (usually LSD) that persists long after drug use has stopped. The basis for this type of reaction is not well understood. Many clinicians speculate that the drug unmasks an intrinsic prepsychotic tendency (see Section **I.B.3**).

C. **Recurrent reactions** ("flashbacks") are the most perplexing variety of adverse reaction. Subjects spontaneously experience hallucinations, intrusive thoughts, or perceptual distortions unassociated with drug-taking (*Am. J. Psychiatry* 126:565, 1969).

III. **Approach to Management of Bad Trips** This section will present some general principles useful in the management of bad trips. Adverse reactions to specific drugs are discussed in Section **IV.**

A. **History** Although most bad trips are frightening to the patient and disquieting to the physician, they are seldom life-threatening. Physicians therefore can take time to obtain a careful history from patient, friends, and family. What drug did he take? How long has he been this way? Has it happened before? Does he have a history of psychiatric disturbance?

B. **Physical examination** should be performed on every patient. Important diagnostic information can be obtained by special attention to the following items:

1. Vital signs: heart rate, blood pressure, core temperature.
2. Skin and mucous membranes: moist or dry? sweating present or absent
3. Eyes: pupil size and reactivity.
4. Abdomen: bowel sounds.
5. Mental status: orientation, reality testing, insight and judgment.

C. **Diagnostic tests** seldom yield useful information beyond what is obtained from history and physical examination. Serum concentration of hallucinogens such as LSD are minute and are not readily detected or quantified. Commercial toxicologic screening of blood and urine can be unreliable, nonspecific, and inordinately delayed. The *methacholine* test (see Section **IV.C**) can help establish the diagnosis of anticholinergic intoxication.

D. **Treatment** is undertaken with the attitude that the patient suffers from drug-induced disease. Since most drugs of abuse are rapidly excreted, bad trips are usually short-lived and do not require pharmacologic treatment. Physicians who aggressively intervene with sedatives and tranquilizers frequently cause unnecessary iatrogenic morbidity.

1. **Reassurance** is by far the most important therapeutic maneuver. The patient should be told that the bizarre things he sees and feels are due to the drug he has taken and that he is not "losing his mind." He can be reassured that drug effects will "wear off" shortly and that no permanent harm will result. Physicians should

be patient and persistent with their reassurance and answer the subject's questions frankly. Individuals who express concern about chromosomal damage due to LSD can be told that there is no substantial evidence that LSD does this in humans (*Teratology* 6:75, 1972; *Conn. Med.* 34:895, 1970).

2. **Sedatives** and **tranquilizers** should be used *only* when agitation or panic is severe or unmanageable and does not respond to reassurance alone. A drug-specific diagnosis is essential before sedatives are given. Phenothiazines, for example, may potentiate agitation and delirium if administered to patients with anticholinergic intoxication. Physicians must be aware of the possible adverse effects of sedative-tranquilizers when used to treat bad trips.

   Major tranquilizers should not be used when nonspecific sedation is desired since they can cause hypotension (chlorpromazine, promazine), extrapyramidal reactions (trifluoperazine, haloperidol), disturbed temperature regulation, or enhanced seizure activity. Barbiturates are also hazardous since they can produce respiratory depression and obtundation unless dosage is carefully titrated. Benzodiazepines are the drugs of choice for nonspecific sedation because they are the safest of the currently available agents. They can be given orally or parenterally. Commonly used derivatives include:

   a. **Diazepam**
      IV: 5 mg/min (maximum dose 20 mg)
      IM: 5 to 15 mg
      PO: 5 to 20 mg

   b. **Chlordiazepoxide**
      IV: 25 mg/min (maximum dose 100 mg)
      IM: 25 to 100 mg
      PO: 25 to 100 mg

   c. **Oxazepam**
      PO: 30 to 120 mg

3. **Specific antidotes** exist in certain situations (see Section **IV**). Their use should be considered if the possible benefits of pharmacologic intervention outweigh the hazards. Examples of specific antidotes are:

   a. **Major tranquilizers** for amphetamine intoxication.

   b. **Propranolol** for adrenergic hyperactivity due to amphetamines or possibly for hallucinogens.

    c. **Physostigmine** for anticholinergic or antihistamine intoxication.

E. **Continued care** The physician's responsibility does not end when the bad trip is terminated. Many drug-takers need followup medical or psychiatric treatment. The availability of facilities for continued treatment should be made clear to the patient.

IV. **Bad Trips Due to Specific Drugs of Abuse**

A. **Hallucinogens** include LSD, mescaline, psilocybin, dimethyltryptamine (DMT), and others. It is not clear whether marijuana deserves to be classified as a hallucinogen, since adverse reactions to this agent appear to be less frequent and less severe. However, bad trips due to marijuana can closely resemble those due to other hallucinogens.

1. **Manifestations** Apprehension, fear, and panic are among the most common adverse reactions. These occur when perceptual distortions and hallucinations are ego-dystonic or intrusive, and subjects fear for their sanity. Less common are the psychotic reactions (e.g., delusions, affective lability) and agitated delirium. Prolonged reactions and flashbacks (see Sections II.B and C) can occur with any hallucinogen, including marijuana. Physical examination often reveals evidence of sympathetic (adrenergic) hyperactivity: diaphoresis, tachycardia, mydriasis (responsive to light), tremulousness, hyperreflexia. Life-threatening manifestations, such as hypertension and hyperpyrexia, are uncommon.

2. **Treatment** There is no specific antidote. Reassurance is the major therapeutic measure. The physician should enlist the help of the patient's colleagues whenever possible. Sedative-tranquilizer therapy should be avoided if possible.

B. **Amphetamines** Abuse of this class of agents can rapidly devastate the drug-taker.

1. **Manifestations** Patients are hyperalert, restless, hyperactive, and talkative, despite having been sleepless and anorectic for days at a time. Stereotyped movements of the face, mouth, or extremities may be obvious. The mental state characteristically is one of psychosis without delirium. The affect is labile and inappropriate. Paranoid manifestations can range from suspiciousness to elaborate systematized delusions; both auditory and visual hallucinations can reinforce these delusions. Adrenergic manifestations (see Section IV.A) are usually present and can be severe. A hypertensive or hyperpyrexic crisis can require emergency treatment. The "crash" following a "speed trip" represents postamphetamine depression, which in some cases can be profound.

2. Treatment

   a. Major tranquilizers are a relatively specific antidote for amphetamine intoxication. Their efficacy is probably due to adrenergic blockade in the central nervous system. As discussed previously, major tranquilizers carry a considerable risk of iatrogenic morbidity; however, they may have to be used if agitation cannot be managed by reassurance or if hypertension or hyperpyrexia is severe. The agents most commonly used are chlorpromazine (25 to 50 mg IM) and haloperidol (2.5 to 5.0 mg IM).

   b. Manifestations of peripheral beta-adrenergic hyperactivity can be safely relieved by propranolol (20 to 40 mg PO or 1 to 2 mg IV). This drug is contraindicated in asthmatics and in persons with uncompensated organic heart disease. Propranolol should also be avoided in insulin-dependent diabetics.

   c. Amphetamine excretion is enhanced by acidification of the urine (*Br. J. Pharmacol.* 24:293, 1965). The duration of amphetamine intoxication can be shortened by administration of oral ammonium chloride. The usual dose is 1 to 2 gm every three to six hours. Urine pH should be measured frequently and kept at 4 to 5.

   d. The postintoxication "crash" should be anticipated, and the availability of psychiatric treatment facilities should be made clear to the patient.

C. Anticholinergics and antihistamines

Intoxication with this class of drugs is common because of their easy availability; they are inexpensive and may be legally obtained. Dozens of over-the-counter hypnotic preparations contain combinations of scopolamine and methapyrilene (see Appendix IV). Antihistamines are contained in many proprietary antiemetics and cold preparations. Antiparkinsonian drugs also are potentially abusable.

1. Manifestations

Dose-dependent peripheral cholinergic blockade is the most consistent sign of intoxication. Tachycardia, mydriasis (unresponsive to light), paralysis of accommodation, absent sweating, dry skin and mucous membranes, flushing, paralytic ileus, and urinary hesitancy are common findings. The mental status can vary from CNS depression to excitement. Fluctuations in mental status are frequent, and agitated toxic delirium is the usual finding. Patients are disoriented, confused, and hyperactive, and appear to hallucinate; they often pick or grasp aimlessly at bedclothes or imaginary objects.

The diagnosis is established by history, physical findings, and by subcutaneous injection of methacholine (10 to 30 mg), an acetylcholine analogue. Normally, methacholine elicits brady-cardia, rhinorrhea, salivation, sweating, and abdominal distress, but this response will not occur if an anticholinergic agent has been ingested.

2. **Treatment** Bad trips due to anticholinergics and antihistamines usually are shortlived and benign, and adverse psychiatric sequelae are rare. Treatment other than observation and reassurance is not often required. The specific antidote is *physostigmine* (1 to 4 mg IM or IV), which will rapidly reverse both peripheral and central manifestations of poisoning. The major indications for its use are uncontrollable agitation and severe hyperpyrexia. Major tran-quilizers potentiate toxicity and should not be used.

D. **Sedative-hypnotics** Bad trips due to CNS depressants usually take the form of obtundation due to overdosage (see Chapter 15). Oc-casionally, however, drug-takers will seek help following smaller doses of sedative-hypnotics because the drug experience has been un-pleasant. In some cases, subjects are brought to medical facilities by their colleagues.

1. **Manifestations** Adverse reactions usually resemble those seen in alcohol intoxication. Patients are ataxic, dysarthric, and drowsy. Garrulousness, aggressive behavior, and combativeness can occur due to a general "disinhibiting" effect. Methaqualone abuse is currently in fashion among drug-takers. In addition to the afore-mentioned effects, methaqualone frequently produces peripheral numbness and paresthesias, described as a "buzz" (*J.A.M.A.* 224: 1512, 1973; 224:1505, 1973; *Arch. Gen. Psychiatry* 28:627, 1973).

2. **Treatment** consists only of observation and reassurance, with patients being allowed to "sleep it off." Obviously, administration of other sedative-tranquilizers should be avoided. The possibility of withdrawal symptoms following drug discontinuation should be considered, since all sedative-hypnotics have an addicting potential.

References

Brawley, B., and Duffield, J. C. The pharmacology of hallucinogens. *Pharmacol. Rev.* 24:31—66, 1972.

Consroe, B. F. Specific pharmacological management of acute toxicity due to "psyched" drugs. *Ariz. Med.* 29:920—925, 1972.

Greenblatt, D. J., and Shader, R. I. Adverse effects of LSD: A current perspective. *Conn. Med.* 34:895—902, 1970.

Greenblatt, D. J., and Shader, R. I. Drug therapy: Anticholinergics. *N. Engl. J. Med.* 288:1215—1219, 1973.

Greenblatt, D. J., and Shader, R. I. Drug abuse and the emergency room physician. *Am. J. Psychiatry* 131:559–562, 1974.

Pillard, R. C. Marihuana. *N. Engl. J. Med.* 283:294–303, 1970.

Schwartz, C. J. The complications of LSD: A review of the literature. *J. Nerv. Ment. Dis.* 146:174–186, 1968.

Shader, R. I., and Greenblatt, D. J. Belladonna alkaloids and synthetic anticholinergics: Uses and toxicity. In R. I. Shader (Ed.), *Psychiatric Complications of Medical Drugs.* New York: Raven, 1972. Pp. 103–147.

Taylor, R. L., Maurer, J. I., and Tinklenberg, J. R. Management of "bad trips" in an evolving drug scene. *J.A.M.A.* 213:422–425, 1970.

Weil, A. T. Adverse reactions to marihuana: Classification and suggested treatment. *N. Engl. J. Med.* 282:997–1000, 1970.

12

Treatment of Dependence on Barbiturates and Sedative-Hypnotics

Richard I. Shader
Eric D. Caine
Roger E. Meyer

General Although concerns about physical dependence are most commonly voiced in relation to middle-aged persons who make indefinite use of "sleeping pills," the population who most often seek or are required to obtain treatment for a drug "habit" of "downs" or "downers" are adolescents and young adults. Short- and intermediate-acting barbiturates and sedative-hypnotics are frequently employed by these young people as mood modifiers, either alone or mixed with amphetamines and opiates. In the language of this set, such illicit drugs are commonly referred to according to the colors of their capsules: "yellow jackets," "red birds," "red devils," "rainbows," and "blue heavens." Dependence on these substances is usually present when the following characteristics obtain: (1) a strong desire or need to continue with the drug or its substitutes; (2) a tendency to increase the dose (usually related to tolerance); (3) psychic dependence; and (4) physical dependence (see WHO Technical Report Series, No. 273, Geneva: WHO, United Nations, 1964, pp. 13–14).

When a patient reporting physical dependence is initially seen by a physician, he must be medically evaluated for symptoms and signs of overdose, intoxication, or abstinence. An accurate history, although often difficult to obtain, can be invaluable; it is important to question the patient about the amount of drug taken and the time of ingestion of the last dose. In addition it is helpful to know the events leading to the referral or admission, what environmental supports are available, and any history of previous psychiatric and drug-related problems. The patient's motivation should be assessed, and it is also useful to examine carefully the realistic quality of the individual's plans.

Among sedative-hypnotic drugs, pentobarbital, secobarbital, methaqualone, and glutethimide are commonly abused, while meprobamate and the benzodiazepines are ingested less often. The barbiturates provide a paradigm for discussing the difficulties encountered when treating persons addicted to these agents.

II. Medical Evaluation

A. **Abstinence** The quality of a person's physical dependence results in part from the type of drug ingested, its dose, and the length of time it was used. Physical dependence usually does not develop unless large doses are ingested over months or years. Thus persons taking nightly doses of 200 mg of a short-acting barbiturate rarely become physically dependent. Routine ingestion of 400 mg a day of pentobarbital or secobarbital can lead to tolerance development and mild withdrawal symptoms after a period of 90 days. Individuals consuming 600 to 800 mg a day of either drug for between 45 and 120 days may have grand mal seizures upon withdrawal, even though they do not usually show symptoms of delirium. Table 12-1 illustrates the relationship between barbiturate dosage level and the intensity of physical dependence (see also *Am. J. Psychiatry* 125:6, 1968; *Fed. Proc.* 15:423, 1956). Table 12-2 summarizes doses of various sedative-hypnotic drugs that reportedly can lead to physical dependence (see *J.A.M.A.* 196:23, 1966; Senate Hearings on Barbiturate Abuse, 1971–1972; *Arch. Gen. Psychiatry* 29:46, 1973). It is important to

Table 12-1. Relationship of Dosage of Secobarbital or Pentobarbital to Abstinence Manifestations*

Daily Dose	Days of Ingestion in Hospital	Percent of Patients Showing:		
		Convulsions	Delirium	Minor Symptoms
200 mg	365	0	0	0
400 mg	90	0	0	5.5
600 mg	35 to 57	11	0	50
800 mg	42 to 57	20	0	100
900 to 2200 mg	32 to 144	78	75	100

*Data derived from 61 patients. Adapted, with permission, from Wikler, A. Diagnosis and treatment of drug dependence of the barbiturate type. *Am. J. Psychiatry* 125: 758–765, 1968. Copyright 1968 by the American Psychiatric Association.

Table 12-2. Nonbarbiturate Sedative-Hypnotic Agents: Dosage and Duration Associated with Withdrawal Symptoms[a]

Generic Name	Dose	Duration
Ethchlorvynol	2.0 to 4.0 gm	7 to 8 months
Glutethimide	2.5 gm	3 months
	5.0 gm	several weeks
Methaqualone	0.6 to 0.9 gm	1 to several months
Meprobamate	2.4 gm	9 months
	3.2 to 6.4 gm	40 days
Chlordiazepoxide	0.3 to 0.6 gm	5 to 6 months
Diazepam	0.1 to 1.5 gm	several months

[a]Derived from case reports.

remember that documented experience with nonbarbiturate sedative-hypnotics is limited.

The syndrome of barbiturate (sedative-hypnotic) abstinence is similar to that seen following alcohol withdrawal and is characterized by tremulousness, anxiety, insomnia, anorexia, nausea, vomiting, diaphoresis, postural hypotension, tendon hyperreflexia, and, in some cases, convulsions and delirium (see Table 12-3) Some authors also include in this list progression to hyperpyrexia, electrolyte abnormalities, cardiovascular collapse, and death. One must carefully separate subjective symptoms from those verified by physical examination. The abstinence syndrome, if it is to occur, usually begins within 72 hours of cessation of drug intake. Grand mal convulsions, when they occur, generally are noted between days three and seven, usually as single episodes but occasionally in multiple bursts (convulsions following benzodiazepine use tend to come late in the abstinence syndrome rather than early). They are accompanied by loss of consciousness and cyanosis, and occasionally by progression to delirium. When present, delirium begins most often between the fourth and sixth days, with fluctuating consciousness, visual and auditory hallucinations, unsystematized delusions, mood fluctuations, restlessness, insomnia, fever, and hyperreflexia with marked blepharospasm. Delirious patients often have no understanding of their situation.

Electroencephalographic (EEG) examination of patients with increased barbiturate blood levels sometimes reveals a "spiky" pattern with abnormal fast activity. Photic stimulation can produce occasional paroxysmal bursts of activity. During abstinence the EEG can become distinctly abnormal. Wulff found that 12 percent of abstinent patients had paroxysmal activity without photic stimulation, while two-thirds showed it with such stimulation (see *Electroencephalogr. Clin. Neurophysiol.*, Suppl. 14, 1–173, 1959).

B. **Intoxication** Intoxicated patients range in appearance from those who are sleeping but easily aroused to those who are alert with fine lateral nystagmus as the only sign of recent use. Moderate intoxication is characterized by drowsiness, slurred speech, coarse nystagmus, hyporeflexia, and ataxia.

C. **Overdose** The treatment of overdosage of sedative-hypnotics is discussed in Chapter 15.

III. **Detoxification: Assessment and Management** When assessing a patient for detoxification, the context of the patient's admission must be carefully examined: the events leading to admission, the availability of social supports, the purpose for which the patient used the drug, his past history of drug detoxification, his expectation of difficulties

Table 12-3. The Barbiturate Abstinence Syndrome[a]

Clinical Phenomenon	Frequency (percent)	Time of Onset	Duration (Days)	Remarks
Apprehension	100	1st day	3 to 14	Vague uneasiness or fear of impending catastrophe
Muscle weakness	100	1st day	3 to 14	Evident on mildest exertion
Tremors	100	1st day	3 to 14	Coarse, rhythmic, nonpatterned, evident during voluntary movement and subside at rest
Postural faintness	100	1st day	3 to 14	Evident on sitting or standing suddenly; associated with marked fall in systolic and diastolic blood pressure and with pronounced tachycardia
Anorexia	100	1st day	3 to 14	Usually associated with repeated vomiting
Twitches	100	1st day	3 to 14	Myoclonic muscle contractions, or spasmodic jerking of one or more extremities; sometimes bizarre patterned movements
Seizures[b]	80	2nd to 3rd day	8	Up to a total of 4 grand mal episodes, with loss of consciousness and postconvulsive stupor
Psychoses and/or delirium[b]	60	3rd to 8th day	3 to 14	Usually resemble "delirium tremens"; occasionally resemble schizophrenic or Korsakoff's syndrome; or acute panic states may occur

[a]After abrupt withdrawal in 19 cases of experimental addiction to secobarbital or pentobarbital employing chronic intoxication at dose levels of 0.8 to 2.2 gm PO per day for 6 weeks or more.

[b]Four developed seizures without subsequent psychosis; one exhibited delirium without antecedent seizures; three escaped both seizures and delirium. Adapted, with permission, from Wikler, A. Diagnosis and treatment of drug dependence of the barbiturate type. *Am. J. Psychiatry* 125:758–765, 1968. Copyright 1968 by the American Psychiatric Association.

without the drug, and the realistic quality of his plans. The attentive physician can foresee from this assessment some of the problems that may arise after the detoxification regimen is begun.

It is possible to detoxify a person on either an inpatient or an outpatient basis. Although the former offers more safety and control, particularly when the reliability of the patient is uncertain, the latter may be the only means of engaging the patient in treatment. A stable environment and strong motivation may permit withdrawal to take place in the context of daily life routines. Detoxification must not be carried out perfunctorily. Information is frequently unavailable or unreliable, and it is essential that the patient's responses be closely observed and that a thorough physical examination be conducted. Individuals respond differently to medication. What may be an adequate withdrawal schedule for one person can heavily sedate another.

With any form of drug detoxification, the patient should be informed at the outset that this is an uncomfortable procedure, often accompanied by malaise, anxiety, "shakiness," insomnia, and nightmares. Nightmares may at times be so distressing that patients will interrupt drug withdrawal to suppress the nightmares by taking more drugs. Some people complain of anorexia, nausea, and mild abdominal cramps. The physician must separate these from symptoms of other physical ailments. The insomnia from sedative-hypnotic abuse frequently lasts for weeks and is associated with a "dream rebound" ("REM rebound"), with many anxious, nightmarish dreams described.

A. Initiation of withdrawal Two methods are available for establishing the patient's level of drug requirement when beginning withdrawal.

1. **Test dose** The patient is given 200 mg of pentobarbital orally and changes in the neurologic exam are assessed after one hour. Table 12-4 presents possible findings on physical examination, the associated degree of tolerance, and estimates of 24-hour pentobarbital requirements (*Dis. Nerv. Syst.* 34:162, 1973). If no physical changes are observed after one hour, the level of the habit is probably above 1200 mg of pentobarbital per day. The test is then repeated three to four hours later using a dose of 300 mg of pentobarbital. No response to the 300 mg dose suggests a habit above 1600 mg per day.

   Either phenobarbital or pentobarbital can be employed for withdrawal, but the course of withdrawal is often smoother with phenobarbital since there are fewer variations of the blood barbiturate level. When employing pentobarbital, the estimated daily requirement is divided into four equal doses and administered orally every six hours. Smaller total doses of phenobarbital are

Table 12-4. Clinical Response Patterns to Test Dose of 200 mg PO of Pentobarbital: Relationship to Tolerance

Patient's Condition One Hour after Test Dose	Degree of Tolerance	Estimated 24-hour Pentobarbital Requirement mg
Asleep, but arousable	None or minimal	None
Drowsy, slurred speech; coarse nystagmus; ataxia; marked intoxication	Definite	400 to 600
Comfortable; fine lateral nystagmus is only sign of intoxication	Marked	800
No signs of drug effects; perhaps persisting signs of abstinence; no intoxication	Extreme	1000 to 1200 or more

required, usually one-third of the amount of pentobarbital due to longer duration of action. Phenobarbital is given in equally divided amounts orally every eight hours. Both the pentobarbital and the phenobarbital can be reduced at a rate of one-tenth the starting dose per day (e.g., an initial daily dose of 600 mg of pentobarbital would be decreased 60 mg per day, and the equivalent 200 mg of phenobarbital would be lowered by 20 mg each day).

2. **Phenobarbital equivalents** Another technique for determining the baseline level of drug required daily was developed for outpatients who refused admission but nonetheless sought detoxification (see *J. Psychedelic Drugs* 3:81—88, 1971). Table 12-5 gives the empirically established amounts of phenobarbital that correspond to some of the abused drugs. It becomes important with this method to know the names and quantities of the drugs frequently abused (see Table 12-6). By totaling the number of daily hypnotic

Table 12-5. Estimated "Phenobarbital Substitution" Withdrawal Dosage Equivalencies for Certain Sedative-Hypnotic Agents

Generic Name	Dosage
Phenobarbital	**30 mg**
Secobarbital	100 mg
Pentobarbital	100 mg
Chloral hydrate	250 mg
Glutethimide	250 mg
Meprobamate	200 mg
Chlordiazepoxide	25 mg
Diazepam	5 mg

Table 12-6. Sedative-Hypnotics: Street Names of Some Commonly Abused Forms

Generic Name	Trade Name	Street Name
Amobarbital	Amytal	Blue heaven Blue velvet
Pentobarbital	Nembutal	Yellows Yellow jackets Nembies
Secobarbital	Seconal Seco-8	Reds Red devils Redbirds Seggy
Amobarbital and secobarbital	Tuinal	Reds and blues Double trouble Rainbows Tooies
Methaqualone	Optimil Parest Quaalude Somnafac Sopor	Sopers

doses, the physician can establish the patient's initial requirement for phenobarbital. Once this is completed, the dose is divided on an every eight hours schedule, with a total daily decrease of about 10 percent.

If withdrawal is impending, the patient may be given a loading dose of phenobarbital, 100 to 200 mg IM. The first oral dose is then begun after the patient has been without significant physical signs of intoxication for several hours.

B. **Mixed addiction** When a patient is dependent on both an opioid and a hypnotic, it is best to withdraw the hypnotic gradually while maintaining the opioid at a constant level (e.g., methadone, usually 20 mg per day, if the patient has verifiable opioid dependence). It is possible to decrease both drugs at once, but occasionally this complicates the clinical picture. A person withdrawing from opioids (see Chapter 13) is found to have dilated, reactive pupils; elevated pulse rate, blood pressure, and respiration; muscle aches and twitches; tremulousness, nausea, vomiting, diarrhea, lacrimation, rhinorrhea, yawning, restlessness, chills, and gooseflesh ("cold turkey"). By carefully examining the patient's eyes, pulse, blood pressure (both lying and standing), reflexes (including blink reflex), and mental status, it should be possible to separate one withdrawal syndrome from the other. Nonetheless, clinical distinction can be difficult. Although opioid withdrawal is uncomfortable, it rarely leads to convulsions, and it is not lethal. Abstinence from a sedative-hypnotic is more dangerous.

IV. **Long-term Therapy** Many individuals who begin detoxification from sedative-hypnotic agents do not complete their course of treatment, and of those who do, many quickly return to a drug-dependent state. Discussions with barbiturate users reveal that many use their drugs as substitutes for unsatisfying or unpredictable interpersonal bonds. A common theme is the avoidance of interpersonal frustration. Some constrict their relationships, avoiding strong ties, while others evolve tortuous, torturous associations.

There are no specific treatments for those who abuse hypnotic drugs. At present there is no "barbiturate maintenance" drug similar to methadone. Therapeutic communities, historically developed for heroin users, often reject the frequently relapsing hypnotic-dependent person. Detoxification centers often serve secondary functions — providing food, shelter, social support in times of crisis, or sometimes even drugs to a patient with no money or connections. Many clinics become "revolving-door" institutions. Whether this is regarded as desirable depends on the philosophy, policy, and goals of the particular treatment center.

Efforts to develop a therapeutic alliance with an addicted individual are often discouraging and frustrating. Attempts are interrupted by multiple readmissions for detoxification. Little is known about interventions that will substantially and reliably alter the natural history of these addictions.

13

Heroin and Methadone Abuse: Acute and Chronic Management

Alan I. Green
Roger E. Mayer
Richard I. Shader

The clinical problems resulting from the abuse of heroin and methadone are regularly presented to physicians. Basic knowledge of the pharmacology of these agents is essential if effective treatment is to be delivered. This manual assumes an understanding of the concepts of tolerance and physical dependence, as well as the basic pharmacological actions of heroin and methadone.

I.   **Acute Overdosage**

A. **Diagnosis** Acute overdosage with heroin or methadone can be deliberate or accidental. The patient will often be young and is usually brought to treatment facilities by colleagues or police. The clinical picture of overdose is similar for heroin and methadone: depressed respiration, depressed consciousness, pinpoint pupils (the pupils may be dilated if severe hypoxia is present or if the narcotic was mixed with other drugs), possibly hypotension, and possibly pulmonary edema (or pulmonary congestion). Old or fresh track marks may be regarded as supplementary evidence of opioid use, but their absence does not refute the diagnosis, since heroin may be taken intranasally, and methadone may be taken orally. The presence of ice packs near the testicles, or milk in the mouth, may also suggest opioid use, since these are sometimes employed as "street" remedies for overdose (*Am. J. Med.* 51:709, 1971). This combination of findings, together with available history, is usually sufficient to establish the diagnosis, although other causes of coma (including multiple drug overdose) must be considered. (See Chapter 15 for a complete discussion of the diagnosis and medical management of the comatose patient.)

B. **Management** Emergency management consists of supporting or restoring vital functions and administering an opioid antagonist.

1. Adequacy of circulation and respiration are immediately assessed. If these functions are inadequate, resuscitation is instituted. Intubation should be performed if clinically indicated

(see Chapter 15, Section 1). If intubation is not performed, care should be taken to prevent aspiration in case of vomiting. Vital functions should continue to be supported while further diagnostic and therapeutic procedures are undertaken.

2. A reliable intravenous route should be established. Blood should be taken for appropriate laboratory determinations (including blood glucose). As a conservative procedure, a 50% glucose solution is then injected rapidly, even when hypoglycemia is not thought to be the primary cause of the coma.

3. Depending on the particular clinical situation, gastric lavage may occasionally be helpful if there is evidence of recent oral ingestion of drugs. However, this procedure should not be undertaken in a patient who has evidence of central nervous system depression unless the airway has been protected by previous intubation.

4. Naloxone is the opioid antagonist of choice for the reversal of the respiratory depression accompanying opioid overdosage. A usual adult dose is 0.4 mg, given intravenously.[*] A response to naloxone is indicated by a reversal of the respiratory depression within minutes. (A lightening of the level of consciousness and a widening of the pupils will also generally be seen.) Repeat doses may be given about every three minutes, but only if the previous dose appears ineffective. If at least some clinical improvement is not observed after two or three doses of naloxone, the clinical condition is usually not due solely to heroin or methadone, and other causes of coma should be considered (e.g., trauma, other drugs).[†] Because patients can be agitated, combative, and violent as they emerge from coma, physical restraints should be in place before naloxone is given. (If the patient is not intubated, however, care must be taken to avoid aspiration in case of vomiting. Therefore a non-intubated patient should only be restrained in a position which would not predispose to aspiration.)

5. Naloxone should be administered cautiously to an opioid-dependent individual, since excessive administration may precipitate withdrawal symptoms. If withdrawal symptoms do appear they may be severe, but should last only as long as this effect of the naloxone (about 30 minutes to 2 hours).

---

[*] The manufacturer's recommended child's dose (below age 12) is 0.01 mg/kg.
[†] Although not documented in the literature, we have received an anecdotal report of rare cases of apparently massive methadone overdoses, which seemed to require further doses of naloxone to produce an initial response (W. Leigh Thompson, M.D., personal communication, 1975).

6. A syndrome of interstitial or alveolar pulmonary congestion can accompany acute overdosage. Manifestations range from asymptomatic congestion seen only by x-ray to severe life-threatening pulmonary edema. The heart is of normal size, and cardiac function is unimpaired. Digitalis and diuretics are of no value and should not be used. Treatment consists of oxygen, positive pressure ventilation, and intubation if necessary (*Am. J. Psychiatry* 131:559–562, 1974).

7. Even following a positive response to naloxone, the physician should remember that the patient may have taken a multiple drug overdose, and the patient should be examined accordingly.

8. Because heroin or methadone may have a longer duration of action than naloxone, serious respiratory depression and coma can recur following the initial doses of naloxone. This is particularly true with an oral methadone overdose, which may produce depressant effects for 24 to 48 hours following the overdose (*N.Y. State J. Med.* 71:542, 1971). The patient should be carefully observed, and naloxone readministered as required following an initial positive response.

9. Patients should be hospitalized (preferably with continuous observation in an intensive care unit) for at least 24 hours following acute overdosage in order to minimize the dangers of relapse into coma and to provide for full medical evaluation (see *Am. J. Med.* 51:704–713, 1971 for a more detailed discussion of the medical aspects of the management of these patients).

10. Before discharge from the hospital, the availability of facilities for followup medical and psychiatric care should be made clear to the patient.

II. Withdrawal

A. **Diagnosis of opioid dependence** The diagnosis of opioid dependence is based on a history or evidence of opioid use followed by abrupt cessation of use and the development of the characteristic symptoms of opioid withdrawal (the abstinence syndrome).

1. **Heroin or morphine abstinence syndrome** The heroin or morphine abstinence syndrome begins approximately 8 to 12 hours following the last dose. Relatively early signs and symptoms include: drug seeking behavior, increased respiratory rate, sweating, lacrimation, yawning, rhinorrhea, piloerection, tremor,

anorexia, irritability, and dilated pupils. More advanced signs and symptoms (which occur within 48-72 hours after the last dose) include insomnia, nausea, diarrhea, weakness, abdominal cramps, vomiting, tachycardia, hypertension, and involuntary muscle spasms. The syndrome subsides gradually over a period of 7 to 10 days (Goodman and Gilman, *The Pharmacological Basis of Therapeutics* [4th ed.]. New York: Macmillan, 1970. Pp. 287–28

2. **Methadone abstinence syndrome** The methadone abstinence syndrome is qualitatively similar to that of morphine or heroin, but follows a different time course. The first signs and symptoms of abstinence are seen within 24 to 48 hours after the last dose. The peak intensity appears on the third day (or later). The syndrome gradually subsides, but may continue for 3 weeks or longer (*Arch. Gen. Psychiatry.* 28:286–295, 1973). Deep bone pain has been reported in the methadone abstinence syndrome (see R. E. Meyer, *Guide to Drug Rehabilitation: A Public Health Approach.* Boston: Beacon, 1972).

B. **Diagnosis of opioid dependence in the neonate** An infant born to a heroin- or methadone-dependent woman may develop a withdrawal syndrome which most commonly occurs within 48 hours after birth. The signs of this reaction include: hypertonicity, tremor, irritability, vomiting, fever, respiratory distress, high-pitched cry, hyperbilirubine and convulsions (*N. Engl. J. Med.* 289:1216–1220, 1973).

C. **Management of withdrawal (detoxification)** An individual who is dependent on heroin or methadone should be withdrawn gradually, using oral methadone, to attenuate the abstinence syndrome. Optimally, detoxification should be performed in conjunction with a complete treatment program in an attempt to prevent recidivism. (Food and Drug Administration regulations [1972] require licensing for facilities using methadone to detoxify opioid addicts.)

1. The initial evaluation of a patient for detoxification should at least include a complete medical and drug abuse history, physical examination, and screening for drugs of abuse in the urine.

2. Attempts to establish the size of an individual's habit are rarely helpful. In addition to the fact that an addict's reporting of drug use may be misleading, any formula for conversion of "bags" of street heroin to methadone dose will vary as a function of the quality of the street drug, which is usually unknown. (More accurate estimates of the level of physical dependence can be made in the case of methadone maintenance patients who are taking a known amount of methadone.)

3. Detoxification may be done on an inpatient or outpatient basis. Some facilities reserve inpatient detoxification for patients who are dependent upon more than one drug, who plan to enter a therapeutic community, who are being withdrawn from high dose methadone maintenance, or who are psychotic. Other facilities favor inpatient detoxification for most addicts.

4. After the appearance of withdrawal symptoms, an initial dose of 10 to 20 mg of oral methadone should be given. Signs of intoxication (such as somnolence) following the intial dose indicate the use of too much methadone. Incremental doses of 5 to 15 mg may be given over the next 24 hours if further signs of abstinence occur, but no more than 20 mg should be required in any 12-hour period (unless the patient has a documented history of tolerance to more than 40 mg of methadone per day). Induction of methadone in an outpatient setting is sometimes done in a more routinized fashion, which usually varies from program to program. Within the first few days of detoxification, the methadone dose is adjusted to reach stabilization. After the first day, the methadone may be administered once a day or in divided doses every 12 hours. Some detoxification programs seldom exceed a stabilization dose of 20 mg per day. It is rarely necessary to use more than 40 mg of oral methadone to reach stabilization (except for patients with a documented history of tolerance to more than 40 mg of methadone per day).

5. Once stabilization is achieved, detoxification can begin. According to the Food and Drug Administration regulations, detoxification must be completed within 21 days. Most schedules call for a reduction of 5 mg per day (or a maximum of 15 to 20 percent reduction per day) and complete withdrawal in 7 to 10 days. Patients should be told that they may experience some mild withdrawal symptoms (similar to a mild case of the "flu") during detoxification. Patients should have their urine monitored for drugs of abuse during detoxification.

6. Following detoxification, patients should be offered continued outpatient or residential rehabilitative care to try to prevent a relapse.

7. Patients being withdrawn from methadone maintenance (especially those on doses of greater than 50 mg per day) are often detoxified over a more prolonged period (over 4 weeks in some clinics). These patients can be detoxified with a reduction of 5 mg per day until the level of 20 mg per day is reached. At this level, they are often detoxified more gradually. Some facilities favor inpatient detoxification once the 20 mg level is reached.

8. The detoxification of patients who are dependent on both heroin or methadone and sedative-hypnotics is discussed in Chapter 12.

9. The infant born to a heroin- or methadone-dependent mother should be observed for signs of withdrawal. Treatments utilized include paregoric, chlorpromazine, methadone, and phenobarbital (see P. G. Bourne [Ed.], *A Treatment Manual for Acute Drug Abuse Emergencies.* Rockville, Md.: National Clearinghouse for Drug Abuse Information, 1974. Pp. 27–33).

III. **Long-Term Treatment**   Long-term treatment involves the rehabilitation of the heroin or methadone addict and the prevention of his recidivism to drug use. Such treatment should be given by organized programs that include at least the following: 1) medical treatment for the complications of addiction; 2) services such as psychotherapy, family counseling, supplementary education, job training and placement, legal aid, and welfare assistance as necessary; and 3) attempts at helping the addict to overcome the drug craving that has been described in addicts following withdrawal. Drug abuse treatment programs can be divided according to their overall approach to treatment as follows:

A. **Drug-free programs**   Drug-free programs are programs that do not use chemotherapy in their treatment regimen. These programs try to stimulate a "change" in the addict that will allow him to remain drug-free. Treatment usually begins following detoxification and often includes a phase of full-time residence in the program. Rehabilitation and return to independent living frequently takes from 9 to 24 months. Such programs are very demanding and experience suggests that only the most highly motivated addicts stay in treatment. However, for the group that does stay in treatment, the outcome may include a significant enhancement of social and psychological functioning. Many graduates of these programs have become effective workers in drug abuse programs.

B. **Methadone maintenance programs**   Methadone maintenance programs provide a daily oral dose of methadone to previously addicted individuals. The methadone is thought to blunt the craving for heroin and diminish the effects of injected heroin. Addicts maintained on methadone become tolerant to most of its effects at the maintenance dosage and carry out their usual functions without any evidence of intoxication (once they are tolerant).

The methadone is begun without prior detoxification. The maintenance dose usually varies from 40 to 120 mg per day, often depending on the treatment philosophy of the particular program. A recent study has indicated that a regimen of 50 mg per day may work as effectively as one of 100 mg per day (Proceedings Fourth National Conference Methadone Treatment, 1972, Pp. 411–414) and it probably has the advantage of fewer side effects and greater ease in ultimate withdrawal. Methadone maintenance is usually provided in an outpatient setting and is augmented by the various rehabilitative services listed earlier. The methadone maintenance approach may be the most widely applicable treatment available today.

The Food and Drug Administration, in 1972, released regulations on the use of methadone maintenance. These regulations define admission standards for methadone maintenance programs, limit the daily dose (120 mg) and the take-home supply (100 mg for 2 days), and specify the need for urine testing, record keeping, and supportive services in a methadone program. Each program must be approved by the FDA before it can use methadone as a maintenance agent.

Some programs maintain heroin-dependent pregnant women on low doses of methadone (20 to 40 mg per day) in order to reduce the likelihood of both continued intravenous heroin use by the mother and severe withdrawal reaction in the infant. Further research studies may give more information on the optimal management of these patients.

C. **Multimodality programs** Many drug abuse treatment programs utilize more than one treatment track or option. Such options might include drug-free residential treatment, methadone maintenance treatment, methadone detoxification with continued outpatient treatment, or various combinations of these. All patients in these different settings have access to common social and rehabilitation services as described earlier.

D. **Experimental chemotherapy programs**

1. **L-alpha acetyl methadol (LAAM)** is a long-acting methadone-like drug that lasts for 72 hours after an oral dose and therefore needs to be taken only three times per week. At the time of this writing it is being studied in experimental programs throughout the country and is not available for general use.

2. **Naltrexone** is a long-acting opioid antagonist. It lasts for more than 24 hours after a single dose and has few side effects (agonist effects). The possible utility of naltrexone as a long-term treatment agent is currently being studied in clinical programs. It is postulated that naltrexone, which would block the effects of an administered opioid, would be taken by the detoxified addict until the likelihood of recidivism to opioid use is diminished. A definitive statement concerning the actual utility of naltrexone (or other long-acting antagonists) must await the results of current studies.

References

Bourne, P. G. (Ed.). *A Treatment Manual for Acute Drug Abuse Emergencies.* Rockville Md.: National Clearinghouse for Drug Abuse Information, 1974.

Brown, B. S. The Treatment and Rehabilitation of Narcotic Addicts in the United States. In *Drug Use in America: Problem in Perspective,* Appendix Vol. IV. Washington, D.C.: U.S. Government Printing Office, 1973. Pp. 127–142.

Glasscote, R., Sussex, J. N., Jaffe, J. H., Ball, J., and Brill, L. *The Treatment of Drug Abuse.* Washington, D.C.: American Psychiatric Association, 1972.

Jaffe, J. H. Narcotic Analgesics. In L. S. Goodman and A. Gilman (Eds.), *The Pharmacological Basis of Therapeutics* (4th ed.). New York: Macmillan, 1970. Pp. 237–275.

Jaffe, J. H. Drug Addiction and Drug Abuse. In L. S. Goodman and A. Gilman (Eds.), *The Pharmacological Basis of Therapeutics* (4th ed.). New York: Macmillan, 1970. Pp. 276–313.

Meyer, R. E. *Guide to Drug Rehabilitation: A Public Health Approach.* Boston: Beacon, 1972.

14

Treatment of the Alcohol Withdrawal Syndrome

David J. Greenblatt
Richard I. Shader

Alcoholism continues to be an "inglorious addiction" and to receive little attention relative to the magnitude of the problem. Alcohol is by far the nation's most important drug of abuse. A significant proportion of general hospital admissions are due to alcoholism and its medical sequelae; at city and municipal hospitals, the proportion can exceed 50 percent. It is therefore essential that hospital physicians be thoroughly familiar with the medical and psychiatric consequences of alcoholism.

I. **Who is an Alcoholic?** Recent exhaustive efforts (*Am. J. Psychiatry* 129:127—134, 1972) to define the term *alcoholism* with some precision suggest that a reliable definition is necessarily a complex one. Physiologic, medical, attitudinal, and behavioral factors all must be considered For hospital physicians, the term alcoholism is applied to three distinct conceptual entities:

A. A pathologic **psychosocial behavior pattern**, characterized by deteriorating function in occupation, family, and citizenship, resulting from excessive alcohol ingestion. Its basis is the alcoholic's inability to resist the craving for alcohol despite the obvious adverse psychosocial sequelae.

B. A **drug addiction** of the classic type. Cessation of alcohol ingestion is followed by a withdrawal syndrome subjectively unpleasant enough to perpetuate continued alcohol use.

C. A **medical disease** with certain characteristic sequelae, such as cirrhosis, nutritional disorders, and neurologic damage.

"Alcoholism" is easy to recognize when the three entities coexist, as they often do. But they do not necessarily coexist. To cite several examples — many skid row chronic alcoholics with multiple hospitalizations for "DTs" never develop medical sequelae (A and B, but not C). The heavy-drinking executive whose drinking pattern never interferes with occupation or family life can develop withdrawal symptoms when hospitalized for elective surgery (B, but not A or C). Certain binge-drinkers never become physiologically addicted to alcohol nor develop medical complications, yet are unemployed, have broken families, and are derelicts because of alcohol abuse (A and C, but not B).

This chapter deals primarily with alcoholism as a drug addiction and the approach to therapy of the withdrawal syndrome. It is difficult to predict which alcohol abusers are candidates to develop withdrawal symptoms. Consumption of the equivalent of a fifth of whiskey daily fc 3 to 4 weeks is usually considered sufficient to produce addiction. How ever, drinking patterns that lead to physiologic dependence vary widely among individuals. Some consume seemingly huge quantities of alcohol in binge fashion — for weeks or months at a time, yet can abruptly go "on the wagon" with no apparent signs of withdrawal. Others who claim to have only "a couple of beers at night" develop full-blown delirium tremens when consumption stops. Alcohol abusers are notably unreliable historians, and physicians often have great difficulty assessing the patient's actual pattern of drinking.

Typically, the withdrawal syndrome develops in chronic alcoholics who have had a recent increase of consumption (binge) and who subsequently stop drinking or reduce their intake, for whatever reason. However, hospital physicians must be aware of the variabilities mentione The occurrence of withdrawal symptoms is *possible* in any individual with any pattern of regular alcohol consumption who ceases drinking or reduces his level of intake.

II. **Signs and Symptoms of Alcohol Withdrawal**   Manifestations are usually divided into two varieties: the *mild, early,* or *prodromal;* and the *late, advanced,* or *severe.* It is thought by some that *mild* manifestations if untreated progress to *severe* ones and that *severe* manifestations are invariably preceded by *mild* ones. However, recent evidence suggests that these relationships are by no means invariable. Physicians who approach all patients expecting this logical progression of disease will make unnecessary errors, since in many cases — perhaps most — no such progression occurs.

A. **Mild or early symptoms** ("impending DTs") can begin any time between a few hours and 10 days after the last drink. Typically, they appear in 6 to 48 hours following cessation of alcohol ingestion. They can be suppressed by continued drinking. Possible manifestatio are listed in Table 14-1.

B. **Advanced or severe manifestations** (Table 14-2) often, but not always are preceded by mild or early ones. "Delirium tremens" is a classic term used to describe the most advanced or severe toxic state. This term is exceedingly vague and carries numerous nondiagnostic connotations.

Table 14-1.   Mild or Early Symptoms of Alcohol Withdrawal

Gastrointestinal disturbances
    Loss of appetite
    Nausea
    Vomiting
    Abdominal discomfort
    Diarrhea
Muscular symptoms
    Weakness
    Cramps
    Tremulousness
Sleep disturbances
    Insomnia
    Nightmares
Autonomic imbalance (excess sympathetic activity)
    Tachycardia
    Systolic hypertension
    Diaphoresis
    Tremulousness
    Fever
Behavioral changes
    Irritability
    Hostility
    Restlessness
    Agitation
    Exaggerated startle response
Impaired cognitive function
    Inability to concentrate
    Easy distractibility
    Impairment of memory
    Impairment of judgment and other higher mental functions

Table 14-2.   Severe or Late Symptoms of Alcohol Withdrawal

Worsening of prodromal manifestations (from Table 14-1)
    Tremor
    Diaphoresis
    Tachycardia
    Agitation
    Marked startle response
Delirium
    Clouding of sensorium
    Fluctuation from hour to hour in nature and severity
    Impairment of cognitive function
    Disorientation as to time and place
Hallucinations
    Can be auditory, visual, or tactile
    Can be threatening in nature
Delusions
    Usually paranoid in nature
    Merge with and are reinforced by hallucinations
    Can create agitation and terror
Seizures
    Usually nonfocal and generalized
    Occasionally have lateralizing or nonfocal beginnings
    Prior seizure disorder not necessary
    Occur within 48 hours of cessation of drinking
    Usually self-limiting
    Always precede severe agitation, delirium, hallucinations

Because of the limitations of these categorizations, diagnosis must be approached with caution and an open mind. Prodromal manifestations can be subtle; slight irritability or intransigence in the patient's demeanor may be the only clue. Severe tremulousness and auditory hallucinosis can develop in some patients without progression to delirium or panic. In others, a grand mal seizure may be the very first manifestation of withdrawal. The alcohol abstinence syndrome *must* be understood as a heterogeneous one with numerous possible combinations of signs and symptoms. Terms such as "impending DTs" or "delirium tremens" should be used only when the aspects of the disease process to which they refer are clearly understood.

III. **Criteria for Hospitalization** Abstinent alcoholics usually present at acute treatment facilities (emergency rooms) of general and psychiatric hospitals with symptoms already in progress. Ideally, all should be hospitalized but because the supply of hospital beds is invariably exceeded by the demand, this is not always possible. Consequently, admitting physicians sometimes must select the most seriously ill to be hospitalized and treat the least ill patients on an outpatient basis. Because of the unpredictable natural history of the withdrawal syndrome, this is not always an easy choice; mistakes can be made in both directions. Table 14-3 lists criteria for hospitalization of the withdrawing alcoholic. Guidelines for management of those who are not hospitalized are given in Table 14-4.

IV. **Hospital Treatment of Alcohol Withdrawal** All newly hospitalized abstinent alcoholics should receive the following minimum evaluation: history (taken from patient, family, friends, and previous hospital record), physical examination, chest x-ray, urinalysis, and determination

Table 14-3. Criteria for Hospitalization of the Withdrawing Alcoholic

Severe tremulousness or hallucinosis
Significant dehydration
Fever above 101°F
A documented seizure in a patient with no known seizure disorder
Clouding of the sensorium
Wernicke's encephalopathy (ataxia, nystagmus, internuclear ophthalmoplegia)
Head trauma with a documented episode of unconsciousness
Presence of major complicating or associated disease:
    Hepatic decompensation
    Respiratory failure
    Respiratory infection
    Gastrointestinal bleeding
    Pancreatitis
    Severe malnutrition
Known history of previous episodes of withdrawal that progressed to full-blown delirium, psychosis, or seizures if untreated

Table 14-4. Emergency Room Treatment of Alcohol Withdrawal

Intramuscular administration of thiamine (100 to 200 mg)
Administration of a sedative or tranquilizer (i.e., chlordiazepoxide, 50 to 100 mg IV or PO)
3- to 6-day supply of a sedative or tranquilizing drug (i.e., chlordiazepoxide, 25 mg PO 4 times a day) provided
Observation for 1 to 2 hours after initial tranquilizer administration
Availability of outpatient facilities for followup made clear to patient

of occult blood in a stool specimen. Venous blood samples should be
sent for determinations of hematocrit reading, white blood cell count
with differential, prothrombin time, BUN, glucose, sodium, potassium,
chloride, and bicarbonate. Measurement of serum calcium, magnesium,
and amylase is often indicated. Further workup is dictated by the
clinical situation. The following aspects of therapy should be considered
fundamental:

A. **Vitamins**   Vitamin deficiencies, either clinical or subclinical, exist
in most if not all chronic alcoholics. Because administration of vitamin supplements carries no hazard, all patients should receive them
whether or not clinical manifestations are present.

1. **Assessment**

    a. Neurologic examination will reveal signs of Wernicke's en-
    cephalopathy if it is present. These are: nystagmus, inter-
    nuclear ophthalmoplegia, cerebellar ataxia, and a characteristic
    pattern of intellectual deterioration. Immediate administration
    of thiamine can prevent irreversible brain damage. All patients
    should receive thiamine (see Section IV.A. 2), even if Wernicke's
    encephalopathy is not detected.

    b. Peripheral neuropathy and megaloblastic anemia characteristic
    of folic acid deficiency are revealed by neurologic exam and
    study of the peripheral blood smear and bone marrow aspirate.

    c. Prolongation of prothrombin time in the absence of cirrhosis
    suggests vitamin K deficiency.

    d. Signs and symptoms of other deficiency states, such as hypovita-
    minosis C or scurvy (corkscrew hairs, perifollicular hemorrhages,
    gingival hemorrhage), are not infrequently encountered.

2. **Treatment**

    a. *All* patients should receive thiamine. The initial dose of 100
    to 200 mg IM or IV should be given immediately. The same
    dose is repeated, parenterally or orally, for at least the next
    three consecutive days.

b. All patients should receive folic acid, 1 to 5 mg daily, IM or PO.

c. All patients should receive a daily multivitamin supplement. Berocca-C can be given intramuscularly or by intravenous infusion. Its equivalent can be given by mouth if oral intake is adequate.

d. If prothrombin time is prolonged more than 3 seconds beyond control, vitamin K (5 to 10 mg) is given as a *single* parenteral dose. Larger doses are of no additional benefit. Failure of this dose to correct the prothrombin time suggests that significant hepatic disease is present.

3. **Hazards** of short-term vitamin treatment are essentially nonexisten. Paradoxical prolongations in prothrombin time have been reported following vitamin K administration in patients with cirrhosis, but these reports are anecdotal, and the actual hazard is not known.

B. Sedation   There is ample evidence that administration of sedatives or tranquilizers to abstinent alcoholics makes the subjective experience less unpleasant, and in general attenuates the severity of the withdrawal syndrome. Treatment is of greatest benefit when begun as early as possible. Most abstinent alcoholics are candidates to receive sedatives. The drugs must be used with caution when significant hepatic disease is present (see Section **VI.A**).

1. **Assessment**   Therapy must be carefully titrated and individualized. No fixed schedule can be considered rational. Larger doses of sedatives and tranquilizers are needed when symptoms are severe than when symptoms are mild. Dosage and frequency of administration should be adjusted and titrated so that symptoms are suppres — a state of light sleep is usually desirable. When therapy is inadequate, symptoms rage on, while overdosage produces obtundation, coma, and respiratory depression. Achieving the desired therapeutic effect, between the two extremes, is not always easy.

2. **Treatment**   A variety of sedatives and tranquilizers have been successfully used in alcohol withdrawal. Each has its benefits and hazards. Pharmacologic properties are discussed in detail in Chapter 1. Whatever drug is chosen, the suggested dosage increment (see Table 14-5) is given every 1 to 2 hours until adequate sedation is achieved. Parenteral therapy is usually necessary at first. When symptoms are suppressed, dosage increments are reduc in size and the time interval between dosage is lengthened, with subsequent drug administration on an as-needed basis.

Table 14-5. Hypnotics, Sedatives, and Tranquilizers Used in the Treatment of Alcohol Withdrawal

Drug	Dose Increment (see text)	Advantages	Disadvantages
Benzodiazepines			
Chlordiazepoxide	50 to 100 mg	Little cardiovascular or respiratory depression	Absorption after IM injection may be unreliable; long duration of action; accumulation of drugs and active metabolites
Diazepam	10 to 20 mg	No REM depression	
Oxazepam	30 to 60 mg	Same as chlordiazepoxide and diazepam	
		Short duration of action	Parenteral preparation not available
Chloral hydrate	1.0 to 2.0 gm	Short duration of action	REM depression
			Gastric irritation
			Parenteral preparation not available
Barbiturates			
Secobarbital Pentobarbital	100 to 300 mg		Cardiovascular and respiratory depression
			REM depression
			Enzyme induction
Phenobarbital	100 to 300 mg		Same as other barbiturates
			Long duration of action
Paraldehyde	10 to 30 ml	Short duration of action	Highly noxious odor
			Large volume needed for parenteral injection — can cause serious injection site complications
Antihistamines			
Hydroxyzine Diphenhydramine	50 to 100 mg		Anticholinergic side effects
Major tranquilizers			
Chlorpromazine Promazine	50 to 100 mg	Potent sedation	Long duration of action
			Postural hypotension
			Lowered seizure threshold
			Impaired temperature regulation

a. **Benzodiazepines** are preferred by many clinicians. They are safe and effective sedatives and produce minimal cardiovascular and respiratory depression. Benzodiazepines have little effect on dreaming (see Chapter 1); therefore, they allow dream recovery or "REM rebound" to occur in the abstinent alcoholic following prolonged dream suppression by alcohol. This seems to be an important aspect of the escape from alcohol dependence.

The long duration of action and cumulative effects of chlordiazepoxide and diazepam must be remembered. Oxazepam is relatively short-acting, but a parenteral form is not available.

b. **Barbiturates** effectively suppress alcohol withdrawal. However they are potent respiratory depressants and REM inhibitors. Barbiturates should be given only with great caution. They are especially hazardous in patients with obstructive pulmonary disease.

c. **Chloral derivatives** are time-tested and effective. Unfortunately parenteral preparations are not available, and administration must be by the oral or rectal route.

d. **Paraldehyde** is an effective short-acting hypnotic. Contrary to popular myths, less than 10 percent is exhaled via the lungs — the rest is metabolized in the liver. The unpleasant odor of paraldehyde is highly noxious to patients and medical staff. Th value of parenteral injections is limited by the large volume required (10 to 30 ml) and by the extremely irritating nature of the liquid, which can cause severe injection site complication Paraldehyde has no place in modern therapeutics.

e. **Sedative antihistamines** (hydroxyzine, diphenhydramine) can produce unwanted complications because of their anticholinergi properties — urinary retention, paralytic ileus, fever, tachycardia, and occasionally exacerbation of delirium and psychosis.

f. **Major tranquilizers** have been extensively used in alcohol withdrawal. There is reliable evidence, however, that major tranquilizers may do more harm than good. Serious and fatal hypotension can occur following administration of such drugs as promazine and chlorpromazine. Major tranquilizers lower the seizure threshold and can precipitate grand mal seizure activity. These drugs are *contraindicated* in patients with a known seizur disorder and in those who have had convulsions in the course of withdrawal.

3. **Hazards** of sedative-tranquilizer drug therapy have been discussed above and are summarized in Table 14-5. Drug dosage must be carefully modified when cirrhosis or hepatic failure is present.

C. **Hydration** It is traditionally taught that withdrawing alcoholics are dehydrated and need large quantities of parenteral fluid. This is undoubtedly true in many cases. When binge drinking precedes withdraw intake of nutrients, solute, and fluid other than alcoholic beverages is poor. Anorexia, nausea, vomiting, and diarrhea are common when alcohol intake ceases. Fever, diaphoresis, and muscle hyperactivity contribute to fluid loss in the later stages of the disease. All of these factors can combine to produce significant volume depletion.

Yet dehydration does not invariably occur, and excessive fluid therapy can be harmful. Many authors point out that overhydration is more common than volume depletion and that parenteral fluid therapy can worsen symptoms by producing cerebral edema — a common finding in fatal cases. Some further suggest that diuretics should be given instead of parenteral fluid and solute. Like sedative-hypnotic therapy, the use of parenteral fluids must be carefully individualized and titrated. No fixed schedule is rational. At all times the hazards of overhydration should be remembered.

1. **Assessment** of the withdrawing alcoholic's state of hydration is notably difficult. The usual reliable indicators can be misleading.

   a. **Skin turgor** assessment must be done with caution. Poorly nourished alcoholics may have reduced subcutaneous connective tissue and may appear to be dehydrated when in fact they are not.

   b. **Body weight** is useful, provided a recent weight is available from a previous admission. However, weight loss may be due to poor nutrition as much as dehydration. Once a baseline weight has been obtained on admission, daily changes in weight are a valuable indicator of the state of hydration. For this reason *all withdrawing alcoholics should be weighed daily.* Unless initial dehydration was severe, weight gain should be no greater than 0.5 to 1.0 kg per day.

   c. **Blood urea nitrogen** also can be deceiving. It may be inappropriately high if renal disease is present or if blood is present in the gastrointestinal tract. Misleadingly low values can occur because of poor protein intake or due to failure of urea synthesis by a diseased liver.

   d. **Thirst or dry mucous membranes** cannot be relied upon. Hyperventilation is common in alcohol withdrawal and can produce drying of mucous membranes in the absence of volume depletion.

   e. **Hematocrit reading** can be normal even with significant dehydration, since many alcoholics are anemic when in a normal state of hydration.

   f. **Urinalysis** is valuable provided renal function is normal. A urine *specific gravity* of greater than 1.025 or a *sodium concentration* of less than 10 mEq/L in a spot urine sample strongly suggests volume depletion.

2. **Treatment** If the patient is not seriously ill and can tolerate oral intake, he will correct fluid deficits and maintain normal hydration if given *ad lib* access to water and a diet containing normal amounts of sodium chloride. Patients who cannot eat or drink must be given parenteral fluids. If history, physical examination, body weight, and laboratory studies suggest that a fluid deficit is present, the deficit must be corrected in addition to administration of the maintenance fluids.

   a. Approximate daily **maintenance requirements** are: water, 30 to 40 ml/kg; sodium, 40 to 80 mEq; potassium, 30 to 60 mEq. These should be given by continuous infusion using appropriate combinations of the following available solutions: 5% dextrose in 0.9% NaCl, 5% dextrose in 0.45% NaCl, 5% dextrose in water, 10% dextrose in water. All infused solutions should contain dextrose so that calories are provided and hypoglycemia is avoided (see Section **V.D.2**). Appropriate quantities of potassium chloride can be added to any of these solutions.

   b. Fluid and electrolyte **deficits** should be corrected as indicated. No more than 50 percent of an initial deficit should be replaced in the first 24 hours, and no more than 6 liters of fluid should be given in a 24-hour period. Deficits developing during hospitalization because of vomiting, fever, diaphoresis, or marked hyperactivity can be avoided by increasing maintenance therapy.

3. **Hazards** were discussed earlier. In general these patients tolerate a mild degree of volume depletion better than overhydration. Fluid therapy therefore should be cautious and, if anything, conservative. The approach to parenteral fluid and electrolyte administration must be modified when cirrhosis is present and sodium metabolism is abnormal (see Section **VI**).

D. **Potassium balance** Even when parenchymal liver disease is not present most chronic alcoholics have a total body potassium deficit. This can contribute to symptoms such as depression, fatigue, and muscle weakness. When the deficit is severe and is superimposed on sympathetic nervous system hyperactivity during alcohol withdrawal, fatal cardiac arrhythmias can ensue. Most patients therefore should receive potassium supplementation.

1. **Assessment** Serum potassium is the only measurement readily available to most clinicians. Potassium is primarily an *intracellular* cation. Of a normal total body potassium content of 3000 to 3500 mEq, less than 1 percent is found in serum. Consequently, serum potassium can be normal despite a tremendous total body

deficit. Patients who have received long-term thiazide diuretic therapy without either potassium supplements or potassium-sparing agents invariably have a large deficit.

The influence of pH on serum potassium must be remembered. Respiratory alkalosis due to hyperventilation is frequently found in alcohol withdrawal. This results in a flux of potassium into cells, lowering the serum concentration without changing the total body store. Systemic acidosis does the reverse, and serum potassium rises.

2. **Treatment** Potassium chloride is *always* the supplement of choice. The kidney cannot conserve administered potassium unless chloride is given concurrently.

   a. If serum potassium is normal, the danger of cardiac arrhythmias is slight. Replacement can proceed slowly, at a rate of 60 to 100 mEq per day. A normal diet contains ample potassium, and supplements are not necessary when oral intake resumes.

   b. A low serum potassium in the absence of alkalosis almost always indicates a large total body deficit. Replacement rate is limited in part by the quantity of fluid given. Potassium chloride concentrations of more than 60 to 80 mEq/L are extremely irritating when given intravenously. The maximum replacement rate is 30 to 40 mEq per hour. The usual replacement dose is 100 to 140 mEq per day. Oral therapy is preferable whenever possible.

3. **Hazards** are those of hyperkalemia. Potassium should *not* be given unless urine output is adequate. Renal insufficiency necessitates caution and reduced dosage. Serum potassium concentrations should be determined at least daily during replacement therapy. Intravenous potassium chloride must be given by continuous infusion, *never* by bolus. The electrocardiogram should be monitored if large amounts of potassium are given intravenously. Administration of potassium chloride together with potassium-sparing diuretics (spironolactone, triamterene) is extremely hazardous even when thiazides are coadministered (*J.A.M.A.* 225:40, 1973).

E. **Magnesium balance** Metabolism of potassium and magnesium is similar. Most alcoholics are magnesium-depleted regardless of serum concentrations. Magnesium deficiency can contribute to symptoms of lethargy and weakness. Hypomagnesemia has also been suggested to lower the seizure threshold. Withdrawing alcoholics should receive 2 to 4 ml of 50% magnesium sulfate by intramuscular injection every 8 hours for at least three doses.

F. **Prophylactic anticonvulsants** The indications for prophylactic anticonvulsant therapy in alcohol withdrawal are very limited. Unfortunately, anticonvulsants are usually given when not needed or are given in such a way that they would do no good.

1. **Assessment** depends largely upon history.

   a. Most patients either have no history of seizures or have had convulsions only during prior episodes of alcohol withdrawal.

   b. A smaller group of patients are known to have grand mal seizures that occur apart from the alcohol abstinence syndrome. Almost all of these individuals are or should be receiving maintenance diphenylhydantoin (DPH) therapy. Either they have continued taking DPH up to the present or they stopped taking DPH 5 or more days earlier.

2. **Treatment** depends on which of these categories the patient falls into.

   a. With no seizure history or seizures during alcohol withdrawal only, there is no evidence that prophylactic DPH will prevent withdrawal seizures. Sedative-hypnotics and minor tranquilizers all have anticonvulsant activity in themselves. Adequate treatment of the abstinence syndrome minimizes the likelihood of seizures.

   b. Patients known to have an underlying seizure disorder are at risk of developing convulsions during alcohol withdrawal. They should be given adequate doses of DPH as rapidly as possible. *Major tranquilizers are contraindicated.*

      (1) If DPH therapy has been continued to the present, then daily maintenance doses should be given. Most patients require 300 to 400 mg per day. The dose can be given all at once. If oral intake is precluded, then maintenance dosage should be given intravenously at a rate not exceeding 50 mg per minute. DPH should never be given by intramuscular injection since it is incompletely absorbed (*Neurology* 23:318, 1973). As soon after admission as possible, serum DPH concentration should be determined and used to guide therapy. The effective serum concentration range is 10 to 20 μg per ml. Dosage should be adjusted to keep serum concentrations in this range, rather than fixed according to an arbitrary schedule.

      (2) If maintenance was stopped 5 or more days prior to admission, then total body DPH stores are essentially

depleted. In this case a *loading dose must be given.* One gram of DPH is mixed with 250 to 500 ml of 5% dextrose in water and given by continuous infusion over 1 to 4 hours. Maintenance therapy is begun on the next day. Starting maintenance therapy without a loading dose produces adequate anticonvulsant blood levels only after 4 to 5 days.

3. **Hazards** Parenteral DPH is given in a propylene glycol solvent vehicle that can cause bradycardia and hypotension if given in a rapid bolus. For this reason intravenous DPH should be given no faster than 50 mg per minute. Long-term administration of DPH can produce malabsorption of folic acid and vitamin D. These possibilities should be considered in newly admitted alcoholics who have received DPH as outpatients.

G. **Prophylactic antibiotics** Prophylactic administration of antibiotics undoubtedly does more harm than good. It insures only that if infection does occur, it will be of the antibiotic-resistant hospital-acquired variety. Infection during alcohol withdrawal is common. The development of fever obligates an exhaustive search for the source of infection (see Sections **V.A** and **V.B**). Antibiotics are not given until the site and nature of the infection are identified or in the uncommon instance that an unidentified infection will be fatal unless treated immediately.

H. **Corticosteroids** There is no evidence that abstinent alcoholics benefit from corticosteroid therapy.

V. **Recognition and Therapy of Complications** Complications of the alcohol withdrawal syndrome must be assessed and dealt with promptly. Sequelae such as infection and metabolic derangements can be rapidly fatal if unrecognized, but are readily reversible with sound medical management.

A. **Fever** Fever during alcohol withdrawal becomes more common with increasing severity of the withdrawal syndrome. Pyrexia per se is a symptom, not a disease. Epidemiologic studies suggest that fever in this setting is due either to dehydration or to pulmonary infection (*Am. J. Med. Sci.* 260:112, 1970). Alcoholic hepatitis is another common cause of low-grade fever (see Section **V.E**). Acute pancreatitis can also be associated with fever. However, statistics do not apply to individual patients. In any abstinent alcoholic, fever greater than 100.6°F means infection until proven otherwise. A systematic search for a source of infection must be undertaken.

1. **Assessment** of fever includes the following:

a. White blood cell count (WBC) *with differential.* Elevated WBC and shift to immature granulocyte forms can occur with sympathetic hyperactivity alone, hence are not diagnostic of infection. On the other hand, since alcohol can impair mobilization of leukocytes in response to infection, a normal WBC does not rule out infection. The appearance of basophilic ("toxic") granulations in neutrophils strongly suggests systemic infection. A *low* WBC in the presence of infection is prognostically grave.

b. Chest x-ray.

c. At least *two* blood cultures obtained from separate venipuncture sites. If fever persists with no source located, followup blood cultures are taken in sets of two at subsequent points in time.

d. A sputum sample is obtained for bacterial culture, acid-fast culture, gram stain, and acid-fast smears. Careful examination of sputum smears is a crucial aspect of the fever workup.

e. A *clean* urine sample is obtained, if necessary by catheterization, and cultured. The sediment must be carefully examined.

f. If the mental status is abnormal, a lumbar puncture must be performed. In addition to culture, cell counts (including differential and gram stain of the spinal fluid are done *by the physician.*

g. If physical examination reveals signs of peritoneal irritation, then x-rays of the abdomen in supine and upright positions are obtained, and four-quadrant diagnostic paracenteses are performed.

h. All indwelling intravenous catheters are removed and sent for culture. A new intravenous route is established at another site, preferably with a Butterfly scalp-vein infusion needle.

2. **Treatment**   Fever per se is not the object of therapy until dangerous levels of pyrexia are reached (greater than 103° to 104° F). Symptomatic therapy of fever includes salicylates, topical cooling measures, and *cautious* use of a phenothiazine such as chlorpromazine, if necessary. Since fever often is associated with volume depletion, the patient's state of hydration should be carefully assessed. If indicated, fluid therapy should be increased. The treatment of pyrexia associated with infection is discussed in Section **V.B.**

3. **Hazards**   Precautions and hazards in the treatment of fever and infection are discussed in Section **V.B.** Physicians can *prevent* or reduce the frequency of certain infections and their sequelae by the following measures:

    a. Butterfly scalp-vein infusion needles should be used for intravenous therapy whenever possible. Infectious complications of longer indwelling catheters are much more frequent and severe. *All* intravenous sites should be examined and palpated daily. The incidence of infection rises sharply when an indwelling intravenous arrangement has been in place more than 24 hours. It almost always is wise to change intravenous sites after 48 hours, even if no infection is evident.

    b. *All* indwelling Foley catheters become septic after being in place for more than 48 hours. This cannot be avoided. However, suppression of bacterial overgrowth in the bladder can prevent spread of infection to renal parenchyma and the systemic circulation. All indwelling catheters should receive *continuous* irrigation with either 0.25% acetic acid or a commercial bladder irrigant containing neomycin and polymyxin.

B. Infection Evaluation of fever as outlined in Section **V.A.1** usually will identify the site of infection if infection is present.

  1. Assessment

    a. **Pulmonary infection** is the most common type. The probability of pulmonary infection is higher in patients with chronic obstructive pulmonary disease (COPD). Cough, purulent sputum production, pleuritic chest pain, tachypnea, and an infiltrate on chest x-ray are common signs. Positive x-ray findings may not appear for up to 24 hours after other clinical manifestations. Not infrequently, the chest film is normal but significant infection is present in the upper tracheobronchial tree. Examination of sputum gram stain and acid-fast stain are the crucial diagnostic techniques.

      (1) **Pneumococcal infection** accounts for the majority of respiratory tract infections. Sudden shaking chills and high fever are common in severe infection. Positive blood cultures are obtained in more than 50 percent of cases. Chest x-ray characteristically shows segmental consolidation. Sputum gram stain reveals large numbers of polymorphonuclear leukocytes and gram-positive cocci, usually in pairs but sometimes in chains or clusters.

      (2) **Hemophilus influenzae** is often seen on gram stain, appearing as small pleomorphic gram-negative coccobacillary forms. It is difficult to tell how often this organism is actually a significant pathogen, especially since other organisms are usually seen as well. No doubt *H. influenzae* is more often a pathogen in withdrawing alcoholics and in patients with COPD.

(3) **Klebsiella pneumoniae** (Friedlander's bacillus) can produce rapidly fatal pulmonary infection in withdrawing alcoholic Chest x-ray shows characteristic dense consolidation with a "sagging" fissure. The sputum is thick and tenacious. Gram stain shows pairs of ovoid gram-negative cocci with thick capsules.

(4) **Mixed bacterial pneumonia** often is the result of aspiration of mouth flora during an episode of unconsciousness. Occasionally a lung abscess can result (seen as an air-fluid level on chest x-ray), but the infiltrate is usually streaky in nature and located in the right upper lobe. Gram stain reveals polymorphonuclear leukocytes and mixed flora.

(5) **Acid-fast infection** is surprisingly common in the alcoholic population. Active infection is diagnosed by identification of the organism on an acid-fast sputum smear. However, failure to locate these organisms does not rule out infection. Cavitation on chest x-ray is seen in advanced cases. Usually there is evidence of previous upper lobe disease on chest x-ray.

b. **Urinary tract infection** is uncommon in males unless there is obstruction due to prostatic hypertrophy. The patient may complain of dysuria or flank pain if infection is present in renal parenchyma.

Culture of clean urine is diagnostic if more than 100,000 organisms are present per milliliter of urine. Coliform organisms are the usual species involved. Urine sediment examination reveals polymorphonuclear leukocytes and gram-negative bacilli.

c. **Meningeal infection** is suggested by fever, altered mental status, seizures, and signs of meningeal irritation. Lumbar puncture should be performed promptly. In obvious cases the spinal fluid is purulent; polymorphonuclear leukocytes and bacteria can be identified on Wright's stain and gram stain, respectively. Usually there has been antecedent pulmonary, middle ear, or sinus infection with the same organism. Pneumococcus, *H. influenzae* and *Neisseria meningitidis* are the most common organisms.

If meningeal infection is not established on an initial lumbar puncture, repeat examination can be performed in 6 to 12 hours if suggestive signs and symptoms persist or become worse.

Spinal fluid white blood cell counts of greater than 7 per cubic mm are abnormal. Acute infection is strongly suggested when neutrophils predominate over lymphocytes in the differential count.

d. **Peritoneal infection** is usually secondary to a perforated abdominal viscus. Free air under the diaphragm on upright abdominal film strongly supports this, in which case surgical consultation should be obtained. Peritoneal infection is established by examination of fluid obtained from four-quadrant paracenteses. Tuberculous peritonitis is not rare in alcoholics.

e. **Intravenous catheter site infection** unfortunately is often over-looked. Severity can range from mild local phlebitis and cellulitis to fatal systemic staphylococcal septicemia. The intravenous catheter should be removed and sent for culture. Any local exudate should be sent for gram stain and culture. Aspiration of erythematous, indurated areas for diagnostic purposes should be attempted using a 25-gauge needle on a tuberculin syringe. If physical examination suggests a collection of pus, then incision and drainage should be performed.

f. Other possible infectious processes include osteomyelitis and septic arthritis.

2. **Treatment**

a. All patients with **pulmonary infection** should receive topical therapy to promote mobilization of secretions. These measures include steam inhalation, intermittent positive pressure breathing (IPPB), chest physical therapy, and postural drainage. The role of expectorants and mucolytics is not established. Choice of antibiotic depends on the organism identified. Intravenous therapy is always preferable initially. The drugs listed below are given in their usual order of choice.

   (1) **Pneumococcus**
   Penicillin G (300,000 units q6h)
   Erythromycin (500 mg q6h)
   Tetracycline (500 mg q6h)
   Cephalothin (1.0 gm q6h)

   (2) **Hemophilus influenzae**
   Ampicillin (1.0 gm q6h)
   Tetracycline (500 mg q6h)

   (3) **Klebsiella**
   • Gentamicin (5 mg/kg in 3 divided IM doses during the first day; then 3 mg/kg per day in 3 divided IM doses)

- Kanamycin (1.0 gm IM as a loading dose, then 500 mg IM q12h; gentamicin can be switched to kanamycin if sensitivity testing reveals kanamycin sensitivity)
- Chloramphenicol (1 gm q4h)

(4) **Mixed flora**   Same as for pneumococcus. When an air-fluid level (abscess cavity) is present, penicillin dose must be increased tenfold. The use of initial double therapy is not recommended.

(5) **Acid-fast infection**   Initial therapy should be with isoniazid (300 mg PO per day), and ethambutol (25 mg/kg daily in one oral dose for the first month, then 15 mg/kg daily). In severe cases, a third drug can be added simultaneously: streptomycin (1.0 gm IM daily for one month, then 1.0 gm IM 3 times per week).

b. **Urinary tract infection**

(1) If an indwelling catheter is present, then systemic therapy is futile. *All* indwelling catheters should receive *continuous* irrigation with either 0.25% acetic acid or a commercial polymyxin-neomycin irrigant.

(2) Noncatheter infection should if possible not be treated until sensitivity patterns are determined. "Outside-hospital" organisms are usually sensitive to any of the following agents:

Sulfisoxazole (1.0 gm PO qid)
Nitrofurantoin (100 mg PO qid)
Ampicillin (500 mg PO qid)
Tetracycline (500 mg PO qid)
Cephalexin (500 mg PO qid)

"Hospital" organisms, however, have multiple antibiotic resistance patterns. Usually one of the following is required

Kanamycin (500 mg IM q12h)
Gentamicin (3 mg/kg IM daily in 3 doses)
Chloramphenicol (500 mg PO qid)

c. **Meningeal infection** requires very high-dose antibiotic therapy. Penicillin derivatives are the agents of choice. Penicillin G (2 million units IV q2h) is suitable for pneumococcus and *N. meningitidis*. Ampicillin (2 gm IV q2h) should be used for *H. influenzae*.

d. **Peritoneal infection** requires two drugs. At least one should be a penicillin or a cephalosporin; the other should be an aminoglycoside or chloramphenicol. The source of infection should be searched for with the assistance of a surgical consultant.

e. **Catheter site infection** should receive local therapy with topical heat and moisture. Incision and drainage are performed if indicated. Septicemia caused by catheter infection should be treated with a penicillinase-resistant penicillin (nafcillin, 12 to 18 gm per day IV) until the organism is identified.

3. **Hazards** of antibiotic therapy are detailed in other sources (*Semin. Drug Treat.* 2:331, 1972; *Calif. Med.* 111:362, 1969). The important hazards can be summarized as follows:

a. **Penicillins:** allergic reactions; seizures (in high doses).

b. **Aminoglycosides:** ototoxicity; nephrotoxicity; weakness and myasthenia due to a curare-like effect.

c. **Chloramphenicol:** bone marrow depression.

d. **Cephalosporins:** nephrotoxicity (cephaloridine); local phlebitis (cephalothin).

e. **Antituberculotic drugs:** hepatotoxicity, peripheral neuropathy (isoniazid); optic neuritis (ethambutol); ototoxicity (streptomycin, an aminoglycoside) (see also *Drug Ther.* 4:39 [Feb.], 1974).

Many antibiotics — primarily aminoglycosides and tetracyclines require dosage adjustment in the presence of renal insufficiency. This is discussed in detail elsewhere (*J.A.M.A.* 214:1468, 1970).

C. **Seizures** Indications for *prophylactic* anticonvulsant therapy were described in Section **IV.F.** Seizure activity, when it occurs, appears within 48 hours of cessation of drinking in 95 percent of cases (*Epilepsia* 8:1, 1967). Seizures are usually grand mal, nonfocal, and one or two in number. They cease without specific treatment. Seizures *precede* the severe manifestations of alcohol withdrawal ("DTs").

1. Assessment

a. Seizures should be carefully observed for lateralizing or focal signs. Neurologic examination, skull films, and lumbar puncture should then be performed. Neurologic or neurosurgical consultation or both are promptly obtained if any of the following findings are present: focal neurologic signs, lateralizing seizures, increased intracranial pressure, skull fracture, non-midline pineal, or blood in the spinal fluid. Meningeal infection as a cause of seizures should also be documented by the lumbar puncture.

b. Metabolic or iatrogenic causes for seizures should be ruled out. These include hypoxia, hypotension (related to phenothiazine use or to volume depletion), hypomagnesemia, hyponatremia or hypernatremia, major tranquilizer treatment, high-dose penicillin treatment, and lidocaine infusion.

2. **Treatment** Seizure activity per se does not require treatment unless convulsions are repeated and life-threatening. Seizures due to alcohol withdrawal alone stop spontaneously and require only adequate treatment with sedative-hypnotics. Once seizures appear, *major tranquilizers are contraindicated.* Underlying causes of seizures should obviously be treated.

a. Subdural hematoma or intracranial hemorrhage requires neuro-surgical evaluation and intervention.

b. Metabolic and iatrogenic causes should be removed. When seizures are life-threatening, therapy should be that outlined for status epilepticus (Chapter 1). Treatment includes diphenyl-hydantoin, 1.0 gm in 250 to 500 ml 5% dextrose in water given intravenously over 1 to 4 hours; diazepam, 5 mg IV per minute until seizures cease or until a total of 25 to 30 mg is given; and phenobarbital, 120 mg IM. If these measures fail, then intra-venous amobarbital (100 mg per minute) can be given, up to a total dose of 1.0 gm. Curarization with assisted ventilation is a last resort.

3. **Hazards** are those of respiratory depression, hypotension, and coma following administration of multiple CNS depressant drugs.

D. **Metabolic disturbances** Recognition and therapy of abnormalities in hydration, potassium balance, and magnesium balance were discussed in Sections **IV.C, D,** and **E.** Other common metabolic disturbances include the following:

1. **Hyponatremia** is usually iatrogenic, due to excessive parenteral administration of sodium-free solutions. Treatment consists of restriction of free water. When hyponatremia is severe (less than 110 mEq/L) or accompanied by objective neuropsychiatric symp-toms, hypertonic sodium chloride solution can be *cautiously* given intravenously.

2. **Hypoglycemia** is a significant danger in abstinent alcoholics. Glycogen depletion, hepatic disease, and poor calorie intake can contribute to hypoglycemia. All parenteral solutions should contain 5% dextrose in addition to other solute. Whenever unexplained obtundation occurs, a blood sample should be drawn for glucose determination, and a 50 ml bolus of 50% glucose solution should be given immediately thereafter.

3. **Alkalosis** usually is due to hyperventilation. Alkalosis is important when it lowers extracellular potassium and magnesium concentrations, causing weakness and possibly a lowered seizure threshold. Therapy consists of sedation and supplements of potassium and magnesium, as described earlier.

E. **Alcoholic hepatitis** Alcoholic hepatitis is a complication not of alcohol withdrawal itself but of the drinking episode prior to abstinence. Clinical characteristics include an enlarged tender liver, low-grade fever, leukocytosis, mild hepatic function abnormalities, and fatty infiltration of the liver on histologic study. The syndrome occurs in all individuals after an alcohol binge and in theory is completely reversible if drinking stops. It is thought that repeated episodes of alcoholic hepatitis in chronic alcoholics may lead eventually to irreversible damage (cirrhosis). The only specific therapy is cessation of drinking. The role of corticosteroids has not been established.

F. **Hematologic disorders** Several hematologic abnormalities occur in alcoholics and can complicate alcohol withdrawal. These include:

1. **Hypoprothrombinemia** This can occur on the basis of liver disease or vitamin K deficiency. When the prothrombin time exceeds control by more than 3 seconds, a trial dose of vitamin K (5 mg) should be given. If this fails to correct the abnormality, further doses will be of no value. Severe hypoprothrombinemia associated with intractable bleeding requires administration of fresh blood or plasma.

2. **Thrombocytopenia** Alcohol ingestion can cause a transient reduction in the platelet count to very low levels. The syndrome is rapidly reversible and probably of no consequence.

3. **Impaired granulocyte function** Alcohol depresses granulocyte function. This may explain the increased susceptibility of alcoholics to bacterial infection and the occasional finding of a low or normal WBC count despite serious systemic infection.

4. **Anemia**

a. Anemia in alcoholics is **assessed** by the following methods:

      (1)   Examination of peripheral blood smear.

      (2)   Reticulocyte count.

      (3)   Wright's stain and iron stain of bone marrow aspirate.

      (4)   More expensive, less essential measures include serum concentration determinations of iron, iron binding capacity, vitamin B_{12}, and folate.

   b. Common **etiologies** of anemia are:

      (1)   Iron deficiency due to chronic gastrointestinal blood losses

      (2)   Megaloblastic process, usually due to folic acid deficiency or malutilization.

      (3)   Idiopathic anemia, apparently due to bone marrow depression by alcohol.

   In most alcoholics, anemia is due to a combination of the three.

   c. Treatment depends on the etiology.

      (1)   If bone marrow aspirate reveals iron deficiency, then iron therapy is given. Oral therapy usually fails because alcohol are notoriously poor pill-takers. *Iron dextran* (1.0 gm in 5 5% dextrose in water) is given intravenously over 1 to 2 ho The physician *must be present* for the beginning of the inf An intravenous catheter (Jelco or Angiocath) is used to pre extravasation and a permanent blue stain. Iron dextran sh not be given intramuscularly. A series of painful injections is necessary, and infection site complications can be severe

      (2)   All alcoholics should be assumed to be folate-deficient whe anemic or not. A dose of 1 mg is given daily.

      (3)   Cessation of alcohol ingestion is the only therapy for acute alcoholic thrombocytopenia and idiopathic alcoholic anem

   d. Hazards   Iron dextran rarely causes anaphylactic reactions. The hazard is minimized if the physician starts the infusion himself and monitors the first 50 to 100 ml himself. Iron dextran given intramuscularly is much more hazardous.

VI. Modification of Therapy when Major Associated Diseases Coexist Severa disease states are notoriously common in alcoholics. Some are a direct consequence of alcoholism (cirrhosis, gastrointestinal bleeding); others are not causally related but are closely associated (chronic obstructive pulmonary disease). Treatment of alcohol withdrawal may have to be modified when one or more of these entities is present. Not infrequently, hospital admission is due to an associated disease and the withdrawal syndrome develops *after* the patient is hospitalized.

   A. Cirrhosis Coexistence of the alcohol withdrawal syndrome with cirrhosis is prognostically grave. It indicates continued alcohol consumption despite irreversible alcohol-induced liver damage. The following modifications in therapy are necessary.

1. **Sedatives and tranquilizers** must be administered with the utmost caution. Very small doses can precipitate hepatic coma. Careful titration is the only rational approach, with underdosage preferred to oversedation. When cirrhosis is present, benzodiazepines are the safest choice of drugs. The belief that paraldehyde is safe in liver disease is unfounded. Only a small proportion of paraldehyde excretion is via the lungs; hepatic detoxification is the major route of elimination (*Toxicol. Appl. Pharmacol.* 15:269, 1969).

2. **Fluid and electrolyte therapy** in cirrhosis must account for abnormalities in sodium metabolism. In cirrhotic patients, sodium retention occurs despite total body sodium overload. Sodium and water excess are stored as ascitic fluid. Massive ascites can be present even when intravascular volume is depleted.

   Salt-poor albumin is the volume-expanding agent of choice, especially when hypoalbuminemia is present. Several units of 12.5 to 25 gm each can be given daily. All intravenous solutions should contain 5% to 10% *dextrose* to provide calories and to avoid hypoglycemia. *Potassium* depletion can be very severe in cirrhosis, and supplements are invariably required. Diuresis of ascitic fluid should be undertaken gently with a weight loss of no more than 1.0 kg per day. *Spironolactone* (100 to 200 mg per day) is the diuretic of choice. Hazards of coadministration of potassium chloride with spironolactone must be remembered.

3. **Infection** can precipitate hepatic coma and must be treated aggressively. Ascitic fluid is an ideal culture medium, and it should always be examined in evaluation of fever.

B. **Chronic obstructive pulmonary disease (COPD)** The nonsmoking alcoholic is a rarity, particularly at city and municipal hospitals. COPD therefore usually coexists with alcoholism. When significant pulmonary disease is present, *arterial blood gas determinations* should be a routine aspect of assessment.

1. **Sedatives and tranquilizers** again require careful titration. Oversedation can precipitate carbon dioxide retention, narcosis, and coma. Benzodiazepines are the safest of available drugs. Barbiturates are hazardous. Hypoxia or carbon dioxide narcosis or both should be considered whenever there is an alteration in mental status. Hypoxia can cause agitation, which is made worse by treatment with sedative drugs rather than oxygen.

2. **Fluid and electrolyte therapy** must account for the possibility of *cor pulmonale.* This entity can be diagnosed by physical examina-

tion, chest x-ray, and electrocardiogram. Sodium must be administered cautiously when cor pulmonale is present.

3. **Infection** is a significant threat to the patient with COPD. Pulmonary infection should be carefully considered as the etiology of fever when it occurs. *Superinfection* with hospital-acquired antibiotic-resistant organisms is prognostically grave. This usually occurs during ongoing antibiotic therapy in patients receiving assisted ventilation through tracheostomies or endotracheal tubes.

C. **Trauma** Head trauma, even if seemingly minor, always raises the possibility of intracranial bleeding. Patients with *any* evidence of head trauma should be observed carefully for the appearance of:

1. Focal neurologic signs (e.g., unilateral mydriasis, lateralizing seizures).

2. Increased intracranial pressure (papilledema, vomiting, hypertension, bradycardia, depression of consciousness).

Findings consistent with either of these entities requires immediate neurologic or neurosurgical consultation or both.

D. **Gastrointestinal bleeding** *Superficial gastritis* due to alcohol or aspirin or both is the usual cause of gastrointestinal bleeding in alcoholics. This usually ceases rapidly following nasogastric suction, antacid administration, and abstinence from alcohol. *Peptic ulcer* disease is the next most common cause. Conservative therapy again is usually successful. Bleeding from *esophageal varices* is unusual. When it does occur, bleeding is catastrophic, intractable, and often fatal.

1. **Sedatives and tranquilizers** should be administered in sufficient doses that the patient will not pull out nasogastric tubes and intravenous catheters.

2. **Fluid and electrolyte therapy** should account for the ongoing volume loss. Blood transfusion is frequently necessary. Hematocrit reading should be checked every 4 hours during active bleeding with frequent assessment continued for at least 24 hours after bleeding has stopped. A *central venous pressure line* is quite helpful in determining the adequacy of fluid therapy. Losses of chloride can be large when nasogastric suction is ongoing. These should be replaced with intravenous potassium chloride.

E. **Pancreatitis** Severe abdominal pain, fever, and leukocytosis should suggest the possibility of acute pancreatitis. Elevated urinary clearance of amylase relative to creatinine is the most reliable diagnostic index.

1. As with gastrointestinal bleeding, **sedatives and tranquilizers** must be given in doses sufficient to prevent the patient from pulling out nasogastric tubes and intravenous catheters. Since most patients will require opiate analgesics as well, the possibility of additive CNS depression should be considered.

2. **Fluid and electrolyte therapy** must be vigorous. Patients with acute pancreatitis can lose large amounts of fluid volume into the retroperitoneal space. The hematocrit reading should be taken frequently; plasma or albumin is given as indicated.

    Hypocalcemia can occur in pancreatitis and can lower the seizure threshold. The serum calcium should be measured in all patients with pancreatitis. Calcium supplements (1.0 gm of calcium chloride or gluconate) are given intravenously as indicated.

3. **Malabsorption** syndromes are common in chronic pancreatitis and can produce deficiencies of vitamins D and K. Hypocalcemia can result from hypovitaminosis D and emphasizes the necessity for measuring serum calcium (see Section **VI.E.2**). Vitamin K deficiency increases the possibility of hypoprothrombinemia and bleeding. The prothrombin time should be measured and parenteral vitamin K (5 mg) given if indicated.

4. **Hyperglycemia** can be associated with acute or chronic pancreatitis on the basis of inadequate insulin secretion. Blood and urinary glucose should be measured in all patients with pancreatitis and insulin given if indicated.

References

Benor, D., and Ditman, K. S. Tranquilizers in the management of alcoholics. A review of the literature to 1964. Part I. *J. New Drugs* 6:319–337, 1966. Part II. *J. Clin. Pharmacol.* 7:17–25, 1967.

Greenblatt, D. J. Inside an inner city alcoholic ward. *Medical Insight* 4:23–29 (Aug.), 1972.

Greenblatt, D. J., and Greenblatt, M. Which drug for alcohol withdrawal? *J. Clin. Pharmacol.* 12:429–431, 1972.

Gross, M. M., Rosenblatt, S. M., Lewis, E., Chartoff, S., and Malenowski, B. Acute alcoholic psychoses and related syndromes: Psychosocial and clinical characteristics and their implications. *Br. J. Addict.* 67:15–31, 1972.

Kaim, S. C., Klett, C. J., and Rothfeld, B. Treatment of the acute alcohol withdrawal state: A comparison of four drugs. *Am. J. Psychiatry* 125:1640–1646, 1969.

Kissin, B., and Gross, M. M. Drug therapy in alcoholism. *Am. J. Psychiatry* 125:31–41, 1968.

Victor, M. The role of hypomagnesemia and respiratory alkalosis in the genesis of alcohol-withdrawal symptoms. *Ann. N. Y. Acad. Sci.* 215:235–248, 1973.

15

Psychotropic Drug Overdosage

David J. Greenblatt
Richard I. Shader

A decade ago, overdosage with barbiturates and glutethimide accounted for the great majority of serious and fatal cases of self-poisoning reaching medical attention. This pattern has not changed appreciably, even though other psychotropic drugs now are much more widely used than barbiturates. At least one in ten American adults, for example, takes chlordiazepoxide or diazepam in a year's time. Yet life-threatening poisoning with either of these drugs is exceedingly rare.

Principles of treatment of barbiturate-like CNS depressant overdosage are applicable with only minor modifications to poisonings with other psychotropic drugs. Physicians who are familiar with these principles, therefore, are well-equipped to deal with most if not all deliberate self-poisonings.

I. **Resuscitation** All physicians who staff emergency room facilities *must* be familiar with techniques of cardiopulmonary resuscitation. Successful resuscitation is unlikely unless help is available — from two or three skilled nurses and at least one other physician. Cardiopulmonary arrest following drug overdosage is uncommon, but by no means rare. Ischemic heart disease usually underlies cardiac arrest. The age and sex of the patient can strongly suggest the etiology.

    A. **Assessment** The patient needing resuscitation is unconscious and cyanotic. Carotid and femoral pulses are palpated for evidence of cardiac action. If heartbeat cannot be felt, then resuscitation is instituted to the exclusion of further assessment.

    B. **Initial treatment**

       1. A brisk **blow to the precordium** with a closed fist can effectively restore cardiac action in some cases.

       2. **Assisted ventilation** is begun by insertion of a cuffed endotracheal tube and ventilation with 100% oxygen via an Ambu bag. The bronchial tree should be thoroughly suctioned.

       3. **Closed chest cardiac massage** is simultaneously begun in coordination with bag ventilation. The adequacy of cardiac massage is

judged by palpability of femoral and carotid pulses and by diminution of pupil size.

4. A reliable **intravenous route** is immediately established. Indwelling plastic catheters (Jelco, Angiocath, or Intracath) should be used rather than Butterfly scalp-vein needles, since the latter frequently dislodge during the chaos of resuscitation. Antecubital or forearm veins can be difficult or impossible to cannulate. Physicians therefore *must* be adept at starting intravenous lines by other routes: antecubital or medical malleolar cutdown, or catheterization of the right subclavian vein. Intravenous routes, once established, should be firmly secured with adhesive tape.

5. Continuous **electrocardiographic (ECG) monitoring** is begun since definitive pharmacologic therapy depends on the mechanism of cardiac arrest.

C. Subsequent assessment and treatment

1. The pH of liquid suctioned from the bronchial tree should be determined using commercial pH paper strips. An acid pH (3 or less) suggests aspiration of acidic gastric contents. The patient should receive a rapid intravenous bolus of hydrocortisone (200 mg or its equivalent.

2. Adequacy of resuscitation is assessed by determination of arterial blood gases pH, PO_2, PCO_2), determined by femoral artery blood samples.

3. Intravenous **sodium bicarbonate** is given to correct metabolic acidosis. Bicarbonate can be given by continuous infusion of a 5% solution or by boluses of commercially available ampules, each containing 43 mEq of $NaHCO_3$. Bolus therapy is preferable since it is easier to titrate. Adequacy of replacement is assessed by arterial pH and PCO_2. The initial dose of 1 or 2 ampules is given to all patients. Followup doses of 1 ampule every 5 to 10 minutes are given until metabolic acidosis is corrected or cardiac action is restored.

4. **Cardiac pharmacotherapy** is begun according to the ECG findings. Therapy usually takes one of two possible directions — *stimulatory* or *suppressive*. However, it is common for cardiac findings to change suddenly, such that frequent jumps between the two treatment approaches are necessary. *Acidosis and hypoxia must be corrected* before any form of pharmacotherapy will restore normal cardiac action.

a. **Suppressive treatment** is given when ventricular tachyarrhythmia (ventricular tachycardia or fibrillation) is the mechanism of arrest.

(1) **Direct-current cardioversion** is the first maneuver. The appropriate energy output is 200 joules per shock. The shock is preceded by an intravenous injection of epinephrine (0.5 mg) when fibrillation is present. Cardioversion is repeated as often as necessary, concurrent with antiarrhythmic therapy.

(2) **Antiarrhythmic drugs** are combined with repeated cardioversion as necessary to suppress ventricular tachyarrhythmias. The appropriate agents in their usual order of choice are:

- Lidocaine, 1 mg/kg bolus followed by infusion at 2 to 4 mg/min
- Procainamide, 50 mg/min infusion up to a total dose of 1.0 gm
- Diphenylhydantoin, 50 mg/min infusion up to a total dose of 500 mg
- Propranolol, 1 to 2 mg/min infusion up to 5 mg
- Bretylium, 5 mg/kg in a 3 to 5 minute infusion

b. **Stimulant treatment** is given when asystole or bradyarrhythmia is the mechanism of arrest. Correction of acidosis and its associated hyperkalemia is the most important measure.

(1) Excess **vagal activity** frequently contributes to bradycardia or heart block; therefore, all patients should receive **atropine,** 1 mg IV.

(2) **Cardiostimulant drugs** are given intravenously to initiate adequate cardiac action. The most commonly used agents are:

- Epinephrine, 0.5 mg bolus
- Calcium chloride or gluconate, 1.0 gm bolus
- Isoproterenol, 0.2 mg bolus or continuous infusion of solution containing 2.0 mg in 500 ml of 5% dextrose in water, or both
- Glucagon, 5.0 mg bolus or continuous infusion of solution containing 30 mg in 500 ml of 5% dextrose in water, or both

(3) If these measures fail to initiate cardiac action, then a **right ventricular pacing wire** is introduced through the

antecubital, jugular, or subclavian vein. Electrical depolarization of the heart almost always can be achieved
if the pacing wire is in contact with the endocardium.
Failure of electrical depolarization to stimulate mechanica
contraction suggests that resuscitation will not succeed.

5. **Hypotension** (systolic blood pressure less than 90 mm Hg) may
persist despite restoration of normal cardiac activity. After drug
overdosage in young individuals with healthy hearts, hypotension
is usually due to relative hypovolemia secondary to pooling of
blood in venous capacitance beds.

    a. A **central venous pressure (CVP)** catheter is introduced into the
right atrium. Therapy is assessed using a combination of the
following three indicators: CVP, systolic blood pressure, and
urine output. Continuous measurement of urine output obviously requires an indwelling Foley catheter. Therapy can be
considered adequate when CVP is 12 to 15 cm H_2O, systolic
blood pressure is 100 mm Hg or higher, and urine output is 20
to 30 ml per hour.

    b. **Intravenous fluids and solute** are the first approach to therapy.
They should be given until the above indicators come into the
"adequate" range. CVP of 15 cm H_2O or more usually indicates
that the limit of volume repletion has been reached. Available
solute and colloid preparations include whole blood, plasma,
human serum albumin, lactated Ringer's solution, and 0.9%
sodium chloride solution.

    c. Failure of fluid therapy to restore blood pressure and urine
output is prognostically unfavorable. In this case, **vasopressor
drugs** are required. They are given by *continuous infusion* at
whatever rate is necessary to keep systolic BP at 100 to 110
mm Hg. The following pressors can be used, with infusion
solutions made up by adding the indicated dose to 500 ml of
5% dextrose in water:

        Norepinephrine, 4 mg
        Metaraminol, 200 mg
        Phenylephrine, 1 mg
        Dopamine, 400 mg

    d. The prognosis is grave when hypotension persists despite these
measures. The patient can be given a bolus of hydrocortisone
(1.0 gm) as a "last-ditch" maneuver.

II. **The Comatose Patient** Unresponsive patients who are breathing spontaneously and have adequate blood pressure and normal skin temperature do not require resuscitation. Yet the need for immediate assessment and treatment is only slightly less urgent. The patient's eventual survival can be determined by the first 30 to 60 minutes' contact with the physician. During this period, physicians must do several things simultaneously: determine the history, perform a rapid physical examination, initiate laboratory studies, and begin emergency treatment.

A. **History** Every effort should be made to determine the drug ingested and the quantity. History can be obtained from family, friends, police, and the patient's personal physician. The patient's clothing, belongings, or dwelling should be searched for bottles of pills, either full or empty. The contents of empty bottles can sometimes be determined by contact with the pharmacy that filled the prescription.

Specific questions should be answered if possible: Is the patient known to have a psychiatric disorder? Is he receiving psychiatric treatment? Are drugs or unfilled prescriptions available to him? Has he attempted suicide previously? Has he been depressed, despondent, or talked of suicide recently? Has there been a recent traumatic event in his life? Is the patient a diabetic? Has he been treated for hypertension or a seizure disorder?

An adequate history is of great clinical importance and can be far more useful than toxicologic drug screening services, which often are inaccurate and nonspecific.

B. **Physical examination** The following aspects of the physical examination should be assessed rapidly:

1. Blood pressure.
2. Heart rate.
3. Rectal temperature.
4. Respirations: rate and character.
5. Skull: evidence of lacerations or trauma.
6. Skin: temperature, hydration, evidence of trauma, necrotic areas, bullae.
7. Pupils: size, reactivity, "doll's eye" movement.
8. Fundi: evidence of increased intracranial pressure.
9. Ears: hematotympanum.
10. Mouth: dentures removed.
11. Neck: carotid pulsations, jugular venous pressure.
12. Chest: aeration of both lungs, rales or rhonchi.
13. Heart: rate, rhythm, murmurs, gallops.
14. Abdomen: evidence of hepatosplenomegaly or other organ enlargement.

15. Rectal: occult blood in stool.
16. Extremities: evidence of self-harm, fractures.
17. Neurologic: spontaneous movement, muscle tone, responsivenes to pain in four extremities and over sternum, deep tendon reflexe superficial reflexes.

C. **Objective tests** The following laboratory studies should be obtained on all patients:

1. Hematocrit reading.
2. White blood count and differential.
3. Blood urea nitrogen.
4. Creatinine.
5. Glucose.
6. Electrolytes (Na^+, K^+, Cl^-, HCO_3^-).
7. Arterial blood (pH, Po_2, Pco_2)
8. Urine specimen for glucose, acetone, and sediment exam (if patie is unresponsive, then Foley catheter is left indwelling).
9. Serum sample for toxicologic screening.
10. X-ray examinations of chest and skull using portable equipment; other areas are x-rayed if fracture is suspected.
11. Lumbar puncture with spinal fluid examined by physician.
12. Electrocardiogram.

D. **Emergency treatment**

1. *All patients must immediately receive intravenous glucose* (50 ml of 50% solution) even if another cause of coma is established. Failure to administer glucose constitutes a grave error.

2. *Antidotes* can be given when specific ones exist. These instances are rare but include:

   a. *Naloxone,* for opiate-induced coma (see Section **V.L**).

   b. *Physostigmine,* in anticholinergic drug-induced coma (see Chapter 11) and in tricyclic antidepressant overdosage (see Section **V.I**).

E. **Precautions** Causes of coma other than drug ingestion *must be ruled out in all patients.* Common etiologies include hypoglycemia, hyperglycemic ketoacidotic coma, head trauma, postictal state, and spontaneous intracranial hemorrhage. Less common causes are accelerated hypertension, cerebrovascular accident, hepatic coma, uremic coma, meningoencephalitis, hypercalcemia or hypocalcemia, hypernatremia or hyponatremia, myxedema, and addisonian crisis.

III. **Removing Ingested Poison** Attempts to accelerate the normal mechanisms that detoxify and excrete psychotropic drugs are justified providing the possible benefits of such measures outweigh the risks. Some procedures (gastric lavage, induced catharsis) carry little hazard and are indicated in most cases. Other interventions (hemodialysis, exchange transfusion) carry significant risk and are used only when poisoning is prolonged or life-threatening. Needless to say, no poison-removal measures can be considered until circulation and respiration are stabilized.

A. **Clearing the stomach** The physician's first thought should be the removal of any drug that remains in the stomach. The value of emptying the stomach rapidly diminishes as the time since drug ingestion grows longer. It is unusual for significant quantities of poison to be removed if more than 4 hours have elapsed since ingestion, or if the patient is comatose. Since clearing the stomach is relatively safe if done properly, it is not unreasonable that stomach-emptying procedures be performed routinely regardless of the time since ingestion.

1. **Induced emesis** is the most efficient and effective means of emptying the stomach. Vomiting should be induced *only in a fully conscious patient* because of the danger of aspiration.

   a. *Apomorphine* (2.5 to 5.0 mg IV) has the advantage of rapid action and nearly 100 percent effectiveness. However, the drug can produce unwanted CNS and respiratory depression. Occasionally vomiting becomes intractable and requires an opiate antagonist (naloxone 0.4 to 0.8 mg IV).

   b. *Syrup of ipecac* (15 to 45 ml PO) is less consistently effective than apomorphine and produces vomiting only after a delay of 10 to 30 min. CNS depression is not a problem. Large volumes of water *should not be given* since this will enhance dissolution of remaining poison and stimulate emptying of stomach. There is no evidence that syrup of ipecac works faster or is more effective when administered with large amounts of water. Fluid extract of ipecac is cardiotoxic and *should never be given.*

   c. **Other emetic agents** used in the past include lobeline, zinc sulfate, copper sulfate, potassium antimony tartrate, sodium chloride, powdered mustard, and soap. Their efficacy is not established; moreover, serious and fatal toxicity can occur if emesis fails.

2. **Gastric lavage** is less effective than emesis in removing stomach contents. Lavage is time-consuming and cannot recover intact pills

or large particles of undissolved poison. Gastric lavage is performed under the following circumstances: (1) when consciousne is depressed, making vomiting hazardous, (2) when induced emesi has failed, (3) when the ingested drug has antiemetic properties (major tranquilizers, tricyclic antidepressants, anticholinergics).

a. A **conscious patient** is placed in the sitting position. The lubricated tip of a Levine tube (size 14 or 16) is inserted through th nose to the posterior pharynx. While the patient swallows a small volume of water, the tube is advanced rapidly to the stomach. Auscultation of the stomach while 50 cc of air is injected into the proximal end of the tube verifies that the distal end is in the stomach.

b. The **unresponsive patient** should have endotracheal intubation prior to lavage, to prevent reflux and aspiration of gastric contents. Passage of the Levine tube is more difficult since the patient is not able to alter the position of the glottis.

Lavage is performed by repeated injection and withdrawal of 50 ml of water or physiologic saline. Hypertonic saline should not be used. A sample of the aspirated fluid can be sent for toxicologic analysis.

B. **Interference with drug absorption**   Measures that empty stomach contents often fail to recover enough drug to alter its clinical course. Following lavage or emesis, physicians can administer one or both of the following substances, which have the potential to inhibit drug absorption from the gastrointestinal tract:

1. **Activated charcoal** can bind and prevent absorption of significant quantities of barbiturates. Fifty to 100 gm is suspended in water and given by mouth or instilled through the nasogastric tube.
   Activated charcoal and *syrup of ipecac* are antagonistic when given concurrently. Since charcoal adsorbs ipecac, the activity of the latter is diminished. Conversely, adsorption of ipecac by charcoal reduces its ability to bind other drugs. *The two agents should not be given together.*

2. **Irritant lipid cathartics** serve two purposes:

   a. They partition highly lipid-soluble drugs (glutethimide, short-acting barbiturates, diazepam) into the lipid substance, thus preventing absorption.

   b. Induced catharsis speeds gastrointestinal transit and reduces the time during which the poison is in contact with absorbing epithelium.

Either *castor oil* or *mineral oil* can be given by mouth or in-stilled through the nasogastric tube. The usual dose is 60 to 120 ml.

C. **Enhancing urinary excretion**   Significant quantities of certain psy-chotropic drugs are excreted unchanged in the urine. They include phenobarbital, butabarbital, meprobamate, tranylcypromine, amphet-amines, and lithium. These drugs are relatively water-soluble and weakly bound to plasma protein. The actual quantity recovered in the urine depends on urine volume and pH. Other drugs (glutethimide, short-acting barbiturates, benzodiazepines, tricyclic antidepressants), which are lipid-soluble, strongly protein-bound, and completely bio-transformed prior to excretion, are not recovered unchanged in the urine to any significant degree.

1. **Forced diuresis** is indicated to enhance removal of any of the first-mentioned group of drugs. An indwelling Foley catheter is inserted, and urine outputs are measured hourly.

   a. Diuresis can be initiated with a small dose of furosemide (20 to 40 mg IV). However, diuretics are *not* needed in a majority of patients with normal renal function.

   b. An appropriate intravenous solution contains 5% dextrose, 0.23 to 0.45% saline, and 10 to 20 mEq of potassium chloride per liter. Premixed intravenous solutions having approximately this concentration are available commercially (Isolyte).

   c. Daily urine output should be 6 to 12 liters.

   d. Serum electrolytes should be measured at least every 12 hours. Adjustments in the composition of intravenous infusions are made as necessary.

2. **Alterations in urine pH** are combined with forced diuresis to further enhance elimination.

   a. **Alkalinization** of the urine markedly enhances phenobarbital excretion. One ampule of sodium bicarbonate (containing 43 mEq) is given by intravenous bolus. Then one ampule is added to each liter of intravenous solution. Urine pH is measured every 2 to 4 hours. Alkalinization is adequate *only when urinary pH is 8.* A lower pH indicates that more bi-carbonate must be given.

   b. **Acidification** enhances urinary excretion of amphetamines and tranylcypromine. Arginine hydrochloride (20 gm) or ascorbic acid (250 to 500 mg) is given as often as necessary to keep urine pH at 4.

D. **Peritoneal dialysis** The technique of peritoneal dialysis is discussed elsewhere (*J. Pharm. Sci.* 60:1767, 1971; *N. Engl. J. Med.* 281:945, 1969; *Br. Med. Bull.* 27:165, 1971). It can be performed by a knowledgeable physician in any community hospital with no special equipment. Peritoneal dialysis enhances removal of drugs that are weakly protein-bound and relatively water-soluble (phenobarbital, meprobamate, lithium). However, for peritoneal dialysis to be of significantly greater benefit than forced diuresis, the procedure must be done repeatedly over a long period of time. This increases the hazards of infection and metabolic complications. The slight incremental benefit from peritoneal dialysis seldom justifies the risk; therefore peritoneal dialysis is not usually indicated in acute poisoning with psychotropic drugs.

E. **Hemodialysis** Facilities and personnel for hemodialysis are generally located only in large urban medical centers. Hemodialysis is performed in cases of severe poisoning that cannot be managed by noninvasive means. Indications are:

1. Ingestion of potentially fatal doses or very high serum concentrations.
2. Prolonged coma.
3. Refractory hypotension.
4. Failure of excretory organs (liver or kidney).

As with forced diuresis and peritoneal dialysis, hemodialysis is most effective in removing relatively water-soluble and weakly protein-bound drugs. Dialysis using oil dialysates has been reported successful in poisoning with highly lipid-soluble drugs (glutethimide, ethchlorvynol).

Hemodialysis is discussed in detail elsewhere (G. L. Bailey, Ed., *Hemodialysis: Principles and Practice,* New York: Academic, 1972).

IV. **Complications of Overdosage** Some of the complications of psychotropic drug poisoning are specific pharmacologic effects of the particular drug ingested. These will be discussed further in Section V in the context of overdosage with specific drugs. Other complications are nonspecific consequences of coma and can occur with prolonged obtundation due to any of a number of causes.

A. **Hypotension** can occur in poisoning with any psychotropic drug.

1. There are two primary **etiologies:**

   a. In poisoning with sedative-hypnotics (barbiturates, glutethimide, meprobamate), hypotension is due to relative hypovolemia caused by pooling of blood volume in venous capacitance beds (*Am. J. Med.* 38:853, 1965).

b. With major tranquilizers (particularly chlorpromazine, promazine, and thioridazine), hypotension is due to decreased peripheral resistance caused by alpha-adrenergic blockade.

2. Manifestations that indicate treatment is necessary include: a low arterial blood pressure (systolic < 90 mm Hg), oliguria (< 20 ml per hour), or the "clinical shock" syndrome of cold, clammy skin and cutaneous vasoconstriction.

3. Treatment is discussed in detail in Section I.C.5. Initial therapy consists of blood volume expansion. If this fails, then pressors are given. Refractory hypotension is prognostically grave and is an indication for hemodialysis.

Phenothiazine-induced hypotension should *not* be treated with sympathomimetic amines having beta-adrenergic activity (epinephrine and isoproterenol). Administration of these drugs can cause a further *fall* in blood pressure.

B. Hypertension usually occurs in poisoning with tricyclic antidepressants or monoamine oxidase (MAO) inhibitors. It can be caused by or can itself produce elevated intracranial pressure.

1. Etiology is not well understood but probably is due to impaired metabolism of endogenous pressor amines. Hypertension can also occur if pressors are given exogenously to treat hypotension, particularly in MAO inhibitor overdosage.

2. Manifestations that indicate treatment is necessary include any of the following:

a. Diastolic pressure > 120 mm Hg.

b. Elevated intracranial pressure (bradycardia, papilledema, seizures, focal neurologic signs).

c. Deterioration of renal function.

d. Congestive heart failure.

3. Treatment of severe hypertension can be approached in numerous ways. We recommend the following methods as the safest and most effective:

a. Vasodilating drugs, one of the following:

(1) *Diazoxide,* 300 mg IV bolus over 10 to 15 sec. This causes a sustained fall in blood pressure lasting 2 to 8 hours. The dose is then repeated as necessary.

    (2) *Sodium nitroprusside,* 50 to 100 mg in 500 ml 5% dextrose in water. The solution must be prepared just prior to use. A *continuous infusion* is used with the effect titrated by constant blood pressure monitoring.

  b. Diuretics must *always* be given concurrently with vasodilators since the latter cause fluid retention. Furosemide (40 mg IV) is given with each bolus of diazoxide or at the start of the nitroprusside drip. Furosemide counteracts fluid retention and also helps reduce blood pressure by reducing intravascular volume.

  c. Reduction of intracranial pressure is undertaken if this is the cause of hypertension (see Section **IV.C**). If intracranial pressure is increased *because of* systemic hypertension, signs will probably remit when blood pressure is lowered.

C. Increased intracranial pressure usually occurs in poisoning with the drugs described in Section **IV.B** but can occur with any psychotropic agent.

  1. Etiologies include:

    a. Systemic hypertension.

    b. Iatrogenic overexpansion of blood volume and subsequent cerebral edema.

    c. Intracranial hemorrhage.

  2. Manifestations indicating that treatment is necessary are:

    a. Systemic hypertension (see Section **IV.B**).

    b. Papilledema.

    c. Projectile vomiting (in a conscious patient).

    d. Seizures.

    e. Focal neurologic signs (such as unilateral mydriasis).

  3. Treatment

    a. Reduction of systemic hypertension (Section **IV.B**).

    b. Reduction of intracranial pressure with *mannitol* (50 gm IV) and *hydrocortisone* (200 mg IV).

D. Pulmonary edema is commonest after sedative-hypnotics (particularly glutethimide) and opiates.

  1. Etiology

    a. Pulmonary edema in sedative-hypnotic poisoning results from nonspecific depression of cardiac function. Iatrogenic overexpansion of intravascular volume often contributes.

b. Opiate-induced pulmonary edema occurs in the presence of normal cardiac function. It is a poorly understood local phenomenon, presumably related to increased permeability of pulmonary capillaries. The heart is not enlarged. (See Chapter 13.)

2. **Manifestations**

   a. Interstitial and alveolar pulmonary edema.
   b. Rales and rhonci on auscultation of the lungs.
   c. Hypoxia.
   d. Metabolic or respiratory acidosis or both.

3. **Treatment** depends on etiology.

   a. Cardiogenic pulmonary edema is treated as follows:

      (1) Sitting posture.
      (2) Positive pressure ventilation with oxygen.
      (3) Reduction of intravascular volume by use of tourniquets, phlebotomy, and intravenous furosemide (40 to 80 mg). Opiates should not be administered.
      (4) If these measures fail, then *digoxin* is given. The initial dose is 0.5 mg IV followed by 0.25 mg IV every 4 hours until a total dose of 1.0 to 1.25 mg is reached. Digoxin should never be given intramuscularly.

   b. Heroin pulmonary edema is noncardiac in origin. Treatment consists of oxygen and positive pressure ventilation. Opiate antagonists (naloxone, 0.4 to 0.8 mg IV) are given as necessary. Digitalis, diuretics, and phlebotomy are of no value and should be avoided.

E. **Respiratory failure** can occur in poisoning with any psychotropic drug.

   1. **Etiology** of respiratory failure is depression of the central ventilatory drive.

   2. **Manifestations** are those caused by or leading to inadequate arterial oxygenation:

      a. Respiratory pattern can range from shallow, irregular, or Cheyne-Stokes respirations to complete apnea.

      b. Cyanosis is a reliable sign if anemia or shock is not present.

      c. *Blood gas determinations are an absolute requirement for adequate assessment.* Assisted ventilation is usually required when blood gas analysis reveals hypoxia ($PO_2 < 60$ mm Hg) or hypercapnia ($PCO_2 > 50$ mm Hg).

3. **Treatment** consists of assisted ventilation.

   a. A cuffed endotracheal tube is inserted through the mouth or nose. The bronchial tree is thoroughly suctioned.

   b. Mechanical ventilation is started, using either a pressure-controlled or a volume-controlled respirator.

   c. Ventilatory parameters are initially set as follows:

   Respiratory rate: 12/min
   Tidal volume: 10 ml/kg
   Inspiratory pressure: 25 cm H_2O
   Inspired oxygen tension: 40%

   These parameters are adjusted and titrated according to frequent blood gas determinations. "Perfect" adjustment yields PO_2 = 100 mm Hg; PCO_2 = 40 mm Hg; pH = 7.4; bicarbonate = 25 mEq/liter. High oxygen tensions should be avoided.

   d. The endotracheal tube cuff should be deflated for at least 5 minutes per hour to prevent tracheal necrosis.

   e. "Weaning" is attempted frequently. If respiratory dependence persists after 48 hours or more, tracheostomy should be considered.

F. **Hypothermia** can occur in poisoning with any drug. Barbiturates, glutethimide, and phenothiazines are most often implicated. Exposure to low environmental temperatures increases the likelihood of hypothermia.

   1. **Etiology** of hypothermia can be both central and peripheral. Phenothiazines specifically impair central temperature-regulating mechanisms. Barbiturates and glutethimide probably also do this on a nonspecific basis. They may also depress cutaneous vascular mechanisms that conserve heat.

   2. **Manifestation** of hypothermia is a low core body temperature. Readings of less than 90° F have been recorded with subsequent survival. Hypothermia may be missed unless thermometers are shaken down all the way.

   3. **Treatment** is purely symptomatic, consisting of topical or core rewarming. Intravenous solutions — *particularly blood* — should be warmed at least to room temperature before they are infused.

G. **Hyperthermia (Fever)**

   1. **Etiology**

      a. Fever caused by infection can complicate poisoning with any psychotropic drug. When fever ($\geq$ 100.6° F) is documented, infection is *always* presumed to be the etiology until this possibility is ruled out.

b. MAO inhibitors, tricyclic antidepressants, and lithium commonly cause high body temperatures in the absence of infection. These drugs probably impair central temperature regulation. Tricyclics in addition can prevent cutaneous heat elimination because of their anticholinergic effects.

2. Elevated core temperature (taken rectally) is the major manifestation.

a. Slight hyperpyrexia (100° to 101° F), particularly when continuous rather than spiking, suggests the following etiologies: mild infection (e.g., catheter site phlebitis, urinary tract infection, tracheobronchitis), dehydration, or pulmonary atalectasis.

b. Fever in the range of 101° to 104° F, particularly when intermittent or spiking, strongly suggests that bacterial infection is the cause. Shaking chills followed by a fever spike suggests gram-negative bacteremia.

c. Very high body temperatures (greater than 104° F) are usually due at least in part to impaired central thermoregulation.

3. Assessment of fever greater than 100.6° F ("fever workup") includes the following in addition to physical examination:

a. White blood cell count and differential.

b. Blood cultures, taken in pairs from two separate sterile venipuncture sites. They are repeated in pairs of two as often as indicated.

c. Chest x-ray.

d. Aspiration of a deep endobronchial sputum specimen, which is gram-stained and examined by the physician.

e. Culture and analysis of a clean urine specimen.

f. Lumbar puncture, with culture, gram stain, and Wright's stain of the cerebrospinal fluid.

g. Inspection and/or removal of all indwelling intravenous catheters. Those that have been in place for 48 hours or more should be removed and cultured even if there is no evidence of local infection or cellulitis.

4. Treatment

    a. If infection is documented or strongly suspected as the cause of fever, specific therapy is instituted (see Section **IV.H**).

    b. High body temperatures (greater than 104° F) can precipitate cardiac arrhythmias and seizures and therefore require symptomatic cooling therapy:

        (1) Antipyretic drugs, such as aspirin or acetaminophen, 10 to 15 grains by mouth or rectum every 3 to 4 hours.

        (2) Topical cooling using mechanical "cold blanket" or alcohol sponging.

        (3) Core cooling using ice water enemas.

        (4) Physostigmine (1 to 4 mg IV or IM) is the specific antidote for hyperpyrexia due to tricyclic antidepressants or anticholinergics.

H. Infection can be a life-threatening complication of psychotropic drug overdosage. The assessment of fever is discussed in Section **IV.G** and elsewhere (Chapter 14). Since certain psychotropic drugs can cause hypothermia (see Section **IV.F**), the absence of fever does not rule out the presence of infection.

    1. Bacteria are the most common and, fortunately, the most treatable etiologic agents. The usual sites of infection and the manifestations of infection in these sites include the following:

        a. **Pulmonary infection** is suggested by purulent sputum production, an infiltrate on chest x-ray, and hypoxia due to large alveolar-arterial oxygen tension differences. Conscious or spontaneously breathing patients may have tachypnea, cough, or pleuritic chest pain.

        (1) **Pneumococcal pneumonia** is the most common pulmonary infection. It is manifested by fever, purulent sputum, chest pain, segmental consolidation on x-ray, and encapsulated gram-positive diplococci on gram stain (see Chapter 14).

        (2) **Mixed bacterial pneumonia** follows aspiration of mouth flora during drug-induced obtundation. X-ray shows "streaky" infiltration in the right upper or middle lobes or both. Mixed flora are seen on gram stain. In some cases, aspiration can lead to lung abscess, seen as an air-fluid cavity on x-ray.

(3) **Gram-negative pneumonias** are usually due to hospital-acquired organisms, occurring in patients with coma and assisted ventilation over prolonged periods. They can also occur as superinfections in patients treated for pneumococcal pneumonia. *Klebsiella* and *Pseudomonas* species are the most common organisms. Unfortunately, they usually are resistant to most commonly used antibiotics.

b. **Urinary tract infection** is inevitable in patients with indwelling Foley catheters in place for 24 to 48 hours or more. *Escherichia coli* and *Proteus* species are the usual organisms. Superinfection or hospital-acquired infection with antibiotic-resistant strains *(Proteus, Klebsiella, or Pseudomonas)* can also occur.

Infection is usually mild and localized in the bladder. Ascending infection that invades renal parenchyma causes pyelonephritis and systemic toxicity (e.g., fever, leukocytosis). Occasionally, seeding of the bloodstream and gram-negative septicemia can occur.

Urine sediment examination reveals many granulocytes and gram-negative bacilli on gram stain. Urea-splitting *Proteus* species can produce an abnormally alkaline urine (pH > 8). The specific organism can usually be identified by culture within 24 hours.

c. **Meningeal infection** is suggested by high fever, changes in mental status, increased intracranial pressure, seizures, nuchal rigidity, or opisthotonos. Pneumococcus and *Nisseriae meningitidis* are the most common organisms. Often meningitis is preceded by pulmonary, sinus, or middle-ear infection.

Diagnosis is made by examination of the spinal fluid. The undiluted specimen is examined for total cells and granulocytes. The sediment is examined using gram stain and Wright's stain. The fluid is also cultured.

A total granulocyte count of more than 7 per cubic mm in a "nontraumatic" spinal fluid specimen strongly suggests meningeal infection, particularly when granulocytes predominate in the differential count.

d. **Intravenous catheter site infection** should always be suspected when fever occurs. The sites are carefully inspected for evidence of erythema, induration, warmth, or tenderness. Catheters are removed and cultured if there is any evidence of infection. Catheters in place for 48 hours should be removed.

2. **Treatment**

   a. All *pulmonary* infections are treated by topical humidification, frequent suctioning, intermittent positive pressure ventilation, and postural drainage. Antibiotic therapy is discussed in Chapter 14, Section **V.B.**

   b. See Section **V.B** of Chapter 14 for therapy of infections of the urinary tract, meninges, and catheter sites.

   c. **Gram-negative bacteremia,** heralded by shaking chills, spiking fever, and sometimes hypotension and shock, must be treated in "shotgun" fashion before the organism is identified. The treatment is:

      (1) *Hydrocortisone,* 1.0 gm IV immediately, then 1.0 gm every 6 to 8 hours for 48 hours.

      (2) *Gentamicin,* 5 mg/kg over 24 hours in 3 divided IM doses (IV if shock is present), then 3 mg/kg per day.

      (3) A *penicillin* or *cephalosporin,* such as cephalothin (2 gm IV every 4 hours), ampicillin (2 gm IV every 4 hours), or nafcillin (3 gm IV every 4 hours).

I. **Oliguria and renal failure**

   1. The **etiology** of oliguria and renal failure in drug overdosage almost always is renal hypoperfusion due to arterial hypotension. Evidence for a direct nephrotoxic effect of any psychotropic drugs is scant. Occasionally, renal insufficiency is iatrogenic, due to antibiotics such as gentamicin or tetracyclines.

   2. **Manifestations** include oliguria (urine output less than 20 ml per hour), as well as rising blood urea nitrogen and creatinine concentrations.

      a. When oliguria is due to volume depletion alone without parenchymal renal damage, salt-conserving and urea-excreting functions are preserved. The urine sodium concentration is less than 10 mEq per liter, and the ratio of urine to serum urea concentration is greater than 15.

      b. Oliguria due to acute renal failure is characterized by salt-wasting and urea retention. Urine sodium concentration is greater than 10 mEq per liter, and the urine-to-plasma urea ratio is less than 1.

   3. **Treatment** is as follows:

      a. **Hypotension** and **volume depletion** are treated as in Sections **I.C.5** and **IV.A.**

b. If this fails to correct oliguria, furosemide (100 mg IV) is given. The dose is doubled every 30 to 60 minutes until a diuresis occurs or until a total of 700 mg has been given.

c. Persistent oliguria strongly suggests that acute renal failure has occurred. Mannitol (50 gm IV) can be tried — in some cases it will cause the kidney to "open up." However, retained mannitol can lead to pulmonary edema.

d. The treatment of acute renal failure is discussed elsewhere (*Mod. Treat.* 6:927, 1969; *Med. Clin. North Am.* 55:1249, 1971; *Med. Clin. North Am.* 55:121, 1971).

J. Cardiac arrhythmias

1. Several **etiologies** are possible:

   a. Fever, hypoxia, hypokalemia, hyperkalemia, and hypomagnesemia are common factors that predispose to arrhythmias in drug intoxication.

   b. Tricyclic antidepressants and phenothiazines can cause tachyarrhythmias because of their anticholinergic effects.

   c. Certain drugs appear to have direct cardiotoxic effects. These include the tricyclic antidepressants and some phenothiazines, particularly thioridazine and chlorpromazine (*Dis. Nerv. Syst.* 31:534, 1970; *Am. Heart J.* 78:757, 1969).

2. **Manifestations** can include almost any possible cardiac arrhythmia. The most common ones are:

   a. Atrial tachyarrhythmias: Sinus tachycardia, atrial premature beats, paroxysmal atrial tachycardia, multifocal atrial tachycardia.

   b. Ventricular tachyarrhythmias: Ventricular premature beats, ventricular tachycardia, ventricular fibrillation.

   c. Conduction disturbances: A-V nodal block, bundle branch blocks, widened QRS complexes.

   d. Bradyarrhythmias: Sinus bradycardia or arrest, junctional rhythm, idioventricular rhythm.

   e. Various combinations of the above.

3. **Treatment**

   a. Continuous electrocardiographic monitoring is mandatory in poisoning with tricyclic antidepressants and phenothiazines.

b. Predisposing causes (Section **IV.J.1.a**) are searched for and treated if present.

c. Atrial tachyarrhythmias are relatively benign and do not necessarily require treatment if cardiac output remains adequat The usual modes of therapy, in their approximate order of choice, are:

(1) Carotid sinus massage. If this measure alone fails to convert the arrhythmia, it is repeated after each of the subsequent measures is tried.

(2) Edrophonium, 10 mg IV over 2 minutes.

(3) Propranolol, 1 mg IV, repeated every 5 to 10 minutes to a maximum dose of 5 mg.

(4) Digitalis glycosides are hazardous but will occasionally convert supraventricular arrhythmias. Digoxin (0.5 mg IV) is given, followed by 0.25 mg IV every 4 hours to a total dose of 1.0 to 1.25 mg.

(5) Physostigmine (1 to 4 mg IV) is among the treatments of choice when supraventricular tachyarrhythmias are du to tricyclic antidepressants.

d. The treatment of ventricular tachyarrhythmias is discussed in Section **I.C.4.a.**

e. Bradyarrhythmias and conduction disturbances are not necessarily life-threatening. Treatment is not obligatory provided cardiac output is adequate. Atropine should not be used if poisoning is due to tricyclic antidepressants or phenothiazines. Sympathomimetic amines are hazardous. Temporary transvenous endocardial pacing is the safest mode of therapy.

K. Agitation and hyperactivity

1. Etiology

a. Tricyclic antidepressants can cause agitation and delirium in part on the basis of CNS anticholinergic effects.

b. Hyperactivity following MAO inhibitors probably reflects CNS adrenergic imbalance, the nature of which is not well understoc

c. Neuroleptic-induced hyperactivity may represent an acute extrapyramidal reaction. The following drugs are usually implicated: prochlorperazine, trifluoperazine, perphenazine, fluphen azine, chlorpromazine, thiothixene, and haloperidol.

d. The mechanism of hyperactivity and hyperreflexia following lithium carbonate overdosage is not clear.

e. Agitation is sometimes associated with sedative-hypnotic overdosage, particularly if the quantity ingested is relatively small. Agitation can also occur during the recovery phase of poisoning with larger quantities.

2. **Manifestations** include agitation, combativeness, delirium, muscular rigidity, twitching, clonic movements, and hyperreflexia.

3. **Treatment**

a. Other causes of agitation, such as hypoxia, hypoglycemia, and somatic pain, should be ruled out.

b. Whenever possible, agitation should be treated with carefully applied and monitored restraints rather than drugs.

c. Physostigmine (1 to 4 mg IV or IM) is the specific antidote for agitation and delirium due to tricyclic antidepressants or anticholinergics.

d. Acute extrapyramidal reactions are treated with intravenous diphenhydramine, 25 mg per minute up to a maximum dose of 100 mg.

e. If a sedative-hypnotic must be used to control agitation, diazepam is the safest of available drugs. The dose is 5 mg per minute IV to a maximum dose of 20 mg.

L. Seizures

1. **Etiology**

a. Hypoxia, cerebral hypoperfusion, increased intracranial pressure, fever, meningeal infection, hypoglycemia, hyponatremia, hypernatremia, and intracranial hemorrhage are among numerous entities that can precipitate or predispose to seizures regardless of the drug ingested.

b. Tricyclic antidepressants, major tranquilizers (neuroleptics), MAO inhibitors, and lithium appear to lower the seizure threshold.

c. Patients who are habituated or addicted to a sedative-hypnotic drug (e.g., ethanol, barbiturates, meprobamate) and are hospitalized with overdosage of a drug from the same class can experience withdrawal seizures during recovery from the overdosage.

2. **Manifestations** are divided into two categories:

   a. Nonfocal seizures, usually major motor or tonic-clonic in nature, with no evidence of lateralization.

   b. Lateralizing or focal seizures, which suggest that increased intracranial pressure or intracerebral hemorrhage must be looked for.

3. **Treatment**

   a. Predisposing causes (Section **IV.L.1.a**) should be ruled out or treated.

   b. Lateralizing or focal seizures are grounds for neurologic or neurosurgical consultation, or both.

   c. Nonfocal generalized seizures without apparent predisposing causes do not necessarily require immediate treatment. Seizures are usually self-limiting and not life-threatening. Treatment is indicated if seizures are repetitive or intractable, or interfere with respiration. The acute treatment of intractable seizures is discussed elsewhere (Chapter 1).

M. **Skin lesions**

1. Skin lesions were once thought to be characteristic only of barbiturate overdosage. However, recent evidence suggests that these lesions are due to pressure or local ischemia, or both, and therefore that they are nonspecific manifestations of coma.

2. Possible **manifestations** include: erythema, blisters, bullae, or necrotic ulcerations.

3. **Treatment** is topical and symptomatic.

N. **Clinical relapse** in psychotropic drug overdosage refers to a phenomenon in which clinical worsening follows a period of improvement. It has been reported with almost every psychotropic drug. Glutethimide, meprobamate, and tricyclic antidepressants are most commonly implicated.

1. The **etiology** of the phenomenon is not clear. At least three mechanisms are possible:

   a. The parent drug and its active metabolites are initially "tied up" in the enterohepatic circulation but are subsequently released into the systemic circulation.

   b. A portion of the ingested agent is initially unabsorbed from the gastrointestinal tract due to poor splanchnic circulation. When hypotension is treated and splanchnic blood flow is restored, the remaining quantity is rapidly absorbed.

c. Highly lipid-soluble drugs (glutethimide, short-acting barbiturates) are initially taken up into lipid storage sites other than the brain. At a later time, after distribution is complete, the drug is released from storage sites into the systemic circulation.

2. **Manifestations** of relapse include worsening of neurologic, hemodynamic, and respiratory status. Serum concentrations of the drug may rise. Deterioration follows a period of clinical improvement, anywhere from a few hours to a few days after drug ingestion.

3. Treatment consists of continued supportive care. Induction of emesis can be attempted if the patient becomes fully conscious. The possibility of relapse underscores the need for continued close monitoring even when clinical improvement occurs.

V. **Poisoning with Specific Psychotropic Drugs** The following section discusses manifestations of and treatment of overdosage with particular psychotropic agents. Frequent reference is made to preceding sections.

A. **Barbiturates** are the most commonly implicated drugs in deliberate self-poisoning.

1. **Epidemiology**

a. The case fatality rate in barbiturate poisoning recently has fallen to the range of 1 percent or less, owing to refinement in principles of supportive care. Still, barbiturate deaths in the United States number in the thousands yearly.

b. Short-acting barbiturates (secobarbital, pentobarbital) are implicated in most cases of serious poisoning. Single doses of 2 to 3 gm (10 to 30 times the usual therapeutic dose) can be life-threatening or fatal. Serum concentrations of 35 μg/ml or greater are usually fatal.

c. Long-acting barbiturates (phenobarbital) have a somewhat wider margin of safety. Single doses of 5 gm or more (approximately 50 times the usual daily dose) are generally fatal. Serum concentrations of 100 to 120 μg/ml usually indicate severe or fatal intoxication.

2. **Manifestations** of poisoning are similar for all types of barbiturates. Drowsiness, nystagmus, ataxia, dysarthria, and somno-

lence occur in early stages of poisoning or in mild cases. The larger the dose, the more profound is general CNS depression. Deep coma, areflexia, muscle hypotonicity, apnea, hypotension, and hypothermia occur in the most serious cases.

3. Treatment

a. In short-acting barbiturate poisoning, treatment is usually limited to supportive care. Forced diuresis is of no value. Unfortunately, secobarbital and pentobarbital are poorly dialyzable so even hemodialysis does not remove large quantities of drug. However, hemodialysis may be the only alternative in severe cases.

b. Forced alkaline diuresis significantly enhances excretion of phenobarbital. This should be started as soon as the diagnosis is made. Peritoneal dialysis is only slightly better than alkaline diuresis, but much larger amounts of phenobarbital can be removed by hemodialysis.

B. Glutethimide is another popular and effective agent for self-poisoning.

1. **Epidemiology**   Because glutethimide is lipid-soluble and has a large volume of distribution, serum concentrations do not correlate well with the depth of coma. However, nearly all individuals with moderate or severe intoxication have serum concentrations greater than 20 μg/ml. Levels greater than 40 or 50 μg/ml almost always are associated with deep coma. Single doses of 10 gm or more (10 to 20 times the usual hypnotic dose) generally produce serious poisoning. A hydroxylated, polar metabolite of glutethimide may contribute to CNS depression.

2. **Manifestations**   Glutethimide produces dose-dependent CNS depression similar to the barbiturates. Glutethimide has anticholinergic properties and frequently produces tachycardia, paralytic ileus, and mydriasis. Cardiovascular depression (hypotension, pulmonary edema) is also common in glutethimide poisoning.

3. **Treatment** should be supportive in nearly all cases. Some authors suggest gastric lavage with castor oil, or instillation of mineral oil in the gastrointestinal tract, or both. Recent evidence suggests that ordinary hemodialysis is of little clinical benefit (*J.A.M.A.* 208:837, 1969). Dialysis using oil dialysates may be of more value (*Trans. Am. Soc. Artif. Intern. Org.* 11:173, 1965). Treatment of hypotension by intravascular volume expansion should be done cautiously because of the hazard of pulmonary edema.

C. **Methyprylon** resembles glutethimide in structure but has greater water-solubility.

1. **Epidemiology**   A single dose of 6 gm usually produces severe intoxication. The largest survived overdosage is 30 gm. Serum concentrations of greater than 40 to 50 μg/ml indicate serious toxicity.

2. **Manifestations** are the same as in poisoning with other barbiturate-like hypnotics.

3. **Treatment**   Supportive care is usually adequate since methyprylon is rapidly biotransformed to inactive metabolites. Forced diuresis is of little benefit. Hemodialysis has been reported in several cases to remove considerable quantities of unchanged methyprylon and produce rapid clinical improvement.

D. **Methaqualone** has become increasingly popular as a drug of abuse and suicide.

1. **Epidemiology**   Most experience with methaqualone overdosage comes from Britain and other parts of Europe, where a combination hypnotic preparation (Mandrax) containing methaqualone (250 mg) and diphenhydramine (25 mg) in each pill is much more widely used than methaqualone alone. Studies of serum concentrations in cases of overdosage are limited. Blood levels greater than 8 μg/ml usually occur in serious poisoning.

2. **Manifestations**

   a. In Mandrax poisoning, anticholinergic manifestations can be prominent. These include mydriasis, tachycardia, muscular rigidity, twitching, hyperreflexia, and seizures.

   b. Overdosage with methaqualone alone usually produces barbiturate-like CNS depression. However, excitatory phenomena (as described for Mandrax) can occur as well.

3. **Treatment** is supportive. The role of hemodialysis is not established.

E. **Ethchlorvynol** can produce serious intoxication but fortunately is an uncommon agent of self-poisoning.

1. **Epidemiology**   Single doses of 15 gm and serum concentrations greater than 100 μg/ml are associated with severe intoxication.

2. **Manifestations**   Ethchlorvynol poisoning can result in prolonged coma, hypothermia, hypotension, and respiratory depression. The characteristic odor of ethchlorvynol detected in body fluids of

intoxicated patients can be compared with the smell of a freshly opened ethchlorvynol capsule.

3. **Treatment**   Since ethchlorvynol appears to be weakly protein-bound, particularly at high serum concentrations, forced diuresis and hemodialysis can enhance drug removal.

F. Meprobamate

1. **Epidemiology**   Serious poisoning occurs after single doses of 20 gm. Fatalities are reported with doses of 12 gm, but ingestions of 40 gm have been survived. The usual daily dose is 1.6 gm. Serum concentrations of 100 μg/ml indicate serious intoxication.

2. **Manifestations** resemble barbiturate-like intoxication.

3. **Treatment**   Meprobamate is weakly protein-bound. Forced diuresis should be started early in the course of treatment. Peritoneal dialysis and hemodialysis enhance the removal rate even further.

G. Benzodiazepines include a number of antianxiety, anticonvulsant, and hypnotic agents. Commonly used drugs are: chlordiazepoxide, diazepam, oxazepam, clorazepate, nitrazepam, flurazepam, and lorazepam. Benzodiazepines are among the most widely used drugs in the world, but they rarely produce serious poisoning.

1. **Epidemiology**   The largest reported overdosage with chlordiazepoxide is 2.25 gm and with diazepam, 1.4 gm. Chlordiazepoxide serum concentrations of 40 to 60 μg/ml occur after large single doses. Fatal overdosage of any benzodiazepine derivative alone is rare.

2. **Manifestations**   Patients can have muscle weakness and hypotonia, ataxia, dysarthria, and somnolence, but they generally remain responsive. Coma, respiratory depression, hypotension, and hypothermia rarely occur even after very large ingestions.

3. **Treatment**   Measures other than supportive care are seldom necessary. Forced diuresis is of no value. The role of hemodialysis is not established. Diazepam is strongly protein-bound and highly lipid-soluble, so hemodialysis is unlikely to enhance its removal. Chlordiazepoxide is water-soluble and less strongly bound to protein; enhanced drug removal by hemodialysis is suggested by one report (*J.A.M.A.* 202:438–440, 1967).

H. Major tranquilizers (neuroleptics)

1. **Epidemiology**   Most reported poisonings involve chlorpromazine. Ingestion of 3 to 4 gm produces serious intoxication. Fatalities

are rare. Adequate serum concentration data are unavailable. Since piperazine phenothiazines (fluphenazine, perphenazine, trifluoperazine) have higher relative potency, intoxication is produced by smaller quantities. Accidental phenothiazine ingestion by children accounts for many cases of poisoning.

2. **Manifestations** depend on the class of drug ingested.

   a. **Aliphatic and piperidine phenothiazines** (chlorpromazine, thioridazine, mesoridazine) tend to produce CNS depression rather than excitation. Coma and unresponsiveness occur after ingestion of large amounts. Seizures can also occur. Because the drugs impair temperature regulation, both hypothermia and hyperthermia can occur. Cholinergic, alpha-adrenergic, and dopaminergic blocking effects result in tachycardia, urinary retention, paralytic ileus, and hypotension. Cardiac manifestations can range from minor ECG abnormalities (QT prolongation, minor ST-T changes) to life-threatening ventricular tachyarrhythmias.

   b. Piperazine phenothiazines (fluphenazine, perphenazine, trifluoperazine), haloperidol, and thioxanthenes can produce CNS excitation: agitation, delirium, muscular rigidity, spasm, twitching, hyperreflexia, tremor, seizures. Some of these neuromuscular manifestations may represent acute dystonic reactions. These drugs can also produce impaired temperature regulation, autonomic nervous system dysfunction, and cardiac arrhythmias.

3. **Treatment**

   a. All phenothiazines (except thioridazine) have antiemetic properties. Since induced emesis is likely to fail, it should not be attempted. Gastric lavage should be performed as soon as possible after ingestion.

   b. All patients should have continuous ECG monitoring because of the possibility of cardiac arrhythmias. When they arise, rhythm disturbances are treated as described in Section **IV.J.**

   c. Hypotension is treated by volume expansion. If pressors are needed, only alpha-adrenergic stimulators (norepinephrine, metaraminol) should be used. Catecholamines having beta-adrenergic activity (isoproterenol, epinephrine) can cause a further *fall* in blood pressure.

   d. Dystonic reactions are treated by intravenous diphenhydramine, 25 mg per minute to a maximum dose of 100 mg.

e. Hypothermia or hyperthermia is treated symptomatically (Sections **IV.F** and **IV.G**).

f. Forced diuresis and dialysis are of little value.

I. Tricyclic antidepressants

1. **Epidemiology** Tricyclic antidepressant poisoning is more grave than major tranquilizer overdosage. Amitriptyline and imipramine are the usual drugs implicated. Single doses of approximately 1.5 to 2.0 gm in adults produce serious intoxication. Numerous fatalities are reported, usually involving doses of more than 2.0 gm. Accidental poisoning in children is reported with increasing frequency.

2. **Manifestations** can include either CNS excitation or CNS depression. Aspects of both can be present, and the overall clinical picture can fluctuate from one to the other.

   a. Excitatory manifestations include: agitation, delirium, hallucinations, twitching, hyperreflexia, muscular rigidity, clonus, seizures.

   b. Anticholinergic effects are prominent. Many of the signs of CNS excitement may represent central cholinergic blockade. Tachycardia, urinary retention, paralytic ileus, mydriasis, and hyperpyrexia are usual peripheral anticholinergic manifestations.

   c. Cardiac arrhythmias due to tricyclic antidepressants are potentially fatal.

   d. CNS depression (coma, hypotension, respiratory depression) occurs with large overdosages. Amitriptyline produces serious coma somewhat more frequently than imipramine.

3. **Treatment**

   a. Gastric lavage should be performed rather than induced emesis, which usually fails.

   b. Forced diuresis and dialysis are of little value.

   c. Continuous ECG monitoring is mandatory.

   d. **Propranolol** (1 to 5 mg IV) is reportedly effective in the treatment of tachyarrhythmias associated with tricyclic antidepressant poisoning.

   e. **Physostigmine** appears to be a specific antidote for anticholinergic manifestations such as delirium, hyperpyrexia, tachycardia, and in some cases, obtundation. An intravenous dose of 1 to 4 mg should be tried early in the course of intoxication. The effective dose can be repeated as often as necessary.

J. Monoamine oxidase inhibitors

1. **Epidemiology** MAO inhibitors are highly toxic drugs. Fatal poisoning has occurred with as little as 170 mg of tranylcypromine or 375 mg of phenelzine.

2. **Manifestations** Clinical signs and symptoms do not appear immediately after ingestion. The lag period can be as long as 12 hours. Signs of CNS excitation then appear rapidly: confusion, agitation, delirium, diaphoresis, tachycardia, hyperreflexia, muscular rigidity, and seizures. Malignant hyperpyrexia is the usual terminal event.

3. **Treatment**

   a. Treatment should begin in the lag period, if possible, before the patient becomes symptomatic.

   b. Gastric lavage should be performed on all patients. The role of dialysis is not established, but it should be considered if potentially fatal doses have been ingested.

   c. Forced diuresis with urinary acidification greatly enhances excretion of tranylcypromine.

   d. Sympathomimetic amines can precipitate hypertensive crises and should be used to treat hypotension only with great caution.

K. Lithium carbonate

1. **Epidemiology** Serum lithium concentrations of greater than 2 mEq/L are toxic. Higher serum concentrations are associated with more severe toxicity. Lithium poisoning can develop slowly during maintenance therapy as well as after acute overdosage. Factors that can lead to insidious lithium toxicity are: failure to monitor serum concentrations, coadministration of diuretics, dietary sodium restriction, and dehydration.

2. **Manifestations** Early signs of lithium toxicity include nausea, tremor, drowsiness, thirst, and muscle irritability. Severe poisoning produces muscle fasciculations, twitching, rigidity, clonus, hyperreflexia, seizures, hyperpyrexia, obtundation, and coma.

3. **Treatment** Lithium is neither biotransformed nor protein-bound. Forced saline diuresis should begin as early as possible. Hemodialysis is highly effective in removing lithium from the body.

L. Opiates

1. **Epidemiology** Opiate overdosage is usually unintentional. It occu when a drug-abuser underestimates the opiate content of a "mainline" dose. It can also occur when an individual who is "tolerant" to high doses ceases drug use, loses his physiologic tolerance, and then returns abruptly to using doses to which he was previously tolerant.

2. **Manifestations**

   a. Acute opiate overdosage produces shallow or absent respirations cyanosis, pupillary meiosis, and unresponsiveness. There is usual evidence of a fresh venipuncture wound as well as "tracks" due to repeated intravenous injections.

   b. "Heroin pulmonary edema" can follow intravenous opiate use, even in a conscious individual. It appears to be a local sensitivity phenomenon producing increased pulmonary vascular permeability. Cardiac function is usually normal, and hemodynamic abnormalities are generally absent.

3. **Treatment**

   a. The trachea is intubated, and assisted ventilation is begun as soon as the patient reaches the treatment area.

   b. Emergence from opiate overdosage is characterized by agitation and combativeness. Patients frequently cause harm to themselves and to medical staff. Therefore *restraints* are carefully applied *before* antidotes are administered.

   c. An intravenous route is established and the patient initially is given naloxone (0.4 to 0.8 mg) and glucose (50 ml of 50% solution). Naloxone can be readministered at 4-hour intervals during the first 24 hours if apnea or coma or both recur.

   d. Pulmonary edema is treated only with oxygen and positive pressure ventilation. Since neither left ventricular failure nor intravascular volume overload is the etiology of pulmonary edema, the usual approaches to treatment (digitalis, diuretics, phlebotomy, tourniquets) are of no value and should be avoided.

   e. All patients must be hospitalized and observed continuously for at least 24 hours. Apnea and coma commonly recur during this period because naloxone is more rapidly eliminated than heroin.

   f. Signs and symptoms of opiate withdrawal can begin as early as 6 hours after the most recent dose.

M.   **Mixed drug overdosage** is almost as common as poisoning with single
drugs. Diagnosis, treatment, and prognostication become somewhat
more complicated. Clinicians dealing with psychotropic drug overdosage must always consider the possibility that more than one
drug is involved. Some of the more common "cocktails" are as
follows:

1. **Alcohol and sedative-hypnotics** are a dangerous combination since
   they cause CNS depression that is at least additive. Recent
   evidence suggests that alcohol can retard the metabolism of other
   CNS depressants, such as chloral hydrate, so the combination can
   be supraadditive.

2. **Amphetamines and sedative-hypnotics** (barbiturates or methaqualone) are combined in many "diet" pill preparations and
   therefore are not infrequently implicated in mixed drug overdosages.

3. **Phenothiazines and tricyclic antidepressants** also occur in fixed
   drug combinations. Anticholinergic manifestations are prominent
   in poisoning with this mixture.

References

Barry, D., Meyskens, F. L., and Becker, C. E.   Phenothiazine poisoning. A review of
48 cases. *Calif. Med.* 118:1–5 (Jan.), 1973.
Chazan, J. A., and Garella, S.   Glutethimide intoxication. *Arch. Intern. Med.* 128:
215–219, 1971.
Davis, J. M., Bartlett, E., and Termini, B. A.   Overdosage of psychotropic drugs: a review.
Dis. Nerv. Syst. 29:157–164, 246–256, 1968.
Gjerris, F.   Poisoning with chlordiazepoxide (Librium). *Dan. Med. Bull.* 13:170–172,
1966.
Greenblatt, D. J., and Shader, R. I.   Acute poisoning with psychotropic drugs. In R. I.
Shader and A. DiMascio, et al., *Psychotropic Drug Side Effects: Clinical and
Theoretical Perspectives.* Baltimore: Williams & Wilkins, 1970. Pp. 214–234.
Hadden, J., Johnson, K., Smith, S., Price, L., and Giardina, E.   Acute barbiturate
intoxication. Concepts of management. *J.A.M.A.* 209:893–900, 1969.
Maddock, R. K., and Bloomer, H. A.   Meprobamate overdosage. *J.A.M.A.* 201:
999–1003, 1967.
Matthew, H. (Ed.)   *Acute Barbiturate Poisoning.* Amsterdam: Excerpta Medica Founda-
tion, 1971.
Matthew, H., Roscoe, P., and Wright, N.   Acute poisoning. A comparison of hypnotic
drugs. *Practitioner* 208:254–258, 1972.
Noble, J., and Matthew, H.   Acute poisoning by tricyclic antidepressants: Clinical
features and management of 100 patients. *Clin. Toxicol.* 2:403–421, 1969.
Rasmussen, J.   Poisoning with amitriptyline, imipramine, and nortriptyline. *Dan. Med.
Bull.* 16:201–203, 1966.
Robinson, R. R., Hayes, C. P., and Gunnells, J. C.   Treatment of barbiturate intoxica-
tion. *Mod. Treat.* 4:679–696, 1967.
Schou, M., Amdisen, A., and Trap-Jensen, J.   Lithium poisoning. *Am. J. Psychiatry*
125:520–527, 1968.
Shubin, H., and Weil, M. H.   Shock associated with barbiturate intoxication. *J.A.M.A.*
215:263–268, 1971.
Slovis, T. L., Ott, J. E., Teitelbaum, D. T., and Lipscomb, W.   Physostigmine therapy in
acute tricyclic antidepressant poisoning. *Clin. Toxicol.* 4:451–459, 1971.
Wilkinson, G. R.   Treatment of drug intoxication: A review of some scientific principles.
Clin. Toxicol. 3:249–265, 1970.

16

Drug Interactions in Psychopharmacology

David J. Greenblatt
Richard I. Shader

A clinically significant drug interaction is identified when the therapeutic or toxic effects, or both, of one pharmacologic agent are altered by coadministration of another. Some interactions are predictable and easily understood, such as the additive CNS depression produced when a sedative-hypnotic drug is taken with alcohol. Others are unpredictable and are discovered only by chance or by large-scale epidemiologic studies. An example of this kind of unforeseen interaction is the potentiation of oral anticoagulant activity produced by chloral hydrate. Regrettably, unexpected interactions sometimes result in serious or fatal drug toxicity.

Pharmacologic agents can interact through a variety of mechanisms. A drug might alter the rate or completeness of *gastrointestinal absorption* or *bioavailability* of another drug by changing its dissolution characteristics, by altering the ambient pH, or by causing variations in gastrointestinal motility. Some agents influence hepatic drug *metabolism,* either stimulating or impairing the liver's ability to detoxify other drugs. Occasionally two drugs potentiate each other's action by competing for the same *metabolic site* in the liver or for the same *binding site* on serum protein. Drug antagonism can occur when one agent prevents another from reaching or acting at its *receptor site.* Some drugs are excreted in significant amounts by the kidney; in some cases their excretion is modified by agents that alter glomerular filtration, tubular function, or urine pH. The most straightforward interactions occur when two drugs exert additive or antagonistic clinical effects through different mechanisms.

A great deal of valuable data on drug interactions has been generated in the past decade. Unfortunately, misinformation has also been perpetuated. Interactions are sometimes suspected on the basis of clinical observation of one or two cases. When these appear in the medical literature as case reports, many readers interpret them as depicting established pharmacologic truth. Systematic study often reveals the apparent interaction to be coincidental or spurious. Animal studies are another potential source of misinformation. Drug interactions that are strikingly evident in animal investigations may be of no clinical significance. Finally, biochemical or pharmacokinetic theory can *predict* many potential interactions. Unfortunately, these theoretical interactions may be depicted as fact even when their reality has not been tested in humans. Thus, uncritical interpretation of case reports, animal studies, and theoretical treatises can generate and perpetuate "facts" that are not really facts. In this chapter reviewing interactions with psychotropic drugs, every effort has been made to evaluate the strength of the evidence and to separate speculation from fact.

I. Hypnotics

A. Bioavailability

1. Limited studies have suggested that administration of hypnotic drugs with meals can slow the *rate* of drug absorption but not necessarily the *completeness* of absorption. One can speculate that lipid substances would bind fat-soluble hypnotics such as glutethimide in the gastrointestinal tract and hence delay absorption. Animal studies show that antacids impair absorption of pentobarbital, but this has not been adequately investigated in humans.

   Recommendation: Although adequate data are not available, it is reasonable to assume that bioavailability of hypnotic drugs is optimal when they are taken on an empty stomach.

2. Limited observations reveal that barbiturates can impair absorption of certain drugs (bishydroxycoumarin, griseofulvin). The mechanism of this interaction is not understood.

B. Metabolism

1. Chronic treatment with certain hypnotics produces hepatic microsomal **enzyme induction** and thus stimulates the metabolism of other drugs.

   a. Enzyme-inducers of *definite clinical importance* are barbiturates (all), glutethimide, and alcohol (see Section III).

   b. *Possible* enzyme-inducers include ethchlorvynol.

   c. Hypnotics with *no clinically important inducing effects* are nitrazepam, flurazepam, and chloral derivatives.

   d. Drugs that are *inadequately evaluated* are methyprylon, methaqualone, and antihistamines.

2. Drugs affected by coadministration of enzyme-inducers undergo more rapid metabolism and hence have a diminished clinical effect. The effect is reversed in several days to several weeks after the enzyme-inducer is stopped.

   a. Drugs *definitely affected* by enzyme-inducers are: oral anticoagulants, vitamin D, corticosteroids, phenylbutazone, and tolbutamide.

    b. Drugs *possibly* affected are digitoxin, diphenylhydantoin, methyldopa, chlorpromazine, tricyclic antidepressants, rifampin, and doxycycline.

    Recommendation: Clinical effects of enzyme induction can be adjusted for by careful titration of dosage and blood concentrations of the agent whose metabolism might have been altered. However, the problem can be avoided altogether if a non-enzyme-inducing hypnotic drug (flurazepam, chloral hydrate) is used whenever the possibility of such an interaction exists.

C. Protein binding All chloral derivatives (chloral hydrate, chloral betaine, triclofos) are metabolized to trichloroacetic acid (TCA). TCA is *strongly bound to albumin* and can displace other protein-bound drugs from their binding sites. The result is *short-term potentiation* of the displaced drug's clinical effect. For example, administration of chloral hydrate to a patient on stable oral anticoagulant therapy with warfarin can result in warfarin potentiation, excessive hypoprothrombinemia, and bleeding.

    1. Drugs *definitely affected* by protein-binding displacement are warfarin and bishydroxycoumarin.

    2. Drugs *possibly* affected are diphenylhydantoin and tolbutamide.

    Recommendation: Flurazepam can be given instead of chloral hydrate in patients receiving drugs whose effect might be influenced by protein-binding displacement.

D. Urinary excretion None of the commonly used hypnotic drugs are excreted unchanged to any significant degree. Therefore, agents that alter urine pH or tubular function have little or no effect on hypnotic drug excretion (see Section **II** for discussion of phenobarbital). Conversely, hypnotics have no known effects on excretion of other drugs.

E. Additive clinical effects with no specific other interaction can be expected to occur when two or more sedative-hypnotic drugs are acutely co-administered. Nonspecific CNS depression associated with other classes of drugs (phenothiazines, antihistamines, opiates, general anesthetics) also is additive to that produced by acute administration of hypnotics. The combined action of sedative-hypnotics and alcohol is at least additive and in some cases can be synergistic or supra-additive (see Section **III**).

    Recommendation: Physicians should warn patients of the potential hazards of combining CNS depressant drugs.

F. Conversely, *clinical antagonism* occurs when hypnotics are coadministered with CNS stimulants such as amphetamines, methylphenidate, or caffeine.

II. Antianxiety Agents

A. Bioavailability The absorption of the systemic antifungal agent griseofulvin is impaired by coadministration of phenobarbital as an antianxiety agent. No other clinically important interactions have been documented.

B. Metabolism

1. **Barbiturates** (phenobarbital, amobarbital, butabarbital), when used as antianxiety agents, are strong enzyme-inducers. See Section I.B for complete discussion.

2. **Meprobamate** causes enzyme induction in animals. In humans, however, the effect has not been demonstrated to be of clinical significance.

3. **Benzodiazepines** (chlordiazepoxide, diazepam, oxazepam, chlorazepate) have no clinically significant hepatic enzyme-inducing effects.

4. The effect of alcohol on antianxiety drug metabolism is discussed in Section III.

Recommendation: Benzodiazepines are generally more effective, although more expensive, than barbiturates when pharmacologic treatment of anxiety is indicated. The use of benzodiazepines is favored when drugs whose effects might be altered by enzyme induction are coadministered. Phenobarbital has the potential to stimulate the metabolism of diphenylhydantoin (DPH), although it is not clear how often and to what degree this happens clinically. In patients receiving DPH and phenobarbital for seizure prophylaxis, DPH dosage should be regulated according to blood concentrations.

C. Urinary excretion

1. **Phenobarbital** is weakly protein-bound and excreted unchanged to a significant degree. Drugs that alkalinize the urine (sodium bicarbonate, acetazolamide) or increase urine volume (diuretics) enhance phenobarbital excretion. The importance of this has been demonstrated only in cases of overdosage.

2. The excretion of unchanged **meprobamate** is enhanced at high urine volumes regardless of pH. The clinical significance of this is unclear except in cases of poisoning.

3. **Benzodiazepines,** in general, are biotransformed rather than excreted unchanged. Changes in urine pH, volume, or tubular function do not influence the disposition of benzodiazepines.

D. **Additive clinical effects** Antianxiety agents are similar to hypnotics in this regard (see Section I.E). Additive CNS depression occurs when they are combined with other drugs having CNS depressant properties

II. **Alcohol** Alcohol shares many properties with the hypnotics and antianxiety agents. However, a separate section is devoted to alcohol because of some important differences of which the clinician should be aware.

A. **Bioavailability** Alcohol is a small molecule that is rapidly absorbed from the proximal gastrointestinal tract. Alcohol's bioavailability does not depend on dissolution, since it is already a liquid. Ingestion can cause gastritis, thereby altering the gastric mucosa. Accordingly, alcohol in theory could alter the bioavailability of drugs that are absorbed in the stomach. Clinical confirmation of this possibility is only anecdotal.

B. **Metabolism** Chronic alcohol ingestion results in significant **enzyme induction.** The clinical consequences of this were discussed in Section I.B. Drugs whose metabolism is *definitely* stimulated by alcohol are oral anticoagulants, diphenylhydantoin, tolbutamide, and meprobamate.

C. **Metabolic site competition** Alcohol and certain other sedative-hypnotics are in part metabolized by the same enzyme system. When alcohol is *acutely* ingested, the metabolism of these drugs is impaired. Drugs *definitely* influenced by this interaction are chloral derivatives, pentobarbital, and meprobamate. The clinical consequences of this interaction are unclear. In theory alcohol and these other CNS depressants should be supraadditive when acutely coadministered, since alcohol impairs their metabolic disposition. However, controlled study reveals synergism to be slight. Dramatic "knockout drops" or "Mickey Finn" effects have not been observed, for example, when therapeutic doses of chloral hydrate are taken with alcohol.

D. **Additive clinical effects**

1. Additive CNS depression occurs when alcohol and other sedative-hypnotics are combined. Clinical synergism predicted from metabolic site interactions (Section III.C) appears to be minor.

   Recommendation: Most patients and physicians are aware of the hazards of combining alcohol with other CNS depressants. It should be remembered that chronic alcoholism causes enzyme *stimulation,* while *acute* alcoholism causes enzyme *inhibition.* The clinical consequences of this dual action cannot be readily predicted.

2. Acute alcohol ingestion can impair glycogen mobilization and caus hypoglycemia. Patients taking oral hypoglycemic agents may be predisposed to alcohol-induced hypoglycemia.

IV. Major Tranquilizers (Neuroleptics, Antipsychotic Agents)

A. Bioavailability

1. Limited studies suggest that coadministration of antacids with chlorpromazine reduces its bioavailability. It is not clear whether the *completeness* of absorption as well as the *rate* of absorption is affected. The significance of the finding is not established.

   Recommendation: Although adequate data are not available, it is reasonable to assume that biologic availability of major tranquilizers is optimal when they are given on an empty stomach

2. The bioavailability of some drugs (digoxin, acetaminophen) can be influenced by changes in gastric motility. Phenothiazines have anticholinergic effects and thus can reduce gastrointestinal motilit The *possibility* that major tranquilizers could change the bio-availability of other drugs on this basis should be considered. At present the reality of this theoretical interaction is not established

B. Metabolism

1. Reports on the effects of major tranquilizers on drug metabolism in humans are few in number. Some studies suggest that pheno-thiazines can *impair* metabolism of certain drugs (tricyclic anti-depressants, antipyrine), resulting in delayed disappearance from the blood. The clinical significance of these findings is not clear.

2. In one study, chlorpromazine metabolism was reported to be stimulated by phenobarbital. In another study, blood concentra-tions of butaperazine in the steady state were higher when subject also received imipramine in doses of 150 mg per day or more. Ag the significance of these findings is not known.

C. Urinary excretion   No interactions have been recognized in humans.

D. Receptor site interactions

1. Major tranquilizers having alpha-adrenergic blocking properties (chlorpromazine, promazine, thioridazine) will produce additive adrenergic antagonism when coadministered with other sympatho plegics. *Potential* interacting drugs are reserpine, phenoxybenzam phentolamine, methyldopa. It is not possible to predict the degre to which this will be of importance in a given patient.

2. Cholinergic blocking effects of major tranquilizers will be additive to those of other anticholinergic drugs. *Potential* interacting drugs are belladonna alkaloids, synthetic anticholinergics, antihistamines, and tricyclic antidepressants. Phenothiazines are contraindicated in cases of anticholinergic drug toxicity because of this interaction.

3. Chlorpromazine prevents guanethidine-like antihypertensive agents from reaching their receptor site of action. The result is antagonism of antihypertensive effects. This is a well-documented interaction. Chlorpromazine and guanethidine should not be coadministered (see also Section **V.D**).

E. **Additive effects** occur when sedating phenothiazines (chlorpromazine, promazine, thioridazine) are given with other CNS depressants.

F. **Clinical antagonism** of anticonvulsant drugs is possible in theory. Some reports suggest that major tranquilizers can lower the seizure threshold and precipitate seizures in certain susceptible individuals. This is well-documented in studies of major tranquilizer therapy in alcohol withdrawal. In other situations the clinical significance of the effect is not clear.

Recommendation: Major tranquilizers should be given with caution to patients with a history of a convulsive disorder. In theory these drugs could cause "breakthrough" seizures in individuals previously controlled with anticonvulsant medications.

V. **Tricyclic Antidepressants**

A. **Bioavailability** Tricyclic antidepressants have strong anticholinergic effects and have the potential to alter the biologic availability of other drugs whose absorption depends on gastrointestinal motility. Delayed or reduced absorption, or both, of phenylbutazone and levodopa has been reported in subjects also receiving tricyclic antidepressants (see also Section **IV.A**).

B. **Metabolism**

1. Reports on the effects of antidepressants on hepatic drug metabolism are conflicting. Various studies have documented *enhancement, impairment,* and *no effect* on metabolism of other drugs. Further work is needed to elucidate the actual extent and clinical significance of such interactions.

2. Tricyclic antidepressant metabolism is reportedly stimulated by barbiturates and inhibited by major tranquilizers. The significance of these interactions is not clear. *Methylphenidate* impairs hepatic metabolism of several drugs, including tricyclic antidepressants.

Coadministration of methylphenidate to antidepressant-treated patients reportedly increases blood concentrations of the antidepressant and potentiates its clinical effect.

3. Conjugated estrogens and oral contraceptive preparations containing high estrogen dosage reportedly enhance the clinical toxicity of imipramine. Inhibition of drug metabolism by steroids is postulated to explain this phenomenon.

C. **Urinary excretion**   Acidification of the urine appears to enhance the urinary excretion of certain tricyclic antidepressants. However, since excretion of unchanged drug is a very minor disposition pathway compared to hepatic metabolism, enhanced excretion is probably of no consequence. No clinically important interactions have been documented.

D. **Receptor site interactions**

1. Tricyclic antidepressants are strong anticholinergics and potentiate the effects of other drugs with similar properties (see Section **IV.D**

2. Tricyclic antidepressants prevent guanethidine-like antihypertensiv agents (guanethidine, bethanidine, clonidine) from reaching their site of action. The result is antagonism of antihypertensive effects (see also Section **IV.D**).

3. Limited studies suggest that tricyclic antidepressants can potentiate the pressor and arrhythmia-producing effects of certain catecholamines (phenylephrine, epinephrine, norepinephrine). The clinical importance of this interaction has not been elucidated. However, the possibility of such an interaction should be considered when antidepressant-treated patients take proprietary cold preparations or receive dental anesthetic mixtures containing catecholamines.

4. Small doses of thyroid hormone potentiate the clinical effect of tricyclic antidepressants in euthyroid patients.

5. Possible clinical interactions between tricyclic antidepressants and monoamine oxidase inhibitors are discussed in Section **VI**.

E. **Clinical antagonism**

1. Several reports suggest that tricyclic drugs can precipitate seizures in certain susceptible individuals. Some of these patients were known to have had a seizure disorder, although others were not. The mechanism of the effect is not known.

   Recommendation: Tricyclics should be given with caution to patients with a history of a convulsive disorder. Antidepressants can cause "breakthrough" seizures even in individuals previously in adequate control with anticonvulsant medications.

2. Some epidemiologic studies show that tricyclic antidepressants are associated with an increased risk of sudden death in patients with ischemic heart disease. Presumably these deaths are due to ventricular arrhythmias. Other studies have not confirmed this.

> **Recommendation:** Until conflicting data are resolved, tricyclic antidepressants should be given with caution to patients with ischemic heart disease. The risk may be greater in those with recurrent ventricular arrhythmias, in patients receiving anti-arrhythmic pharmacotherapy, or in those receiving cardiostimulant catecholamines (see also Section **V.D.3**).

VI. Monoamine Oxidase (MAO) Inhibitors

A. **Bioavailability**   No interactions are documented.

B. **Metabolism**   MAO inhibitors have the potential to antagonize many enzyme systems. A variety of drugs are reportedly potentiated by MAO inhibitors. Most of these observations of potentiation are anecdotal. Because of the seriousness of many of the adverse re-actions, and because of the limited clinical utility of MAO inhibitors, systematic studies in humans are few in number. In many cases, potentiation could be due to receptor site interaction (see Section **VI.D**) as well as impairment of metabolism. Drugs reportedly potentiated by MAO inhibitor coadministration are alcohol, sedative-hypnotics, general anesthetics, analgesics, including opiates, and phenothiazines.

C. **Urinary excretion**   Acidification of the urine enhances the excretion of tranylcypromine. The clinical importance of this is limited to cases of tranylcypromine poisoning.

D. **Receptor site interactions**

1. MAO inhibitors inhibit the degradation of catecholamines. There-fore, coadministration of other substances that contain or release catecholamines can potentially result in adrenergic crises. It is not clear how often such reactions occur, but they can be serious or fatal. Manifestations include hypertension, tachycardia, hyper-pyrexia, diaphoresis, agitation, and delirium.
   Adrenergic crises due to interaction with MAO inhibitors have been reported with the following substances:

   a. Foods containing tyramine, dopa, or serotonin. These include bananas, beer, figs, cheese, liver, pickled herring, wine, yeast products, and yogurt (see Chapter 19).

b. Reserpine.

c. Tricyclic antidepressants.

d. L-dopa.

e. Sympathomimetic amines. These include amphetamines, methyl phenidate, metaraminol, mephentermine, ephedrine, phenyleph rine, and phenylpropanolamine. Many proprietary cold and antiallergy preparations contain sympathomimetics that can interact with MAO inhibitors.

Recommendation: MAO inhibitors add little to the pharma cotherapy of depression or hypertension. Hazards, toxic effects and potential drug interactions are numerous. The use of MAO inhibitors in clinical medicine therefore is seldom justified. If they are used, the possible interactions as outlined above should be clear to both patient and physician.

2. Marked hyperpyrexia has been reported with the combination of MAO inhibitors and meperidine, possibly mediated by serotonin.

VII. Lithium

A. **Bioavailability** Preliminary studies indicate that large variations in biologic availability exist among different brands of lithium. This emphasizes the need for frequent determinations of serum lithium concentrations to guide therapy.

B. **Metabolism** Lithium is not metabolized by the human body. It is not known to alter the metabolism of other drugs.

C. **Urinary excretion** Lithium is excreted unchanged by the kidney. The determinants of its excretion rate are similar to those that govern sodium excretion. The following factors lead to impaired excretion of lithium:

1. **Dehydration,** usually due to chronic diuretic use, poor fluid intake, or fever.

2. Dietary salt restriction (see Chapter 19).

References

Conney, A. H. Pharmacological implications of microsomal enzyme induction. *Pharmacol Rev.* 19:317–366, 1967.
Davis, J. M., Sekerke, J., and Janowsky, D. S. Drug interactions involving the drugs of abuse. *Drug Intel. Clin. Pharm.* 8:120–142, 1974.
Fann, W. E. Some clinically important interactions of psychotropic drugs. *South. Med. J.* 66:661–665, 1973.
Greenblatt, D. J., and Shader, R. I. The clinical choice of sedative-hypnotics. *Ann. Intern. Med.* 77:91–100, 1972.

Greenblatt, D. J., and Shader, R. I. *Benzodiazepines in Clinical Practice.* New York: Raven, 1974. Pp. 245—250.

Hansten, P. D. *Drug Interactions.* Philadelphia: Lea & Febiger, 1971.

Koch-Weser, J., and Sellers, E. M. Drug interactions with coumarin anticoagulants. *N. Engl. J. Med.* 285:487—498, 547—558, 1971.

Morrelli, H. F., and Melmon, K. L. The clinician's approach to drug interactions. *Calif. Med.* 109:380—389, 1968.

Roisfold, I. H Clinical pharmacology of drug interactions. *Annu. Rev. Med.* 24: 385—418, 1973.

Sher, S. P. Drug enzyme induction and drug interactions: Literature tabulation. *Toxicol. Appl. Pharmacol.* 18:780—834, 1973.

Swidler, G. *Handbook of Drug Interactions.* New York: Wiley-Interscience, 1971.

17

The Borderline State: Psychopharmacologic Treatment Approaches to the Undiagnosed Case

Donald F. Klein
Richard I. Shader

The meaning of the label "borderline patient" continues to be a subject of debate. Terms such as *latent schizophrenia* and *pseudoneurotic schizophrenia* are often considered synonymous. The implication is usually that the patient is bordering on psychosis, although he does not manifest clearcut Kraepelinian signs of schizophrenia (delusions, hallucinations) or psychotic degrees of depression. In support of this opinion the diagnostician frequently detects a "soft" thought disorder. However, some psychiatric patients do communicate peculiarly (e.g., rambling, tangential, concrete, overabstract, circumstantial, blocked, or unusual associations without being delusional), and unfortunately there is no systematic body of data relating such features to course or prognosis.

The term *borderline* is most commonly used when the (sometimes inadequately investigated) patient does not neatly fit a common diagnostic stereotype but instead shows features reminiscent of several diagnoses. Indeed, some patients present such a welter of unique familial relationships, developmental idiosyncrasies, social aberrations, affective states, cognitive disturbances, symptoms, defects, and maladaptations that the information overload on the diagnostician is acute, and he is often led to premature mind closure and blindness to the data.

Since the borderline state does not have a neat set of psychopathologic descriptors, development of a drug treatment program for these patients is a complex task. How can the physician develop such a program for a patient he cannot diagnose? One way to pursue this issue is to identify and consider separately a number of syndromes frequently associated with patients labeled borderline and to outline the medications appropriate in the treatment of each of these syndromes. It is important to note that some of our medication recommendations are based on clinical experience rather than on controlled studies, of which there is a notable paucity.

It has been hypothesized that the effects of most major psychotropic agents are related to their capacity to modify states of dysregulation of affect and activation (D. F. Klein and J. M. Davis, *Diagnosis and Treatment of Psychiatric Disorders,* Baltimore: Williams & Wilkins, 1969). It follows from this theory that psychotropic agents work through modification of activation-affective dysregulation and that conditions not characterized by these defects should be refractory to these drugs. On the whole this is accurate; dyssocial, antisocial, passive-aggressive, and narcissistic character disorders, perversions, obsessive-compulsive states, mental deficiency, conversion and hypochondriacal reactions, and chronic "burned-out" schizophrenics are all relatively refractory to antipsychotic and antidepressant-like drugs. Whenever drugs have proved useful in these conditions, it is in the treatment of an intercurrent affective derangement without alteration of the patient's chronic difficulty.

Therefore, it is good strategy, when confronted with a case that does not fit neatly into any diagnostic rubric, to look first for evidence that the patient's psychopathology can be attributed to an affective or activation disorder. Unfortunately such signs may not be immediately apparent nor, for that matter, complained of by the patient, since patients frequently express their difficulties wholly in terms of interpersonal and intrapsychic conflicts. The contribution of the patient's activation and affective status to the patient's distress can be completely overlooked and therefore must be specifically explored. Even if during his mental status examination the patient gives much evidence of affective disturbance, there can be a problem in "figure-ground discrimination" such that the examiner may, like the patient, see the affective disturbance as secondary and "understandable," with the result that these disturbances are quickly relegated to the background.

I.   **Emotional Lability** One central psychopathologic trait that is often overlooked or underemphasized is marked emotional lability. In their detailed study of the borderline syndrome, Grinker and his coauthors (*The Borderline Syndrome,* New York: Basic Books, 1968) found that their sample of 51 patients all fell into one of four groups. Group II, which they described as the core borderline syndrome, contained patients who were characterized by pervasive negative affect. Outwardly they displayed vacillating involvement with others, overt anger, depression, and absence of indications of consistent self-identity. However, their depression was lifted if they acted out and participated in activities or rebelled against the environment. This group distinctly resembles the labile emotionally unstable character disorder described by Klein and Davis (*Diagnosis and Drug Treatment of Psychiatric Disorders*). Such patients are frequently misdiagnosed. In a followup study of emotionally unstable character disorders by Rifkin and colleagues, these patients were frequently considered schizophrenic by their hospital psychiatrists, although they in fact had a relatively benign clinical course similar to that of the borderline patients described in the Grinker project (*J. Biol. Psych.* 4:65, 1972; *J. Biol. Psychiatry* 4:81, 1972).

A. **Description** Such labile, emotionally unstable patients, predominantly female adolescents, are frequently treated with intensive exploratory psychotherapy because of their interesting personalities, high degree of interaction with the therapist, marked introspective capacities, manifest psychological distress, and dramatic life experiences. It is often noted that such patients overreact to the point that some would call them psychotic when they are frustrated by or lose an object relationship on which they have been exceedingly dependent. Although capable of forming intense but brittle attachments to their therapists and displaying much verbal insight, significant modification of their affective behavior patterns is not regularly achieved. Some therapists believe that by age 30 these patients become more mature, with or without treatment. It is often the case that the emotionally chaotic state of these patients makes it impossible for them to utilize their new insights or to plan constructively and engage in a career development program.

B. **Impact of medication** Antipsychotic (neuroleptic) agents are valuable in the treatment of this syndrome and can alleviate both the high, giddy, excitable, impulsive, hedonistic phase and the sullen, hostile, depressive, withdrawn phase. Often feelings of confusion, perplexity, anxiety, and depression are replaced by a manner that is bland, placid, friendly, and ingratiating. Moreover, a reduction in feelings of role diffusion and goallessness may occur, even in the absence of specific solutions. In their psychotherapy, the patients move away from introspection toward a concern with day-to-day events and developing active and friendly peer relationships. They do not, however, demonstrate any increased concern with long-range planning.

Interestingly, some psychotherapists may be distressed by the change in communications from apparent attempts at insight to minimization, denial, and lack of interest in introspection. The therapist will frequently attribute the change in lability to better environmental structuring, ignoring the fact that previous structuring attempts had resulted in negativistic, impulsive actions. Sometimes therapists will conclude that medication is interfering with psychotherapy and will discontinue it, and their patients then promptly regress to emotional lability and episodic impulsiveness.

Such patients also encourage medication discontinuation themselves, since they usually do not like being on an even keel and frequently complain of feeling a lack of spontaneity and a certain deadness. However, external behavioral observation of these patients, who are often active and lively, does not bear this out. Perhaps their complaints can be understood as expression of regret that they no longer experience their high, giddy periods. It may be that such patients are addicted to their elated stages, miss them, and derogate their comparatively normal states. Alternatively, it is possible that the neuroleptics actually do produce a feeling tone somewhat different from normal for these patients during their even periods, possibly related to parkinsonian akinesia. Such complaints may lead patients to discontinue medication surreptitiously.

C. Treatment

1. **Neuroleptics** Thioridazine, in doses of approximately 300 mg hs, is effective and acceptable in this patient group. Larger doses are rarely necessary. While it is our impression that nonaliphatic phenothiazines (e.g., trifluoperazine and fluphenazine) occasionally produce irritability in these patients, they are, on the other hand, often effective and have a somewhat lower degree of lethargy and akinesia associated with their use.

2. **Lithium carbonate** A double-blind placebo controlled study has demonstrated that lithium carbonate is both very acceptable to such patients and of distinct value in damping mood swings, supporting the belief that the patient's drug rejection is related to extrapyramidal disorder (*Arch. Gen. Psychiatry* 27:519, 1972). Lithium may well turn out to be the drug of choice (dosage adjusted to achieve blood levels between 0.75 and 1.2 mEq/L), with occasional supplementation by small doses (50 mg hs) of thioridazine. However, the practicing clinician should take note that the use of lithium carbonate in such borderline patients is not currently sanctioned by the Food and Drug Administration. Single case reports have appeared suggesting that lithium carbonate may also be helpful in diminishing self-destructive (e.g., wrist cutting) and assaultive behaviors (Psychopharmacologia 40:17–24, 1974).

3. **Antidepressants** have diverse effects in this group. Some patients respond very well, with a marked increase in affective stability, whereas others become increasingly angry, irritable, and aggressive although manic episodes are rare. These effects may occur in sequence.

II. **Rejection-Sensitive Dysphoria** One subgroup of patients frequently considered to have either a neurotic depressive reaction or hysterical-hysteroid character disorder is worthy of special notice, since specific medication response patterns occur.

A. Description

1. **Early development** It is postulated that in early development, probably during the period psychoanalytically referred to as the oral phase, an innate affective control mechanism develops with

respect to the experience of social approval, applause, and admiration. We do not consider that these experiences derive their effectiveness from being linked to primary tissue need gratifications (i.e., as secondary reinforcers), although this process also occurs. Rather, we hold such experiences to be primary, innately determined reinforcers. The experience of social approval results in a pleasurable mood, accompanied by self-satisfaction, whereas social disapproval produces marked anhedonia and distress. This distress does not result in paralysis but rather in active efforts to regain the pleasurable state of approval. The precise efforts used will depend on what rewards the family and society usually offer, or, to use operant conditioning language, the reinforcement contingencies.

If a child is afflicted with a marked mood instability that is reactive to social approval and disapproval, it is understandable that he would shortly become overtrained in methods for eliciting approving feedback from the environment. Naturally the exact method used will depend on the reinforcement contingencies offered by the family. Many of these patients have been treated as little princesses by their father and have a narcissistic, self-indulgent mother as a female model. Thus, being reassured of their physical or sexual attractiveness is of remarkable consequence to their feelings of self-worth. Similarly, other patients whose primary parental approval has been for their academic or artistic achievement are overwhelmed with a sense of failure at the slightest hint that they have failed to maintain their excellence. Their efforts are not aimed at developing many capacities for obtaining their own *internal* satisfaction and happiness but at the central goal of obtaining the *external* applause of others.

2. **Mood level** The general psychopathologic state of these patients is an extremely brittle, shallow mood ranging from giddy elation to desperate unhappiness and markedly responsive to external sources of admiration and approval. Such a patient may appear hopelessly bereft when a love affair terminates, but upon meeting a new attentive man, she may feel perfectly fine and even slightly elated within a few days. Similarly, failure to win high praise for their work may devastate them, but the trauma is quickly forgotten if this gap is filled by commendation for another project. This emotionality markedly effects their judgment. When euphoric, they minimize and deny shortcomings of a situation or personal relationship, idealizing all achievements and love objects. But when they are at the opposite emotional pole, feelings of desperation dispro-

portionate to actual circumstances are expressed. While such patients refer to their dysphoric mood as "depression," some of the characteristic features of endogenous depressive states are not observed. Patients are prone to oversleep and overeat, and although they may express themselves despairingly, they are activity oriented and often strive successfully to engage in new, rewarding situations.

3. **Traits** The pattern of their characteristic traits allows an inference concerning the emotional dynamics of these patients. In general, the hysteroid patients are fickle, emotionally labile, irresponsible, shallow, love-intoxicated, giddy, and shortsighted. They tend in many instances to be egocentric, narcissistic, exhibitionistic, vain, and clothes-crazy. In addition, they are seductive, manipulative, exploitive, sexually provocative, and emotional and illogical in their thinking; they are easy prey to flattery and compliments. Their general manner is histrionic and flamboyant. In their sexual relations they are possessive, grasping, demanding, romantic, and foreplay-centered. When frustrated or disappointed, they become reproachful, tearful, abusive, and vindictive, and often resort to alcohol.

Those who seem neurotic depressive are frequently obsessional, accept considerable dissatisfaction and pain to maintain the security of dependent relationships, and, not unlike the hysteric, may complain of a loss of all feeling at moments when self-esteem is most threatened.

These statements concerning the hysteroid patient may appear to be a misogynous characterization of women — a caricature of femininity — and require explanation. In our society, as probably in most others, a primary goal in the life of many women is to attract and retain a supporting male figure. Such sex typing occurs very early in life, possibly within the first two years. Among the social tactics available to women, and approved of as peculiarly feminine, are exhibitionistic, seductive displays of their charms. Women with a normal range of emotional response utilize a wide variety of exhibitionistic and seductive social tactics with discretion and accuracy. The female hysteroid dysphoric patient is a caricature of femininity because her disorder drives her to attempt to repair her dysphoria by exaggerating the social, seductive, exhibitionistic tactics allowable to women in our society. It is the driven quality and repetitiousness of behavior that indicates the underlying affective disorder. Such patients often appear intact when they are able to "latch on" to someone, receiving what might be called "lend-lease" ego functions from the relationship, so that they are not swamped by their affective dysregulation.

Finding a generally acceptable label for these patients would be most useful. They have been referred to as hysteroid characters because of their histrionic emotionality and opposite-sex-centered concerns. This term seems unfortunate in that it emphasizes their interpersonal tactics and fantasy goals. We view these character traits as secondary to the primary affective disturbance. This shift in focus is not accidental but reflects our growing therapeutic armamentarium. Until very recently the psychotherapist's natural focus was on those aspects of the patient that seemed modifiable by psychotherapy: their object relations and interpersonal tactics. Their affective lability and dependence on external sources of narcissistic supplies were considered secondary, reparative, anxiety-binding defenses that were not open to direct intervention. The ability of medication to change directly the affective reactivity of these patients now makes it appear that the interpersonal tactics and object relationships may be viewed as secondary reverberations of the basic affective difficulty.

4. **Clinical characteristics** One can review each group of clinical characteristics as derived from these patients' basic affective vulnerability or as a method by which they have compensated for this defect. For instance, the fickle, shallow, love-intoxicated, giddy nature of the hysteroid dysphoric patient may be viewed as a direct expression of his or her specific variety of reactive affective lability. The shortsightedness, emotional reasoning, illogical and irresponsible attitudes can be viewed as a domination of thinking and judgment process by mood state, and the exhibitionism, clothes-craziness, seductiveness, manipulativeness, sexual pro-vocativeness, and narcissism as devices for eliciting admiring masculine attention. Similarly, the obsessional, task-oriented patterns of the neurotic depressive are buffers against dealing with possible failures in intellectual and artistic arenas.

The egocentrism of the rejection-sensitive dysphoric results from their very narrow perceptual focus; that is, people are viewed essentially as mood-adjusting agents — perhaps consistent with concepts such as part-objects or transitional objects. Therefore, these patients do not develop a discriminating appreciation of the real complexity of others; when the other person is no longer a source of admiration, or the first spontaneous admiring response wears thin, there is no felt reason to continue the relationship. Their reproachfulness, tearfulness, abusiveness, and vindictiveness are viewed as the other pole of their emotional lability compounded by an aggressive response to frustration. These patients do not have a psychopathic coldness and indifference to rejection by a love object.

Although such patients, when deprived, speak fervently of the possibility of suicide, the act seems quite uncommon. Furthermore, although they speak frequently of loneliness, they are not dominated by separation anxiety. That is, they do not develop agoraphobic or travel phobic trends. If in the company of a man who is dull and unadmiring, such a woman will remove herself as quickly as possible, whereas the patient dominated by separation anxiety will accept any type of companionship. The development of psychotic depressive states in these patients can occur but is most unusual. They can be distinguished from patients with an emotionally unstable character disorder by the clearcut "reactive" nature of their dysphoria.

B. Treatment

1. **Psychotherapy** Uncontrolled clinical experience with hysteroid dysphoric patients indicates that supportive and directive psychotherapy is of some moderate value in getting them to organize their lives better, meet deadlines, and fulfill responsibilities. This would seem to result from the patient's attempt to gain the therapist's approbation by accepting the therapist's values. In many instances, the affective disorder seems little changed by psychotherapy. Some skilled therapists are able to help such patients grow emotionally. The therapy often involves a careful alternation between some gratification of the patient's dependency needs and subsequent gradual frustration of these needs to promote progressive autonomy and self-reliance. The patient can be educated to recognize the object-related nature of the dysphoria.

2. **Antidepressants**

   a. **Imipramine** The use of imipramine often has negative effects. These patients may develop racing thoughts, somatic distress, feelings of depersonalization, or manic states. However, an occasional patient seems to respond to imipramine.

   b. **MAO inhibitors** can be of marked value, although they are rarely used by most therapists since the dysphoric states are fleeting, and it is often a matter of weeks before there is an effect from antidepressants. However, one should not ignore the prophylactic effect of MAO inhibitors in this disorder. The patient's marked lability is modified in both directions, still tending to overevaluate, in a giddy fashion, the value of approval and admiration, but able to make a more rational judgment of the situation. A crucial consequence of putting these patients on MAO inhibitors is that they do not then become dysphoric upon deprivation or loss of admiration. This affective modification makes it no longer necessary for them to fling themselves into fruitless, self-destructive, or unrewarding romantic involvements. Also, their frequent use of alcohol becomes markedly diminished. Phenelzine (15 mg tid) is an effective MAO inhibitor for this group. Higher doses (60 to 90 mg/day) may be needed but may cause an irritable hypomania; of course, this may be easily treated by reinstituting a lower dosage schedule. Prolonged treatment is necessary since drug termination regularly leads to a recurrence of emotional lability. A rational goal is to maintain medication until the patient's life is organized well enough to ensure adequate external supplies of self-esteem. At this point weaning from medication may be attempted; this often fails, however. Dietary constraints must be carefully observed in patients taking MAO inhibitors (see Chapter 19).

3. **Alcohol** The practice by these patients of utilizing alcohol may stem from two sources. Alcohol seems to work primarily on anticipatory anxiety, and since these patients are in a chronic anxious state concerning the possibility of being rejected or failing, alcohol serves as a source of courage to them. It is also interesting that alcohol has been shown to operate as an MAO inhibitor. Thus it is possible that alcohol has some specific pharmacologic value for such patients.

4. Soporific neuroleptics are not well tolerated by these patients. A nonsedative neuroleptic may be of some value as an adjunct when used in small doses (e.g., 2 to 5 mg/day of trifluoperazine). In this dose range the patient appears more relaxed, less labile, and less hostile or irritable.

II. Chronic Anxiety-Tension States

A. **Description** The borderline patient also often presents with marked anxiety and tension, overshadowed by other, more salient complaints. In particular, many patients have a syndrome that resembles mild agitated depression but are not diagnosed as such because of their numerous interpersonal difficulties.

B. **Treatment** In primarily anxious-tense patients, without evidence of psychosis or panic attacks, the use of minor tranquilizers appears to have a role. It is current practice to give such patients a benzodiazepine (see Chapter 2), although evidence that these medications are particularly valuable in the complex borderline case with chronic anxiety is hard to come by.

It is even conceivable that some patients react negatively to these agents, developing increased hostility or dysphoric complaints that are not recognized as attributable to their "tranquilizer." It is perhaps wise to minimize the use of such medications until other, possibly more definitive, interventions, such as those provided by the tricyclic antidepressants, MAO inhibitors, phenothiazine-like drugs, and lithium have been exhausted. If the patient is suffering from a pervasive inability to enjoy himself that is quite unreactive to changes in his personal surroundings, associated with sleep disturbances, a loss of interest, and feeling overwhelmed, then the utility of antidepressants rather than minor tranquilizers becomes more evident. Some patients have a pattern characterized by severe anticipatory and phobic anxiety and spontaneous panic attacks. Their treatment is discussed in Chapter 2.

IV. Histrionic States

A. Description
One patient group causing grave problems in clinical management is comprised of tense histrionic patients, who are characteristically labile, episodically agitated, erratic, unpredictable, and manipulative. Although they are usually rational, relevant, and coherent, they express occasional paranoid and hallucinatory verbalizations. It is their ability to change that is so startling; they can act frightened and panicky to the point of suicide and several minutes later be affably laughing with others. Thus, while these individuals maintain a high degree of interaction with others, being at times sociable, friendly, and supportive, they are at other times disturbing, hostile, argumentative, and demanding, yet pleading for help and direction. Such patients express great investment in their doctors and psychotherapy, endowing them with miraculous potentialities. Similarly, their therapists readily become emotionally involved and are frequently frustrated and perplexed by the inability to predict or modify the patient's behavior. In addition, these patients have a tendency to become mute under close questioning. This passive-aggressive maneuver is often inaccurately referred to as catatonic or micropsychotic. The diagnosis of histrionic reaction is difficult to defend in the face of skepticism among colleagues as to one's diagnostic acumen. The apparent fluctuations in states of consciousness that occur with this illness should prompt a thorough neurologic and electroencephalographic investigation.

This grouping was reintroduced into American nosology by

DSM-II (American Psychiatric Association, *Diagnostic and Statistical Manual of Mental Disorders,* 2nd ed.) as "hysterical personality, histrionic personality disorder." However, this category also includes the previous diagnosis "emotionally unstable personality," thus obscuring a valuable distinction.

1. **Impact of environment** One clinical feature of predictive value and theoretical import is the marked relationship of these patients' symptoms to environmental impact. Unlike depressed patients, who may increase the vigor of their complaints in the presence of psychiatric staff in an attempt to obtain maximum caring from them, but who remain inactive or unproductively agitated when not under staff observation, this group of refractory patients may appear in good spirits when apparently unobserved by staff, engage in social games and gossip pleasantly with others, even shortly after an explosive affective display.

   The key issue may be histrionic role playing and symptom imitation. In other words, these patients' symptoms may not be the direct external manifestations of intolerable affective states, but rather may be environmentally oriented, learned manipulative devices associated with loss of role distance. Agitation and depressive complaints in this group are not the same as similarly labeled phenomena in other patients. Interestingly, the conversion reactions of the nineteenth century, as described by Charcot, Freud, and others, consisted mainly of pseudoneurologic syndromes such as convulsions, anesthesia, paralyses, blindness, deafness, and dyskinesia. These behavioral syndromes were noted at a time when hysterical patients were housed in hospital wards along with neurologic and epileptic patients, as in the Salpetriere. Hysteroepilepsy may well have been an artifact of exposure.

2. **Hysteroschizophrenia** It is frequently stated that classic grand hysteria is no longer seen. However, the diagnosis of schizophrenia has become more and more prevalent, and atypical, borderline, or pseudoneurotic schizophrenias are widely reported. Since the knowledge of schizophrenic behavior is widespread via books, television, and movies, and it is common practice to house all patients with emotional disorders together, we speculate that hysteroschizophrenics are being produced in much the same fashion as the nineteenth-century hysteroepileptic.

   The differential diagnosis of hysteroschizophrenia from true schizophrenia presents knotty problems. The major distinguishing feature would seem to be a variant of the well-known hysterical phenomenon, *la belle indifférence.* Hysterics may have the most crippling disorders and yet not display appropriate concern or emotional reaction to their infirmities. If it is their motivation to attain the sick role, one can well understand this phenomenon as resulting from their natural satisfaction with attaining their goal. An analogous phenomenon occurs in patients with hysteroschizophrenia. The attainment of the sick role is dependent on their imitation of extreme emotional distress, including psychotic symptomatology. Therefore, in the initial stages of disorder, there is, rather than *la belle indifférence,* a histrionic accentuation of numerous psychotic features in a confusing jumble. However, once the patient is adjudged psychiatrically ill, as by hospitalization, one is struck by the marked fluctuations in psychiatric status and by the patient's apparent indifference to the content of his expressed delusions. For instance, a schizophrenic may express the belief that the food is poisoned and promptly give up eating. A hysteroschizophrenic may express the same belief and then eat with a good appetite 30 minutes later. Similarly, a schizophrenic who expresses suicidal ideation, because he is convinced that his persecutors are about to close in on him, is in an extremely dangerous state and must be kept under constant observation. His affective state remains constant — fear and agitation. A hysteroschizophrenic may express the same delusional content and then, when away from the immediate observation of professional staff, engage in conversation and banter with other patients. Marked fluctuations in symptomatic behavior, depending on their impact on the environment, are common with hysteroschizophrenics. Furthermore, these patients frequently resort to the use of sedatives, intoxicants, narcotics, and stimulants, thus obscuring their status.

B. **Treatment** Hysteroschizophrenic patients are refractory or respond negatively to psychotropic medication and tend to abuse the use of stimulants and sedatives. Intolerance of distressing side effects due to medication is expressed dramatically. Because of the lability of these patients there is much uncertainty as to the effectiveness of medication, so they tend to receive long treatment courses before medication is found ineffective. However, if the patient responds in a somatizing fashion, medication is terminated promptly.

The disorganization of hysteroschizophrenic patients is so severe that outpatient therapy can rarely be accomplished. On the other hand, inpatient therapy in permissive settings regularly offers these patients such regressive temptations that they are unable to progress toward accepting adult responsibilities. These patients present an unsolved problem.

There is no firm evidence concerning the utility of either short-term or long-term hospitalization in the treatment of this heterogeneous collection of patients. As indicated in the discussion of hysteroschizophrenia, hospitalization is not an innocuous procedure and may serve to solidify demoralized, dependent, exploitive adaptations. However, hospitalization in a high level facility does have a role in arriving at a clearcut diagnostic formulation when this had seemed impossible. Hospitalization affords an opportunity to see the borderline patient "in the round." One is continually amazed to see patients demonstrate glaring defects in affective regulation and cognitive ability that were simply undetectable from the patient's testimony and behavior in the office. Further, hospitalization can afford a full overview of the patient's response to treatment that often cannot be gained in out-patient practice. For these reasons, short-term participation in a well-structured day hospital program may afford a good diagnostic and therapeutic compromise.

Long-term intensive psychotherapy during hospitalization as a sole means of effectively dealing with this heterogeneous group is not supported by experience. Although it is possible that for some patients this may be the treatment of choice, before engaging in such a major, possibly regression-producing and dependency-affirming intervention, it would seem useful to be sure that all lesser interventions have proved failures.

Selected case histories illustrating the types of patients described can be read for further understanding of these clinical and diagnostic concepts (D. F. Klein, *Psychiatric Case Studies: Treatment, Drugs and Outcome,* Baltimore: Williams & Wilkins, 1972).

18

Hypnosis

David Spiegel
Richard I. Shader

Although controversy abounds about its nature, hypnosis can be conceptualized as a state of intense focal concentration with diminished peripheral awareness. When appropriately applied, it can usefully facilitate diagnostic and therapeutic procedures in clinical psychiatry.

I. **The Trance State** The trance state is an altered but natural state of consciousness. Susceptible individuals can enter this state in a matter of seconds, and good hypnotic subjects often slip in and out of trance states without realizing it. One common kind of trance experience is being totally absorbed in reading to the extent that one is unaware of peripheral distractions. This intense concentration on a focal issue permits subjects to "ignore" unwanted stimuli such as noise or pain. Moreover, it is possible to suspend critical judgment or to focus selectively on alternative feelings or behaviors. Typically, a person in a hypnotic trance wants to comply and cooperate with the suggestions offered by the *operator* who induces the trance. However, if the subject profoundly objects to a suggestion, he will certainly fail to comply with it.

II. **The Trance Induction** All hypnosis is in reality self-hypnosis, whereby the subject allows himself to slip into a mode of intense concentration. The operator can systematically teach the subject or patient how to use this capacity, stressing from the beginning that nothing will be "projected" onto the subject. An atmosphere of repose, free of coercion, enabling the operator and subject to choose a focus of fixed concentration, is very important. The particular ritual or technique of trance induction is far less important than the subject's conviction of its efficacy.

III. **Diagnostic Uses** Because patients vary in their ability to undergo a hypnotic trance, there is a growing body of experience that recommends a systematic assessment of this trance capacity as a way of quickly providing useful diagnostic information. The trance experiences of persons who are either healthy or neurotic seem clearly distinguishable from those of persons with severe character disorders, schizophrenia, or organic syndromes. Those with the latter, more severe problems can enter the trance state only erratically, and they commonly break off the trance after a minute or two. For example, hypnosis may assist in the difficult differential diagnosis of hysterical states from other, possibly psychotic conditions. The induction of the trance may be expected to differ strikingly in these two clinical situations. While a hysteric should be more readily hypnotized and cooperative with the operator's suggestions over a 10-minute period, a schizophrenic, by contrast, will break out of the trance in a minute or so. Although hypnosis has yet to be studied adequately in toxic conditions, difficulties similar to those experienced with schizophrenics may reasonably be expected.

A brief, 10-minute assessment of trance capacity, which may be incorporated as part of the induction procedure, is known as the "eye-roll hand levitation" method. It correlates a physiologic sign known as the "eye-roll" with some behavioral instructions. A subject's ability to look up while slowly closing his eyes is associated with his hypnotizability. A series of behavioral instructions can be given. For instance, the operator may suggest that a subject's hand will remain light and in an upright position. The subject evidences his hypnotizability by the degree to which he acts in accordance with this instruction, as well as by the degree to which the eye sign is present. An inconsistency between these two indices may have pathologic significance.

The operator should be alert to at least two sources of artifact in this assessment. If the patient feels coerced or untrusting, his response may be below his real capacity. In addition to this problem of motivation, it is likely that sedatives and tranquilizers will interfere with trance capacity.

IV. **Contraindications to Hypnosis** Hypnosis should never be attempted under threat or coercion. The clinician should attempt to explain the nature of hypnosis, emphasizing that all hypnosis is really self-hypnosis, that the subject or patient is aware of what is happening, and that he is free to break with the trance state at any time. The purpose of the hypnotic intervention should be explained clearly and the nature of the induction procedure reviewed.

A. **Severe depression** A person who is severely depressed and suicidal might have his hopes for a magical cure raised and then dashed by an attempt at a hypnotic induction. He could view this as one more failure in his life, and if he is suicidal already, he could well use this experience as an excuse for an attempt. *Careful assessment of level of depression, expectations, and suicidal tendencies is critical.*

B. **Paranoid thinking of psychotic proportions** A person who has developed a projective framework of thinking is not likely to appreciate the subtleties of self-hypnosis as distinct from mind control. He may attribute great powers to the hypnotist and may get quite angry at what seems to be a loss of control. However, this need not be the case, and a paranoid person may discover, to his surprise, that he retains control. *But care must be taken.* Most paranoid persons will make the operator's decision an unnecessary one in that they simply refuse the technique.

V. **Therapeutic Applications** Psychiatric inpatients are rarely capable of sustained trance experiences. However, in general medical settings and in outpatient treatment, hypnosis can facilitate a variety of therapeutic strategies.

A. **Pain control** Hypnosis can be remarkably effective in controlling pain whether of organic or psychogenic origin. In the last century, Esdaile reported better than 80 percent surgical anesthesia with hypnosis, and it has been used successfully as the sole anesthesia in major surgery. Often better hypnotic subjects can produce full anesthesia; persons with lesser responsiveness can learn to divert their attention from the pain. Hypnosis may be underrecognized as a factor in natural childbirth, and it is also potentially useful for relief of preoperative anxiety. Furthermore, patients with postsurgical or trauma-induced pain, as well as some with chronic distress, may be taught to hypnotize themselves to cope better with pain. It is important to note that opiates and sedatives, by clouding the sensorium, interfere with this hypnotic capacity.

B. **Anxiety control** Patients with recurrent anxiety attacks often experience a tendency to "snowball": incipient anxiety comes to be associated with a dread of being overwhelmed or flooded by the anxiety. In such cases hypnosis can encourage relaxation and lead to a sense of mastery in certain difficult situations. The initial stimulus to anxiety may remain, but corresponding helplessness and immobilization can be contained. However, the success of this technique can be compromised by the anxious patient's inability to bind his anxiety long enough to permit focused concentration. See also Chapter 2.

C. **Habit control** Hypnosis can facilitate a strategy of self-affirmation in dealing with difficult problems such as smoking and obesity. Little success has been shown with alcohol and drug addictions.

D. **Phobias** These conditions respond well to behavior modification and also to the less structured, less time-consuming approach of hypnosis. The patient is taught to bring on a sense of relaxation and well-being and to gradually use this to overcome his fears. The focus again is on mastery.

E. **Conversion symptoms** Here the diagnostic potential of hypnosis can be particularly useful, helping the clinician to sort out functional from organic problems. Very hypnotizable people may be prone to conversion symptoms. It is hypothesized that such patients may be "willing" to alter or eliminate conversion symptoms if the secondary loss has exceeded the gain. A person with an erratic hypnotic performance is more likely to have a hypochondriasis of psychotic proportions or an organic problem.

F. **Psychosomatic illnesses** Some medical conditions with large affective and stress-related components, such as asthma, can be susceptible to intervention with hypnosis. The technique is similar to that used for anxiety, teaching the patient to master his somatic responses in the face of an atopic or emotional stress to prevent further decompensatio

G. **Spontaneous hypnosis** A certain percentage of patients require training in how *not* to enter the trance mode. They are extremely hypnotizable people who are constantly being "entranced" by others, working to please them and suspending their own critical judgment. Here the trance induction is used as a demonstration of how susceptib the subject is, and he is taught how to control his own tendency to slip into trance states.

References

Esdaile, J. *Hypnosis in Medicine and Surgery.* New York: Julian Press and the Institute for Research in Hypnosis, 1957.

Gill, M. M., and Brenman, M. *Hypnosis and Related States: Psychoanalytic Studies in Regression.* New York: International Universities Press, 1959.

Meares, A. *A System of Medical Hypnosis.* Philadelphia: Saunders, 1960.

Speigel, H. Hypnosis: An Adjunct to Psychotherapy. In A. M. Freedman and H. I. Kaplan (Eds.), *Comprehensive Textbook of Psychiatry.* Baltimore: Williams & Wilkins, 1967. Pp. 1228–1233.

Speigel, H. *Manual for Hypnotic Induction Profile.* New York: Soni Medica, 1973.

19

Practical Dietary Considerations

Richard I. Shader
Jerold S. Harnatz

Nutritional status can be an important consideration in evaluating patients. A total treatment approach must include attention to diet and vitamin intake. Beyond these general concerns, however, specific treatment regimens may require special attention to diet, and some of these are reviewed in this chapter.

I. **Monoamine Oxidase (MAO) Inhibitors** Sudden, life-threatening hypertension can occur in patients treated with these agents. These hypertensive episodes reportedly follow ingestion of certain foodstuffs containing bioamines such as tyramine or dopa. Monoamine oxidase inhibiting drugs block the oxidative deamination of endogenous tyramine stores. Several foods are known to contain substantial amounts of tyramine resulting from tyrosine decarboxylation, and in many foods, tyramine is continually produced, especially foods allowed to age or subjected to accidental spoilage.

   Cheese is commonly implicated in these crises. The amount of tyramine in cheese can vary strikingly *from type to type* and *from sample to sample.* Only fresh cream and cottage cheese, and properly stored processed American, parmesan, and gouda seem reasonably safe when ingested in the presence of MAO inhibitors. All other cheeses must be suspected of substantial tyramine levels.

   Several wines have been evaluated for their tyramine content, and some (e.g., chianti) have been singled out for dangerous levels of tyramine. Idiosyncrasies of manufacture and storage, however, admit some risk in drinking any wine. Beer, similarly, ought to be proscribed.

   The following foods have also been implicated: coffee, chocolate, licorice, pickles, sauerkraut, pickled herring, salted herring, lox (smoked salmon), chicken livers, snails, raisins, canned figs, banana peels, and yeast products such as yogurt. Soy sauce is to be avoided, as are fava beans, on account of their dopa content.

II. **The Role of Vitamin B_6 (Pyridoxine)**

   A. **B_6 and L-dopa** Pyridoxine is important to the biotransformation of compounds identified as neurotransmitters. Pyridoxine is also mutually antagonistic to L-dopa. Outside the CNS, pyridoxine has been observed to increase dopa-decarboxylation. In the presence of a dopa-decarboxylase inhibitor, pyridoxine fails to reverse the effect of L-dopa. Patients with parkinsonism or other disorders treated with L-dopa may deplete their B_6 stores and risk neuropathy, which may be mistaken for the somatic concerns encountered in a depressive syndrome. It is also possible that patients deficient in B_6, such as those with diabetes mellitus, chronic alcoholism, malnutrition, or malignancy will develop a peripheral neuropathy when administered L-dopa.

B. **B_6 and MAO inhibitors**   Acetylation is fundamental to the metabolism of monoamine oxidase inhibiting substances, and acetylation varies phenotypically across individuals. For instance, N-acetyl-transferase (NAT) is important to the metabolism of isoniazid (INH). Excessive INH levels result from administration of more than 8 mg/kg of this drug to persons with low titers of NAT. Functionally, more drug will be available to compete with pyridoxal phosphate, thereby imposing a risk of peripheral neuropathy. In such circumstances, 100 mg of B_6 is a useful prophylaxis. Some 20 percent of patients given the monoamine oxidase inhibiting agent iproniazid evidence peripheral neuropathy. Concurrent administration of B_6 both prevents and treats this neuropathy. In general, the frequency of B_6 deficiency neuropathy with MAO inhibitors is not established.

C. **Oral contraceptives and B_6 mediated depression**   Increased depression is consistently observed in some proportion of women who make use of oral contraceptives. Problems of measurement as well as evidence of interindividual and intraindividual variability have compromised accurate incidence and prevalence figures. In one study some 6.6 percent of the women receiving oral contraceptives had more severe depressive ratings. This figure has been cited repeatedly as if it were an incidence statistic. In any event, the sheer number of reports strongly suggests that certain susceptible women become depressed when on "the pill."

The experienced depression is unusual because sleep disturbance is not a typical complaint. Nonetheless, the mechanisms postulated resemble those being investigated in other depressive conditions. These mechanisms represent disturbances along the nicotinic acid ribonucleotide and possibly indole pathways, alterations creating a reduction of 5-hydroxytryptamine (serotonin) and perhaps other bioamines necessary for normal brain biosynthesis.

Estrogen has been demonstrated to reduce the availability of serotonin and other amines. By cortisol induction and other mechanisms, tryptophan metabolism is increased by estrogen, with less available for serotonin production. Augmented tryptophan metabolites are thought to inhibit efficient blood-brain tryptophan transport. In addition, estrogen competitively interferes with pyridoxal phosphate binding to its apoenzyme, such as occurs in normal 5-hydroxytryptophan decarboxylation. Pyridoxal phosphate is a coenzyme of B_6. Pyridoxal phosphate similarly has been studied for its effect on dopa decarboxylation.

Supporting the importance of pyridoxine for women using oral contraceptives is one study claiming evidence for an 80 percent incidence of relative B_6 deficiency. Estrogenic steroids may be expected to produce functional vitamin deficiencies, although it is not clear that such deficiencies are directly linked to depression or any other adverse reaction.

The consequences of estrogen intake may be a function of hormonal and enzymatic states at the time of administration. It may be noted, however, that progesterone seems to have been ruled out as a single causal factor; its importance for individually characteristic ratios with estrogen remains to be explored. Indeed, individual susceptibility may be more important than the amount of estrogen in a given oral contraceptive formulation.

Supplementary B_6 administration may well be of help for some women. It has usually been given (25 mg qd) to provide increased pyridoxal phosphate. However, recent evidence suggests routine prophylactic B_6 administration is contraindicated, since some women become more troubled and only particular women, possibly those with absolute B_6 deficiency, derive benefit.

Given the importance of these processes, it is surprising not to see more than effects on depression. Individual regulating mechanisms probably characterize a group of special B_6 responders. These have been identified as presenting a history of depression and evidence of augmented depressive symptoms when beginning birth control pills. By itself, a history of premenstrual depression is insufficient for this characterization. Moreover, it would seem helpful to examine the possibility of B_6 deficiency in women complaining of side effects of the pill. Typically, the woman with estrogen- and pyridoxine-mediated depression is pessimistic, anxious, dissatisfied, lethargic, and with decreased libido, and she does not show disturbances of sleep or irritable affect. A consistent observation is that women on "the pill" may evidence depression without an accompanying irritability.

III. **Sodium Intake and Lithium Administration** Lithium reabsorption and excretion is intimately and complexly bound to that of sodium. Well recognized, if incompletely understood, are the profound effects of varying levels of dietary sodium on lithium efficacy and toxicity. Inadequate lithium excretion is a likely consequence of restricted sodium intake, and reduced efficacy may follow sodium loading. The latter has been demonstrated for levels of 152 mEq/day. For many patients, excessive sodium intake expedites the excretion of lithium ion and lowers serum levels below what is required to reduce the symptoms of mania. For some patients with reappearing manic symptomatology, no reduction in serum levels is evidenced. Increased intracellular sodium stores have been implicated since the depletion of these stores is hypothesized as one principal mechanism of lithium activity. The physician prescribing lithium is obliged to remain alert to dietary idiosyncrasies encouraging sodium loading or depletion. The patient may valuably share in the responsibility for maintaining his daily sodium intake in the range of 3 to 6 gm of Na^+. Normal hydration and the special hazards of persistent diarrhea must also be recognized.

It is helpful to review a patient's habitual food preferences, with special focus on sodium sources, such as preserved foods, organ meats, and shellfish, in addition to obvious sodium additives and seasoning. Supplemental sodium sources such as water softeners and everyday medicaments such as aspirin and baking soda ought not to be overlooked. Normal sodium intake can be as little as 0.8 gm of Na^+. A typical menu yielding 4.4 gm (Na^+) is presented in Table 19-1.

Table 19-1. A Menu that Illustrates the Sodium Content of Foods (Total Na⁺ = 4.4 gm)

	Measure	Na^+ (mg)
Breakfast		
Orange juice	1 cup	3
2 eggs (fried)	100 gm	338
3 slices bacon	21 gm	228
2 slices toast	46 gm	234
1 pat butter	10 gm	99
Coffee with cream	1 cup	13
Lunch		
Hamburger (on roll with catsup)	1/4 lb	369
French fries	50 gm	3
Table salt	1/4 tsp	500
Coca-Cola[a]	6 oz	2
Supper		
Ham (cured)[b]	1/4 lb	1320
Baby lima beans (cooked frozen)[c]	5/8 cup	101
2 biscuits (baking powder)[d]	70 gm	438
2 pats butter	20 gm	198
Table salt	1/4 tsp	500
1 cup noodles (cooked)	200 gm	4
Vanilla ice cream	90 gm	55
Coffee with cream	1 cup	13

[a]Commercial preparations can vary greatly and may differ in preservative added; Pepsi contains 13 times as much Na^+ as Coca-Cola.

[b]Note that processing (curing) can substantially increment sodium load.

[c]Frozen lima beans and peas are separated by brine immersions. Contrast with cooked *fresh* lima beans, which contain 1 mg for the same measure.

[d]Added sodium bicarbonate, like table salt, constitutes a principal part of the average person's overall sodium intake.

20

Assessment of Suicide Risk

Richard I. Shader

As with other human behaviors, suicide (attempted or completed) can reflect several motivational determinants, personal and interpersonal as well as cultural. Self-immolation is a well-known *religious* (or nationalistic or political) phenomenon. At the same time, death can be seen as a *release* from despair, pain, old age, or a sense of a barren future, or as a means of *rebirth*. It can be experienced as *revenge* (e.g., "you'll be sorry when I'm dead") or as *reunification* with a lost loved one. Suicide also can be a *response* to the disordered thinking of a psychotic decompensation (e.g., hearing a voice directing one to die) or to the disordered thinking of a toxic state (e.g., stepping out of a window and falling to one's death in a response to a belief that one can walk on air or fly).

Just as vital signs are a fundamental part of a physical examination, in a psychiatric examination an assessment of suicidal risk is fundamental. It should not be restricted solely to those appearing depressed. Since suicidal impulses may wax and wane and may be more or less evident, continuing reassessment may be required for some patients. Inquiry about suicidal concerns and impulses can be conducted in a systematic manner, progressing from more general to more specific questions, such as: "How depressed do you feel?" "Do you ever want to die?" "What was going on in your life when you were thinking about killing yourself?" "Did you have a plan?" Clinical experience does not support the fear that asking patients about suicide will put the idea into their minds. Observation of the patient for facial, postural, and other nonverbal clues also is an important part of suicide risk assessment. It may be important with some patients to question family members or other informants about their sense of the patient's suicide potential.

Since the assessment of an individual patient's potential for suicide is a complex and difficult task, attention must be paid to what is said (and *not* said), what has happened (or *not* happened), who is available to the patient (with particular attention to those who feel no one is available or who have just lost or been separated from their last or only caring relationship), and what has been done (or *not* done). The mélange of suicidal variants — attempts, manipulative gestures, thoughts, preoccupations and obsessive ruminations, and the act per se — must be sorted out. Examples are the hurt and angry young child who says "You'll be sorry when I die myself"; the young woman who tries to hold onto her lover by ingesting a nonlethal dose of aspirin; the smoker who says "I wonder why I'm paying someone to kill me"; the recentl widowed, 60-year-old man who wants to die; or the middle-aged man who sho himself when he learns that he has an inoperable carcinoma.

It is important to learn how the patient feels about the future. Does he have evidence of an orientation toward the future? Does he entertain realiz-able goals and realistic expectations, or is he setting himself up for disappoint ment and loss? Assessment must be a continuing process, and one must rema alert to newly appearing stresses in the patient's life and to changes in the patient's available interpersonal and material resources.

No single sign or set of signs is a reliable indicator of a patient's suicide potential. Attention must be paid to the patient's appearance, mood, and thought content and to the overall significance of biographic elements (e.g., the fact that a patient is known to have put his affairs in order* may suggest a plan for suicide). It is likely that the recognized incidence of suicide (20,000 to 25,000 suicides annually reported in the United States) is an underestimate ignoring the suicidal implications of numerous automobile accidents, home fii and such. At least transient suicidal thoughts are reported in some surveys to in about 15 percent of the general population. The following section details specific factors that may serve to increase the clinician's index of suspicion.

I. **Biographic Factors Relevant to Suicide Risk Assessment**

   A. **History of previous attempts**

   1. A pattern of repeated threats or attempts is common. Depending on samples and methods of study, from 20 to 60 percent of suicides have tried before. Known attempts are about ten times more frequent than successful suicides.

   2. Those who have attempted suicide before are more likely to succeed than nonattempters.

   3. Second attempts commonly come within three months after the first attempt.

   B. **Occupational status**

   1. The unemployed and the unskilled have higher suicide rates than those who are skilled and employed.

   2. By profession, higher suicide rates occur in policemen, musicians, dentists, insurance agents, physicians (especially psychiatrists, ophthamologists, and anesthesiologists), and lawyers.

   3. A sense of failure in fulfilling one's occupational role (e.g., in job or as wife-mother) is a common factor in suicides.

*Examples are writing of or changes in last will and testament; buying a burial plot; or making a plan for the disposition of one's remains or effects.

C. Marital status Single (never married) persons are at greatest risk for suicide, followed in rank order by persons widowed, separated and divorced, married without children, and married with children. Those who live "all alone in the world," or who feel alone (with no one who cares or no one to care about), and those who have recently lost a loved one or failed in a love relationship (particularly within the preceding six months to a year) always must be considered serious suicide risks.

D. Sex

1. Men successfully *commit* suicide more frequently than women, perhaps three times as often. Perhaps at highest risk for suicide is the middle-aged male with a recent life crisis (e.g., a health problem, such as myocardial infarction, carcinoma, or kidney disease; a major financial setback; a significant loss of a loved one) who makes use of alcohol and tends to deny depression.

2. Women *attempt* suicide more often (two or three times) than men.

E. Age

1. Suicides may occur in the young, but they are uncommon prior to adolescense.

2. The frequency of suicide increases with age for men until the seventh decade; a decline begins in the 75 to 85 age range.

3. In women the peak frequency for suicide is between 55 and 65 years of age.

F. Family history Successful and attempted suicides are more common among those with a family history of attempts or suicides.

G. Emotional factors

1. Depression (grief, hypochondriasis, insomnia, guilt, gloominess, despair about the future) is a major factor in suicides.

2. Psychosis — particularly with associated terror, suspiciousness, persecutory delusions, hallucinations urging suicide or reasons for dying. Psychotic depressives and young catatonics are especially high risk groups.

3. Acute and chronic alcoholism and other forms of drug-dependency.

4. For women of childbearing age, postpartum months and the pre-menstrual week are high risk times.

H. Health factors

1. Patients who have undergone recent surgery are at special risk.

2. Patients with intractable pain.

3. Chronic or protracted diseases.

4. Terminal illnesses.

I. **Help-seeking** Although many suicides have sought medical or psychiatric care within the year preceding an attempt, help-seeking is not a reliable factor, as illustrated by a study of suicides among college students in which none had sought help nor had they appeared depressed to those who knew them.

J. **Race** Within the United States, recorded suicide rates are higher for whites than for nonwhites.

K. **Geographic location** Rates are higher in urban as compared to rural settings.

II. **Treatment** Unfortunately, assessment of suicide risk and treatment planning may be influenced by clinicians' varied reactions to suicidal patients. Some, for example, imply or openly state that they cannot take responsibility for someone else's life. This attitude often confuses feelings of helplessness, anger, and disappointment-rejection with civil liberties and philosophical positions about individuals' rights. It is important to realize that in all states suicide has legal implications, and commitment laws may allow the hospitalization of those who are considered a danger to themselves. Some clinicians banter with suicide attempters, trying to minimize or undercut the seriousness of the attempt. Some clinicians restrict banter to those who have made repeated attempts. This therapeutic style often assumes a manipulative aspect to the attempt. There are, by contrast, clinicians who hospitalize suicide attempters and then are reluctant to discharge them, feeling uncertain about judging patients' freedom from suicidal impulses.

Although it is beyond the scope of this chapter to offer guidelines for treatment of individual patients, consideration of aspects of one approach to treatment may be helpful. The author approaches most suicidal patients with a bias based on clinical experience — *the majority of suicidal patients change their minds.* When patients have suicidal thoughts or behavior associated with endogenous depressive syndromes, effective treatment of the depression usually is sufficient. Similarly, in suicidal behavior secondary to the hallucinations or delusions of a psychotic state, adequate treatment of the psychosis should be effective. Borderline patients with intense dysphoria also may respond to therapeutic strategies. The recently widowed may be helped to grieve and may find support and companionship from association with others who are successfully handling widowhood.

With each patient, however, the aim is to come to understand and have the patient understand why he wants to die and what might help to make life more worthwhile. Some key elements in working with suicidal patients are: listening to the patient, being open to hearing their often ambivalently expressed cries for help and their deep despair or loneliness; understanding and managing one's own countertransference reactions, such as helplessness, anger, or rejection; *taking seriously all threats of suicide,* providing a safe, nonrejecting environment — this may range from helping the patient to reveal his feelings and impulses to family and friends so that they will be more open and, if necessary, spend increased time with the patient, to hospitalization with continuous observation; the patient's person and his immediate environment may require attention to minimize destructive opportunities — safety screens for hospital windows must not be overlooked; use of appropriate interpersonal and somatic therapies (see Chapters 1, 3, 4, 5, 6, 17); an awareness that improvement in the patient's mood may reflect a decision to try again — continued support and involvement during this phase are essential; taking the crucial risk of reducing suicide precautions and permitting the patient more freedom — the timing of this shift must include consideration of the amount of improvement in the patient's suicidal thoughts, depressed mood, or withdrawal, evidence of an orientation toward the future, and a sense that the patient is engaged with staff in some form of therapeutic alliance; involvement of family members and friends, when appropriate, so that the patient does not return to the same circumstances that contributed to the patient's decision to die; working out with the patient a plan for aftercare and followup — such planning should take into consideration that some patients feel less suicidal when a therapist temporarily fills some void, and that this can lead to a re-emergence of suicidal impulses when treatment termination or interruption is discussed — therapeutic planning must face this possibility, and the therapist must be aware of the quality of other relationships available to the patient; the absence of other available object relationships must be considered, and part of treatment planning should include helping the patient to develop them — group therapy may be beneficial; involvement of community resource persons (e.g., teacher, family, physician, clergyman) may be beneficial to some patients.

A second bias has emerged from the author's clinical experience — *patients who continue to want to die will usually find a way.* We can delay death and provide an opportunity for the patient to improve from a particular episode of depression, demoralization, grief, or psychosis. Some patients, however, find life so empty or painful that a second chance to them means a second chance to die, not a second chance to find something to live for or to work out their disappointment in themselves. A word of caution is in order — the clinician must not let his own feeling that he would not want to live under a particular set of conditions dictate his care of the patient. For example, this can be especially difficult when working with a patient with inoperable and painful metastatic carcinoma.

Suicidal patients should be viewed as medical emergencies, and program planning must recognize the need for 24-hour services.

References

Dublin, L. I. *Suicide.* New York: Ronald, 1963.

Durkheim, E. *Le Suicide.* Glencoe, Ill.: Free Press, 1950.

Farberow, N. L., and Schneidman, E. S. *The Cry for Help.* New York: McGraw-Hill, 1961.

Schneidman, E. S., and Farberow, N. L. *Clues to Suicide.* New York: McGraw-Hill, 1957.

Appendixes

Pertinent Data on Hypnotic Drugs

Generic Name	Trade Name	Preparations Available	Usual Dose Range	Recommended Initial Dose	Effect on REM Sleep	Drug Interactions
Barbiturates, short-acting						
Secobarbital	Seconal Seco-8	Capsules: 50 mg, 100 mg Elixir: 22 mg/5 ml Injection: 50 mg/ml Suppositories: 30 mg, 60 mg, 120 mg, 200 mg	50 to 200 mg	100 mg	REM sleep depressed by all barbiturates	Enzyme induction by all barbiturates
Pentobarbital	Nembutal	Capsules: 30 mg, 50 mg, 100 mg Elixir: 20 mg/5 ml Injection: 50 mg/ml Suppositories: 30 mg, 60 mg, 120 mg, 200 mg	50 to 200 mg	100 mg	REM sleep depressed by all barbiturates	Enzyme induction by all barbiturates
Barbiturates, intermediate-acting						
Amobarbital	Amytal	Capsules: 15 mg, 30 mg, 50 mg, 65 mg, 100 mg, 200 mg Elixir: 22 mg/ml, 44 mg/ml Injection: Unit doses of 65 mg, 125 mg, 250 mg, 500 mg	65 to 200 mg	100 mg	REM sleep depressed by all barbiturates	Enzyme induction by all barbiturates
Butabarbital	Butisol	Tablets or capsules: 15 mg, 30 mg, 50 mg, 60 mg, 100 mg Elixir: 30 mg/5 ml	50 to 100 mg	100 mg	REM sleep depressed by all barbitu-	Enzyme induction by all barbiturates

		Dosage forms			REM sleep depressed by all barbiturates	Enzyme induction by all barbiturates
Phenobarbital Luminal (many others)		Tablets: 15 mg, 30 mg, 60 mg, 100 mg; Elixir: 20 mg/5 ml; Injection: Unit doses of 130 and 320 mg; Solutions of 130 mg/ml	60 to 300 mg	100 to 120 mg	REM sleep depressed by all barbiturates	Enzyme induction by all barbiturates
Benzodiazepines						
Flurazepam	Dalmane	Capsules: 15 mg, 30 mg	15 to 30 mg	15 mg	Probably no effect	None
Nitrazepam[a]	Mogadon	Tablets: 5 mg, 10 mg	5 to 10 mg	5 mg	REM depression	None
Antihistamines						
Diphenhydramine	Benadryl	Capsules: 50 mg, 100 mg; Elixir: 12.5 mg/5 ml; Injection: 10 mg/ml, 50 mg/ml	25 to 100 mg	50 to 100 mg		Potentiation of anticholinergic drugs
Promethazine	Phenergan Remsed	Tablets or capsules: 12.5 mg, 25 mg, 50 mg, 100 mg, 200 mg; Syrup: 6.25 mg/5 ml, 25 mg/5 ml; Injection: 25 mg/ml, 50 mg/ml; Suppositories: 25 mg, 50 mg	50 to 200 mg	50 to 100 mg	?	Potentiation of anticholinergic drugs

[a]Not available in the United States at the present time.

Generic Name	Trade Name	Preparations Available	Usual Dose Range	Recommended Initial Dose	Effect on REM Sleep	Drug Interactions
Hydroxyzine	Atarax Vistaril	Tablets or capsules: 10 mg, 25 mg, 50 mg, 100 mg; Syrup: 10 mg/5 ml, 25 mg/5 ml; Injection: 25 mg/ml, 50 mg/ml	50 to 100 mg	50 to 100 mg	?	**Potentiation of anticholinergic drugs**
Chloral derivatives						
Chloral hydrate	Noctec Somnos Kessodrate Felsules Rectules (suppositories)	Capsules: 250 mg, 500 mg, 1.0 gm; Syrup: 500 mg/5 ml; Suppositories: 650 mg, 1.3 gm	500 mg to 2.0 gm	1.0 gm	Probable REM depression	Protein binding displacement
Chloral betaine	Beta-Chlor	Tablets: 870 mg	870 mg to 3.48 gm	1.74 gm		
Trichloroethyl phosphate (triclofos)	Triclos	Tablets: 750 mg; Liquid: 500 mg/5 ml	750 mg to 3.0 gm	1.5 gm		
Piperidinedione derivatives						
Glutethimide	Doriden	Tablets or capsules: 125 mg, 250 mg, 500 mg	500 mg to 1.0 gm	500 mg	REM depression	Enzyme induction
Methyprylon	Noludar	Tablets or capsules: 200 mg, 300 mg	200 to 400 mg	300 mg	REM depression	?

						Enzyme induction?
Acetylinic alcohols						
Ethchlorvynol	Placidyl	Capsules: 100 mg, 200 mg, 500 mg, 750 mg	500 mg to 1.0 gm	750 mg	?	?
Quinazolines						
Methaqualone	Quaalude Parest Optimil Sopor Somnafac (many others)	Tablets or capsules: 75 mg, 150 mg, 175 mg, 300 mg, 350 mg, 400 mg	150 to 400 mg	300 mg	Probable REM depression	?

Pertinent Data on Sedative Drugs (Antianxiety Agents)

Generic Name	Trade Name	Preparations Available	Daily Dose Range	Duration of Action[a]	Active Metabolites
Barbiturates					
Amobarbital	Amytal	See Appendix I	45 to 200 mg	I	No
Butabarbital	Butisol	See Appendix I	45 to 200 mg	I	No
Phenobarbital	Luminal (many others)	See Appendix I	45 to 200 mg	L	No
Propanediols					
Meprobamate	Equanil Miltown Kesso-Bamate SK-Bamate (many others)	Tablets or capsules: 200 mg, 400 mg, 600 mg Suspension: 200 mg/ 5 ml	1.2 to 1.6 gm	S—I	No
Tybamate	Solacen Tybatran	Capsules: 125 mg, 250 mg, 350 mg	750 mg to 2.0 gm	?	?
Benzodiazepines					
Chlordiazepoxide	Librium	Tablets or capsules: 5 mg, 10 mg, 25 mg	15 to 100 mg/day	L	Yes
Diazepam	Valium	Tablets: 2 mg, 5 mg, 10 mg Injection: 5 mg/ml	6 to 40 mg/day	L	Yes
Oxazepam	Serax	Tablets or capsules: 10 mg, 15 mg, 30 mg	30 to 120 mg/day	S—I	No
Clorazepate	Tranxene	Capsules: 3.75 mg, 7.5 mg, 15 mg	11.25 to 60.00 mg/day	L	Yes
Antihistamines					
Hydroxyzine	Atarax Vistaril	See Appendix I	30 to 200 mg/day	?	?
Beta-adrenergic antagonists					
Propranolol[b]	Inderal	Tablets: 10 mg, 40 mg, 80 mg Injection: 1 mg/ml	30 to 120 mg/day	S	Yes

Pertinent Data on Major Tranquilizers (Antipsychotic Drugs, Neuroleptics)

Generic Name	Trade Name	Preparations Available	Usual Initial Dose
Dimethylaminopropyl phenothiazines			
Chlorpromazine	Thorazine Chlor-PZ	Tablets: 10 mg, 25 mg, 50 mg, 100 mg, 200 mg Sustained-action capsules: 30 mg, 75 mg, 150 mg, 200 mg, 300 mg Syrup: 25 mg/5 ml Concentrate: 100 mg/5 ml, 500 mg/5 ml Injection: 25 mg/ml Suppositories: 25 mg, 100 mg	25 to 100 mg PO 25 to 50 mg IM
Promazine	Sparine	Tablets: 10 mg, 25 mg, 50 mg, 100 mg, 200 mg Syrup: 10 mg/5 ml Concentrate: 150 mg/5 ml, 500 mg/5 ml Injection: 25 mg/ml	25 to 50 mg
Triflupromazine	Vesprin	Tablets: 10 mg, 25 mg, 50 mg Injection: 10 mg/ml, 20 mg/ml Suspension: 50 mg/5 ml	20 to 50 mg
Piperidine phenothiazines			
Thioridazine	Mellaril	Tablets: 10 mg, 15 mg, 25 mg, 50 mg, 100 mg, 150 mg, 200 mg Concentrate: 150 mg/5 ml	25 to 100 mg
Mesoridazine	Serentil	Tablets: 10 mg, 25 mg, 50 mg, 100 mg Concentrate: 25 mg/ml Injection: 25 mg/ml	30 to 50 mg
Piperacetazine	Quide	Tablets: 10 mg, 25 mg Injection: 2 mg/ml	20 to 50 mg
Piperazine phenothiazines			
Prochlorperazine	Compazine	Tablets: 5 mg, 10 mg, 25 mg Concentrate: 50 mg/5 ml Injection: 5 mg/ml Suppositories: 2.5 mg, 5 mg, 25 mg	5 to 10 mg

Generic Name	Trade Name	Preparations Available	Usual Initial Dose
Trifluoperazine	Stelazine	Tablets: 1 mg, 2 mg, 5 mg, 10 mg Concentrate: 50 mg/5 ml Injection: 2 mg/ml	2 to 4 mg
Butaperazine Perphenazine	Repoise Trilafon	Tablets: 5 mg, 10 mg, 25 mg Tablets: 2 mg, 4 mg, 8 mg, 16 mg Concentrate: 16 mg/5 ml Injection: 5 mg/ml	10 to 20 mg 5 to 10 mg
Fluphenazine	Prolixin Permitil	Tablets: 0.25 mg, 1 mg, 2.5 mg, 5 mg, 10 mg Elixir: 2.5 mg/5 ml Concentrate: 25 mg/5 ml Injection: 2.5 mg/ml Delayed-release injection (fluphenazine enanthate, fluphenazine decanoate): 25 mg/ml	2.5 to 5.0 mg
Acetophenazine Carphenazine	Tindal Proketazine	Tablets: 20 mg Tablets: 12.5 mg, 25 mg, 50 mg Concentrate: 250 mg/5 ml	20 to 40 mg 25 to 50 mg
Butyrophenones Haloperidol	Haldol	Tablets: 0.5 mg, 1 mg, 2 mg, 5 mg, 10 mg Concentrate: 10 mg/5 ml Injection: 5 mg/ml	2.5 to 5.0 mg
Droperidol	Inapsine	Injection: 2.5 mg/ml	2.5 to 10 mg
Thioxanthenes Chlorprothixene	Taractan	Tablets: 10 mg, 25 mg, 50 mg, 100 mg Concentrate: 100 mg/5 ml Injection: 12.5 mg/ml	PO: 25 to 50 mg IM: 12.5 to 25 mg
Thiothixene	Navane	Capsules: 1 mg, 2 mg, 5 mg, 10 mg, 20 mg Concentrate: 25 mg/5 ml Injection: 2 mg/ml	2 to 4 mg
Dihydroindolones Molindone	Moban	Tablets: 5 mg, 10 mg, 25 mg	5 to 10 mg
Dibenzoxazepines Loxapine	Loxitane	Capsules: 10 mg, 25 mg, 50 mg	10 to 20 mg

IV

Over-the-Counter Hypnotic Preparations that Contain Anticholinergic Substances

Preparation	Ingredients	Amount	
Alva Tranquil	Methapyrilene HCl	.1	mg
	KBr	.195	mg
	K-salicylate	.85	mg
	Niacinamide	.004	mg
	Thiamine HCl	.002	mg
	Niacin	.004	mg
Asper-Sleep	Methapyrilene HCl	25	mg
	Scopolamine aminoxide HBr	.15	mg
Compoz	Methapyrilene HCl	15	mg
	Pyrilamine maleate	10	mg
	Scopolamine aminoxide HBr	.15	mg
CVS Sleep Capsules	Methapyrilene HCl	25	mg
	Scopolamine aminoxide HBr	.2	mg
Devarex	Methapyrilene HCl	12	mg
	Scopolamine aminoxide HBr	.15	mg
Dormin	Methapyrilene HBr	25	mg
Dormirex	Methapyrilene HCl	25	mg
	Scopolamine aminoxide HBr	.2	mg
Dormutol	Methapyrilene HCl	25	mg
	Scopolamine aminoxide HBr	.2	mg
Dozar	Methapyrilene HCl	25	mg
Ex Tension	Methapyrilene HCl	25	mg
	Scopolamine aminoxide HBr	.2	mg
Masons Timed Sleeping Capsules	Methapyrilene HCl	50	mg
	Scopolamine aminoxide HBr	.25	mg
McKesson Sleep Tablets	Methapyrilene HCl	25	mg
	Salicylamide	216	mg
	Scopolamine aminoxide HBr	.25	mg
Neo Nyte	Methapyrilene HCl	25	mg
	Scopolamine aminoxide HBr	.125	mg
Nite Rest	Methapyrilene HCl	50	mg
	Scopolamine aminoxide HBr	.25	mg
Nytol	Methapyrilene HCl	25	mg
	Salicylamide	Not listed	
Osco Sleep Tablets	Methapyrilene HCl	25	mg
	Salicylamide	200	mg
Paradorm	Methapyrilene HCl	25	mg
	Salicylamide	250	mg
	Ascorbic acid	20	mg
	Pyridoxine HCl	.5	mg
	Thiamine mononitrate	5	mg

Preparation	Ingredients	Amount	
Quietabs	Methapyrilene HCl	15	mg
	Pyrilamine maleate	10	mg
	Salicylamide	120	mg
	Scopolamine aminoxide HBr	.15	mg
	Passion flower	7.5	mg
	Niacinamide	20	mg
	Pyridoxine	.5	mg
	Riboflavin	2	mg
	Thiamine HCl	5	mg
Quiet World	Acetaminophen	2½ grains	
	Acetylsalicylic acid	Not listed	
	Methapyrilene HCl	16.67	mg
	Scopolamine HBr	.83	mg
Rexall Sleep Capsules	Methapyrilene HCl	Not listed	
	Scopolamine HBr	Not listed	
Rexall Sleep Tablets	Ammonium HBr	1½ grains	
	Methapyrilene HCl	25	mg
	Potassium HBr	3 grains	
	Sodium HBr	3 grains	
Sedacaps	Methapyrilene HCl	25	mg
Seda Tabs	Glyceryl guiacolate ether	100	mg
	Methapyrilene HCl	25	mg
	Salicylamide	200	mg
Seedate	Methapyrilene HCl	25	mg
	Scopolamine aminoxide HBr	.125	mg
Sleep-Aid	Methapyrilene HCl	25	mg
Sleep Eze	Methapyrilene HCl	25	mg
	Scopolamine HBr	.125	mg
Sleeping Pill— Professional	Ascorbic acid	25	mg
	Methapyrilene HCl	25	mg
Sleeprin	Acetylsalicylic acid	5 grains	
	Methapyrilene HCl	25	mg
	Scopolamine aminoxide HBr	.15	mg
Slumba-Plus Time Capsules	Methapyrilene HCl	50	mg
	Scopolamine aminoxide HBr	.25	mg
Slumba-Tabs	Methapyrilene HCl	25	mg
	Salicylamide	200	mg
	Scopolamine aminoxide HBr	.25	mg
Somets	Methapyrilene HCl	25	mg
	Scopolamine aminoxide HBr	.20	mg
Sominex	Methapyrilene HCl	25	mg
	Scopolamine aminoxide HBr	.25	mg
	Salicylamide	200	mg
Sominex Capsules	Methapyrilene HCl	50	mg
	Salicylamide	200	mg
	Scopolamine aminoxide HBr	.5	mg
Somnicaps	Methapyrilene HCl	25	mg
Sta-Kalm	Methapyrilene HCl	14	mg
	Pyrilamine maleate	18	mg
	Scopolamine aminoxide HBr	.45	mg

V

Comparison of Classes of Major Tranquilizers

	Relative Potency	Sedative Effects	Antiemetic Effects	Adrenergic Antagonism	Extrapyramidal Effects[a]
Phenothiazines					
Dimethylaminopropyl	Low	Strong	Moderate	Strong	Type I
Piperidine	Low	Moderate	Weak	Moderate	Infrequent
Piperazine	High	Weak	Strong	Weak	Types I and II
Butyrophenones					
Haloperidol[b]	High	Weak	Strong	Weak	Types I and II
Thioxanthenes					
Dimethylaminopropyl	Low	Strong	Strong	Strong	Type I
Piperazine	High	Weak	Moderate	Weak	Types I and II
Dihydroindolones					
Molindone[b]	High	Weak	Strong[c]	Weak	Type I
Dibenzoxazepines					
Loxapine[b]	High	Moderate	Strong[c]	Moderate	Types I and II

[a]Categories of extrapyramidal effects:
Type I: Motor restlessness or parkinsonism or both after weeks or months of therapy.
Type II: Acute dystonic muscle spasms, particularly in young individuals early in treatment.
[b]Only one drug is currently available, so this drug rather than the subclass is given.
[c]Animal data only.

Index